Down Syndrome

*An Introduction for Parents
and Carers*

CLIFF CUNNINGHAM

SOUVENIR PRESS

To you — because you are involved

Contents

Section Three: Characteristics of Down Syndrome

Section Four: Practical Aspects and Future Directions

Prefaces

To the Third Edition

When I first wrote this book I knew of only two others for parents, and one only covered medical aspects, At the time Down Syndrome Associations were just becoming established in a few places. Since the last edition there has been a considerable increase in books for parents and journal articles about Down syndrome. Many countries now have their own Down Syndrome Associations, with their own publications and websites, linked into a European and World Association. This gave me an excuse not to up-date the book. It has taken the encouragement, and gentle pressure, of many parents and colleagues to shake me out of my natural lethargy. I must thank Paul Williams of Disability News who reviewed the last reprint and strongly stated we had taken the easy way with new photographs and that the book was worth up dating. I must particularly thank those parents who selected and translated it into Spanish, Dutch, Polish and most recently Slovenian, as part of their setting up of new Associations in their own countries. I found this very supportive. Special thanks go to Marzenna Rogala who did a fine translation into Polish and then persuaded me to finally start this new edition. Above all, however, I needed to re-write the book to acknowledge the effort and support of the families and young people with Down syndrome who make up the Manchester Down Syndrome Cohort. When we started with the babies in 1973 it never occurred to me that I would have the opportunity and privilege to watch them grow into young adults and find out first hand the sort of people they had become. My overwhelming picture is of young, positive, optimistic people enjoying and getting on with their lives. They, and their families, have provided the inspirations and foundation for any understanding I have achieved about Down syndrome.

I have needed a lot of help from friends and colleagues to re-write the book. I have also contacted many other people to clarify issues and recent work – too many to name – but all were most helpful, something that I have come to expect in the world of Down syndrome. Without Alan Fryer of the Department of Clinical Genetics, Royal Liverpool Children's Hospital I would not have coped with the genetics; as usual Richard Newton guided me through the medical aspects as well as giving me *carte blanche* to freely take from his own new edition; Vee Prasher did the same on aspects of health in adults with Down syndrome; Maggie Woodhouse of the University of Cardiff on visual problems, and Bethan Davies as ever kept me sensibly up to date on hearing dif-ficulties. Tricia Sloper, Steve Turner and Alison Alvarez largely undertook the studies with the cohort during the teenage years. Sheila Glenn and I have continued the research into Down syn-drome over the last ten years, and she has been very helpful with Chapters 8, 9 and 10.

Special thanks go to Ernest Hecht of Souvenir Press. It was he who started the Human Horizon Series that has had such an impact on the lives of people with disability, and has ensured this third edi-tion has finally been published.

I must thank Tamsin Ford, not just for my grandchildren, but the illustrations; Sue Hill, my ever-enthusiastic neighbour for typing and sorting out the book when I was flagging and Gerry Cooney for editing. My son Barnaby, who unlike myself works in the front line with people with disability, kept me abreast of new develop-ments and person-centred planning. My final thanks are for Marta, my wife, for her support, proof reading, research assisting, profes-sional experience and, as usual, honest positive criticism.

Cliff Cunningham, Spring 2006

To the First (1982) Edition

Thanks to Dana Brynelsen for her supportive comments on drafts; Margaret Flynn for her help on the section dealing with brothers and sisters; Robert Craven for his help with the illustrations. For the photographs thanks go to David Griffths, June Hayes-Light and the many parents who keep sending me photographs and allow me to use them. Special thanks are extended to Dian Donnai and the Department of Medical Genetics at St.Mary's Hospital, Manchester for help with the chapter on chromosomes. My most grateful thanks are extended to Ellen Cullen for the typing and layout of the book and her endless patience with the redrafts. Finally, I must thank my wife Marta, who as ever has combined honest criticism with patience and support. My children will be glad to know 'the chapters' are finished and, once again, they can dominate my time and play elephants outside the study. I have been supported over the last eight years by research grants from the Social Science Research Council and the Department of Health and Social Security.

To the Second (1988) Edition

It is an indication of the amount of activity related to Down's syndrome that I have needed to update this book only five years after the first edition. I am indebted to all the parents and professionals who have written to me and given me ideas for changes and additions and the encouragement to revise the book. I am again grateful to Dr. Dian Donnai, and to Dr. Richard Newton of the Royal Manchester Children's Hospital for help on the medical aspects. I am indebted to Dr. Jennifer Dennis of the Park Hospital for Children, Oxford, and Dr. David Southall of the Cardiothoracic Institute, London, for allowing me to describe their work on upper airway obstruction and to Dr. Joyce Ludlow for generously allowing me to incorporate her work. I, of course, take responsibility for errors. I must thank my colleagues who, at various times, have been members of the Manchester Down Syndrome Cohort team: Tricia Sloper, Meg Aumonier, Jiri Berger, Sheila Glenn, Liz Byrne, Anne Rangecroft, Christina Knussen and Chris Lennings, and also the associated students who have made a large contribution: Margret Arnlsdottir, Gyda Haroldsdottir, Vicki Gibbs and Stephanie Lorenz. The Research has been funded by the DHSS.

Note to the 1997 Reprint

Thanks again to all the parents who sent in photographs for the new picture selection, and to the DSA, Belinda Whiting and Stephen Leighton for kindly giving me permission to reproduce photographs from their collections.

What is Down syndrome?

Down – after Dr. Langdon Down who first recognised the distinctive characteristics of Down syndrome.

Syndrome – a collection of distinctive characteristics or symptoms.

It results from extra genetic material from chromosome 21 (Chapter 4). Not every person with it has every characteristic, or the same level of a characteristic. There are great differences between people with Down syndrome in terms of their intellectual abilities, sociability, height, weight, health, personality and so on – just as great, in fact, as the differences between the rest of us.

If you tell me that your child has Down syndrome all I know for a fact is that they have some extra chromosome 21 material. I know they will have similar and distinctive facial features to other people with the syndrome – but for some it is not that obvious. I know they will have some intellectual disability, but again some function as well as people we think of as 'normal'. From then on it is about **'probability'**. He or she will probably be . . .; The chances of XXX are 60% . . .; Four out ten will have . . . etc. etc.

For me, **Down syndrome is not a fixed label, but a statement of probability about another human being. It is not a just a condition but a complex phenomenon.**

The purpose of this book is to provide as up-to-date information as possible about all these probabilities. The hope is that it will help parents and carers understand the uniqueness of the person with the syndrome, and make more informed decisions as to how best to help them lead a fulfilled life.

When I refer to parent I often mean all carers. When I refer to family, I don't just mean the biological mother and father, but to the people with whom the child lives, who care for the child and who are the main advocates and guardians of the child.

Dear Parent,

I ask you to read this page before you read the book. I request this because of a problem I cannot resolve.

If a baby is born and appears quite normal, we parents are not given a detailed catalogue of information on what might go wrong in the future. We are not told about the chances that medical or psychological problems may appear. We are not given lists of statistics about the risk of delinquency, drug abuse or success at school or work. We go home with the baby and dream our dreams for a happy future. If we were given such a list, we would need to learn to live with the information and control our imaginings of what might happen.

But if you have a baby born with a condition like Down syndrome, which is recognisable from birth or shortly after, then many facts and figures are available. Much of the information is about possible medical and developmental problems and how they can be helped. But the majority of children with Down syndrome do not have many of these problems. Therefore you will not need all the information.

However, you will hear and be given a lot of information and advice that is wrong and misleading; you will need factual information in order to weed out what you do not need and to keep what might be helpful. My problem is that I do not know what you know; I do not know your child or your family. I do not know what information you want or need.

You will have to decide just how much information you want and how much you can cope with at a time. You will need to keep it in perspective. One of the parents in our research whose son was six years old, summed this up better than I can:

'You just have to get as many answers to the questions that go around in your head as you can . . . you need to do this as soon as you can so that you can get over a lot of the worrying and puzzling . . . you find when you get some information you can see just how silly the worrying was, but mind you, you can have too much . . . if you keep thinking about the future and all the things that can happen you'd go mad. Best thing to do, is get all that over with as quick as you can, then love him and do what you have to help . . . just take things from day to day as they come up . . . you know, once I got over all the shock and worrying and just helped him and that, things changed. I got to know him and I can truthfully say I've had a lot of joy these last years'.

Whether we are parents, professionals or members of the general public, the danger we all face is that our knowledge of a disability will cloud our vision of the baby, child or adult as he or she really is. We need to be constantly on the alert to this danger and must make efforts to stop focusing solely on the disability or handicap. I feel parents often learn to do this better than professionals.

For most parents who have just learnt that their baby has Down syndrome, this is not an easy process. Fortunately, according to research, and the large majority of parents I have known, as they begin to get over their grief and shock, they begin to see the baby and not the condition. They begin to learn to live with and in most cases, to enjoy the new member of their family.

I sincerely hope that you find this book – with all its limitations – of some help with this process.

Cliff Cunningham

Introduction

'I Used to Think of Her as a Stranger'

'As I learnt more about Down syndrome I felt I understood her better and somehow it helped me get closer to her . . . you know for quite a time I used to think of her as a stranger . . . like someone from a different country . . . not one of us'.

The words of this mother of a three-year old girl with Down syndrome succinctly highlight one of the reasons why parents, or anyone involved, needs information about Down syndrome. Understanding can bring us all closer to the child. Knowledge can reduce the fears and uncertainties that get between us and the other person.

A father of a ten-day old baby with Down syndrome forced this point upon me. I was on my first visit to the family home and had been answering questions such as: 'How was it caused?' 'How will the child develop – physically and mentally?' 'What are the chances of future babies having Down syndrome?' 'Are the other children in the family likely to be affected?' 'Will relatives have more risk of having a child with Down syndrome?' 'What will he be like when he grows up?' 'What can we do to help?' 'What help can we expect?' 'Where can we get help from?' Afterwards, the father said:

'I wish you had come yesterday. My brother and his family were here and kept asking what was wrong with the baby and I couldn't tell them. I felt a right fool. He's my son and I didn't even know anything about him'.

About our research

Both these families are part of a group of nearly 200 who have a child with Down syndrome and who are, or have been, involved in our research. In the late 1960's I was approached by the local parents of children with intellectual disability to do something with families of very young children. At the time they seemed to leave hospital with many unanswered questions and no support or direction. We set up some parent workshops, meeting one evening a week over ten weeks.

Our aim was simply to share with parents our knowledge on early child development and methods of stimulating and teaching young children. These parents quickly taught me how little we understood about the early development of children with Down syndrome and the needs of the family.

In the early 1970's I began to recruit families who had just had a baby with Down syndrome. We visited the home soon after the birth and then every six weeks for the first two years of life, then every six months until they were five. After that, we have managed to see them on several occasions for formal research projects, and keep in touch with many informally. The last research project was in the late 1990's when they were young adults. Around eighty were still available and willing to put up with our intrusions.

It is their questions and needs that have driven and directed the research. Throughout, parents have told us they want accurate, up-to-date, truthful and unbiased information about Down syndrome. They often demanded that it was written down for future reference and to share with relatives and professionals. Looking back, I realise they needed this information in order to make choices and decisions without being always dependent upon some professional or expert – who unfortunately they did not always trust. They had to become experts in order to take control of their lives and that of their child with Down syndrome.

But it was not just about facts. Feelings about having a child with Down syndrome are just as important. The parents have made it quite clear to me that information about how other parents felt when the baby was born and how they coped was a great help. Several parents have told me that when they were given the diagnosis they 'were scared to death', 'just became totally numb', or 'I had no idea what it all meant and couldn't think straight for days'.

In recent years we have begun to talk to the young people themselves about how they feel about having Down syndrome and their hopes and aspirations. Many expressed how they also valued being able to talk to someone about such things, and as with most teenagers and young adults, not always to their parents. Many want information but can easily become 'cocooned' within the protective shell of their family.

About this book

The content of this book is grounded in these experiences, and the many formal and informal discussions with people caring for or involved with children and adults with Down syndrome in many countries. It is also grounded in the work of hundreds of other people who have written about Down syndrome and published their research.

It has been over 140 years since Dr Langdon Down described the special characteristics that make up the syndrome. In those first years there were less than a half a dozen papers or reports on Down syndrome published each year. Last year I traced over 1000 published since 2000. I have over 50 books or monographs just on Down syndrome. Some are written by parents, two by people with Down syndrome and others by professionals from many disciplines – medicine, psychology, education, sociology, politics, health, nutrition, speech and language therapy and physiotherapy.

My point is if you are a parent of a baby with Down syndrome you need not feel alone. There are many thousands of parents and professionals actively engaged with people with Down syndrome or the subject of Down syndrome. This rapid expansion in information, activity and help is overwhelming for professionals who try to keep up to date, and certainly must be bewildering for new parents.

One message in this book is not to try to learn everything too soon. Much of it will not be directly helpful to the development and happiness of your child. Another is not to get too drawn into the views and demands of professionals in doing everything that is suggested to help the baby develop. You can take your time and work out what is best for you and your family.

The book aims to give you enough of an overview so that you can make the decisions about what you need. Most parents soon learn to live with the unique new person and realise that the 'Down syndrome' label is not very useful. Instead, they focus on doing the best they can to meet the needs of the child and family, and hopefully enjoy life. Some get fascinated like I did, and have been for over 30 years. It has led me into all aspects of the human condition from genetics to social policy and big questions like – What do we want from life? Why do we have children? What sort of society do we want to live in?

In using all these sources I have tried to ensure that all the 'facts' are taken from quality research. When there is dispute and controversy I have tried to make this plain. When I give an opinion that may bias my conclusions from such research, I have tried to make this clear.

What I do not have is any direct experience of being a parent of a child with Down syndrome. But, the experience and knowledge I have gained over the years make me feel that, whilst I do not wish any child to be conceived with Down syndrome, if it had happened to me, it would not have been the tragedy that I used to imagine. In this I am like many parents who have had a child with Down syndrome:

> 'When they told me he had Down syndrome I thought it was the biggest tragedy that had ever happened. If only we had known then what it is really like . . . the joy he brings . . . we wouldn't have been nearly as sad. But looking back at those first weeks no one really mentioned the positive things. They just made us feel more depressed and sad. I had this longing to run away from it all'.

I am not in a position to truly understand the feelings of parents who have a baby with Down syndrome. In Chapter 2 I have drawn together what parents have told me, and the observations of other professionals. I have tried to show the feelings that parents seem to have in common and make some sense of them.

Not surprisingly, I find that writing the information in a book is not as easy as giving it face-to-face. The reader can't direct me to their most urgent questions and how much detail they want. I can't shape my answers to meet what I see as their particular needs at that time, and of course to their baby. All children with Down syndrome are very different and it is almost impossible to make any general statements without noting a list of exceptions. The same applies to their families, who are equally unique.

How to use this book

I am conscious that parents often become frustrated when trying to extract answers from long and complicated general explanations. They also get distressed with textbooks that concentrate on the pathological and abnormal characteristics of the condition and use extreme examples and photographs. I have therefore tried to focus on the people and the human story, but provide all the facts from which you can select those you want.

The book is in four parts that follow what I see as the journey to becoming a parent of a child with Down syndrome. The first section is about learning the diagnosis, sorting out the feelings and reactions that are triggered by this, coping and trying to get the family and your life back on course. Section two is about causes and risks; what caused the Down syndrome? how prevalent it is and prenatal testing? Section three is about the characteristics of Down syndrome and what we can do to reduce the chances that they may cause additional problems. Section four looks at treatments, early interventions and other practical things that might help you to feel confident with the baby and in setting up future plans.

The book is not a comprehensive textbook. It is a collection of questions and answers that have built up over the years, an introduction for new parents, relatives, carers and anyone with an interest. I have often got stuck in deciding what to put in and how much detail to include. At these times I asked myself what is it that I need to feel I understand Down syndrome in all its aspects? What information would allow me to make decisions about what might be important to follow-up? What questions might I have to ask others for further information?

To help you find your way through the detail of the book, I have:

- Provided a list of contents and an index.
- Listed the main issues covered in each chapter as questions at the start.
- Tried to make each chapter and some sections stand on their own. This has led to lots of cross-references and some repetition but, as a teacher, I have learnt that repetition is not always detrimental. You can read the book from cover to cover, or dip in as you wish.
- Avoided extremes in selecting photographs and quotes, and used those that seem typical of children and families with Down syndrome.

Much of what is in the book you can probably put aside. This will leave you time to focus on the new person in your life, who happens to have Down syndrome. I hope this will help you develop your own understanding of this person and of the effects that he or she may have on you or your family – happy, sad, joyful, difficult.

Finally, to repeat myself, each child with Down syndrome is unique and as different from others as any child is. Your reactions and feelings are unique to you, as are those of family and friends. All we can do is to try to understand and reduce the fear and lack of confidence that result from our lack of knowledge and the uncertainty of this phenomenon called Down syndrome. Then, having sorted out the unique needs of the child and family, we can plan how to meet them.

Becoming a Family of a Child with Down Syndrome

CHAPTER 1
Will we cope? What can we expect and
how do we tell people?

CHAPTER 2
Coming to terms with the diagnosis – feelings,
reactions and adapting

CHAPTER 3
What effect will it have on the family?

If you have recently been told your baby has Down syndrome you probably have many painful and confused feelings, and feel overwhelmed. Parents have told me it helps to know others have similar feelings. You may prefer to read Chapter 2 first.

1

Will we cope? What can we expect and how do we tell people?

- Will we cope with the baby? – with the family, relatives and friends?
- What are these children like? What sort of people do they become?
- What do I have to do to be a 'good enough' parent for them?
- How do I tell the other children, or grandma, or friends?

This whole book is an attempt to answer these questions. This first chapter tries to give some brief answers. Hopefully, they will be reassuring, and you will feel more ready to read other chapters. A starting point is to sort out the tasks that may lie ahead.

What tasks face the parent of a new baby with Down syndrome?

Being told your baby has Down syndrome is like being given a new identity – the family of a baby with Down syndrome. This usually involves great emotional and psychological changes for the parent and family. It is not surprising that most parents become over-whelmed and feel lost (Chapter 2).

It is true that 'time is a great healer' but it is not just time. It is not just about a passive period waiting for things to get better. Your mind is active. Although you may feel numb and in shock, or in total turmoil and getting nowhere, your mind is trying to make sense of this unexpected event. In a sense, this is a process of **active coping.** Understanding the process has been found to be a very helpful coping strategy. A first step is to identify key questions and tasks. I think these are:

- **Understanding yourself, your feelings and reactions as a parent of a child with Down syndrome (Chapter 2).**
- **Understanding how others feel (Chapter 2), and the effect the birth may have on them (Chapter 3).**
- **Understanding Down syndrome, its causes, characteristics, what to do and what the future might hold (Sections two, three and four).**
- **Understanding your new baby with Down syndrome. This is something you and the baby do together. You, your baby, and your family are unique. All the information about Down syndrome is general and gives background. You get to know the baby and your relationship with the baby through everyday experiences.**

I hope this does not sound too simple. It is not a stress free process. These tasks are not done quickly or in order. The first weeks after a birth are busy and tiring. Sometimes there is just not enough time and energy to sort everything out. I hope to show that most parents do sort it out within the first months.

A first action is to decide which tasks are important at this time, and to work on these. Put the others in a box and leave them until there is energy and opportunity to take them out and examine them. But please don't ignore them – too often all the focus is on the baby and less time is given to think about other things, especially your feelings and keeping family life balanced and working.

Will we cope?

Books and articles by parents, and many studies of families who have a baby with Down syndrome, confirm that the chances of coping are far greater than the chances that you will not. I interpret this as showing that most of us have resources we are not aware of until faced with a challenge.

When the children in our research were 7 to 14 years old, we asked the parents to reflect back on their experiences and feelings of being a parent of a child with Down syndrome. Just over half said

---

**WHAT RESOURCES DO WE NEED TO HELP
OUR FAMILY COPE?**

The key resources can be put into five groups:
- Practical things – like sufficient money, adequate housing, a car or access to transport, energy saving devices like washing machines.
- Health and energy levels – these are particularly important with young lively children and/or those with some physical problems.
- Personal skills – such as being able to solve problems or find information and get help. Knowledge and understanding can make us feel more competent and strong when faced with a challenge. Resilience – being able to bounce back – is important.
- Social support networks – including emotional support and practical help from partners, relatives and friends or from support services or groups. Talking to people in similar circumstances not only gives reassurance, it can also challenge our ideas and give us new ways of thinking about things.
- Beliefs, attitudes, values and aspirations – including beliefs about ourselves, what we want out of life, for our children and ourselves, and attitudes and beliefs about disability. Living somewhere where there are very negative views of disability can make coping more difficult.

it was rewarding and strengthening, a quarter felt it was the same as with their other children, and a quarter were more negative. This last group usually had other problems, and their child with Down syndrome had additional problems (Chapter 9) that made great demands on family resources.

Some studies have asked mothers of young children with and without Down syndrome about how they coped with the baby and young child. Over two-thirds of both groups said they coped, the rest had experienced difficulties and again, this was usually because they lacked some resource.

If we have a problem but not the resources to try to reduce it, we have a need. The task is to work out what are our needs and then seek out the resources. Services should be doing this as part of the support they give to parents – accurate information, practical and financial help, for example. But parents and families can examine their own strengths and needs, make plans and develop their own resources. Leaving it all to one parent, usually the mother, is not likely to help the family cope. The benefits are not just to the child. Many parents state that having a child with Down syndrome has brought the family closer together and helped them to be stronger and more tolerant people. My observations are that this happens in those families that look at individual strengths and weakness, respect each other, work together and marshal their resources. They appear to experience less stress and more *pleasure* in parenting a child with Down syndrome.

As usual parents speak better for themselves:

'When we found out she was a Down syndrome, I thought it would just be an endless burden . . . I didn't expect any joy or anything good. Of course we didn't know any better. We had no experience and the way we were told just made you think of all the problems . . . Over the years that changed. She did things and every little gain was such a joy . . . I felt so proud, like the day she walked straight into the playgroup, head held high and just started to play like any kid . . . none of the other children bothered . . . it was really me feeling all up tight. That's all gone now. She's herself and one of the family. She's sort of brought us all closer together and whenever she's around somehow she soon cheers you up and gets people friendly.'

FAMILIES WHO COPE APPEAR TO:

- Work together – split jobs according to their strengths
- Seek information – make a file of resources, names and addresses
- Be assertive – parents need to learn to fight for their rights and services for their child
- Learn new skills – such as how to interact with the child, understand learning difficulties, managing the child's behaviour and potential health problems
- Rethink their beliefs and values
- Accept the child as he or she is – give unconditional love and come to terms with the disability.

Most families eventually feel the 'tragedy' was not catastrophic, and many feel their lives have changed for the better. Many of these understandings and reflections come slowly, often many months and even years after the diagnosis:

> 'if we hadn't had a handicapped child we would have had two children, everything pre-planned, under control. Instead we have four kids and a lively time . . . the carpet was yanked from under our feet by his birth but it has given us a tremendous amount of pleasure. It brought out our fighting qualities, has given us lots of friends – affiliations that are stronger than non-handicapped friends; it makes us value the important things in life as opposed to achievement and financial success . . . we are less inclined to worry about silly things.'

In other words, the member of the family with Down syndrome is not just a passive recipient of family resources and help. These members can make their own contribution to the quality of the life of the family.

What factors are associated with stress in parents of children with Down syndrome?

About a third of families find coping very difficult and experience persistent high levels of stress. This is more likely when the child has severe behaviour problems, which affects only a minority (Chapter 9). Even with these children, many parents develop ways to cope and find pleasure in their child. However, many studies of families have shown coping becomes more and more difficult if the following other factors are present:

- High levels of stressful life-events – especially if they involve family relationships.
- Financial problems – linked to inadequate housing and transport or employment difficulties. Poorer family relationships may be caused by money worries, which then affect how we manage the children, they develop behaviour problems and this increases the stress for the parents.
- Personality of parents – those more likely to feel anxious and less competent experience more stress.
- Inadequate coping strategies – 'wishful' thinking is associated with stress and health problems, whereas active coping and problem solving appears to reduce stress in many situations.
- Poor adjustment to the disability is associated with stress, lower levels of well- being and failure to enjoy and value the child.

These are all discussed in more detail in later chapters. As noted above, the way to try to reduce the stress and strain is to identify the need and then find a resource. Most people feel better as soon as they have made a plan to do this.

Demands, needs and resources

From my reading and experience, I have found that problems are usually associated with a lack of resources to deal with the child's caretaking demands, or his or her need for supervision. The other category concerns the parent's feelings about being a parent of the child.

Caretaking Demands

These are about the physical needs such as dressing, bathing, feeding, lifting, and taking children to school, hospital, leisure activities and so on. Most children with Down syndrome, even those with mild intellectual disability, never attain all the life-skills and achieve total independence. They do make above average caretaker demands, but only a minority fall into the category of profound disability with very complex needs (Chapter 10). Some have additional health needs that increase caretaking demands such as special diets, need to be kept warm, medicines and preparations for dry skin (Chapter 7).

Faced with such demands, healthy and energetic parents are less likely to feel pressure and strain. Resources such as washing machines, disposable nappies, cars or help with transport, modified housing and practical support like shopping, travel, baby-sitting or respite care, can all reduce or prevent strain and support coping. A lot of this is to do with having enough money. Parents who feel supported emotionally and practically by each other, and by relatives and friends experience less stress.

Supervision demands

This is about having to keep a constant watch on the child. It is a big demand on time and restricts what the family can do. Children who develop slowly need similar levels of supervision as the typical young child, but for longer. As he child matures and develops, supervision demands usually reduce. Most families cope with this 'normal but slower' development (Chapter 9).

A minority of children with Down syndrome are excitable, hyperactive and attention seeking (Chapter 9). Their supervision demands are likely to drain family resources and cause stress and problems within the family. Again, stamina, health and energy are important coping resources for family members. Practical resources like modifications to the house such as an enclosed garden or safety locks can help, as can practical support and respite care. Good management practice can prevent problems and should be established early in life (Chapter 9).

Parental fulfilment

This is about getting pleasure out of being the parent of the child. It is about feeling you are doing a good enough job as a parent, valuing your child and their achievements, and about the child's ability to show affection. Some children with severe intellectual impairment never really recognize their parent, or understand what a parent is – they are happy with any person they feel they can trust. Others have problems with social understanding, interacting with others and showing affection. These difficulties are rare in children with Down syndrome who often show high levels of affection, and for whom social development is their strongest area (Chapter 8).

Parents who have not come to terms with the disability or find it difficult to value their child do not feel fulfilment. These parents often give the child less attention and praise, make more negative comments when talking about the child, and show the child less affection. These children often have more behaviour problems. Whether the lack of attachment is the cause – or the result – of the child's behaviour is difficult to know. Fortunately, this is a small group and we have consistently found that well over three-quarters of parents have good relationships with their children.

Other parents appear to focus all their attention on trying to remedy the child's disability; they may lose sight of their parenting role, and with it fulfilment in parenting the child (see later).

If parents find they cannot value the child, they need to examine their beliefs and feelings and possibly seek professional help or talk to others. It can help to learn about the complexity of child development, how to observe the child, and ways of encouraging their development. With such knowledge, some parents begin to focus on the possible and take pride in their own and their child's achievements – simple things for typical children gained after considerable effort. In the first parent workshop we ran, we gave parents a development checklist like those used by professionals in assessments. They went home and ticked off things they saw their child do. At the next meeting nearly all the parents talked about how much the child could do and how surprised and proud they felt.

What can we expect?

Studies based on groups that include the full range of children and adults with Down syndrome (Chapter 10), have shown:

- There is a greater chance of them growing up as pleasant and amiable people than having major behaviour problems and being difficult to manage. But the management techniques and resource demands are different (Chapters 8 and 9).
- Before the age of five years they are very likely to be able to walk (most have started to walk around 2 years of age), feed themselves (but not cut with a knife), be toilet trained with a few mishaps (although wiping oneself properly can take a long time to learn), to have some words and phrases and to be able to communicate basic needs (Chapter 10).
- Some speak very well and have started reading before five years of age; most have a small vocabulary and, together with gestures and signs can communicate for everyday purposes. A few fail to develop reasonable communication skills (Chapters 8 and 10).
- As young adults it is more likely that they will be able to hold conversations, have friends (in some cases intimate friendships), and a range of interests, than that they will be profoundly intellectually disabled with little communication, poor self-help skills and few interests (Chapter 10).
- There is a greater chance that they will be good natured and attractive young people, than that they will be hostile, aggressive, sullen and difficult (Chapter 8).

Attitudes, expectations and opportunities

The above description is about people with Down syndrome today who have benefited from changes in society's attitudes, beliefs and expectations of them, and who consequently have greater opportunities to engage in life from birth (Chapter 8). In the early part of the 20th Century, many people with Down syndrome lived in large institutions and were deemed unable to profit from life experiences and education (Chapter 10). Even by the 1950's, an eminent researcher stated that after adolescence they lose all the characteristics that made them delightful children, and that they become listless, uninvolved, silent and dull. Some do 'lose their spark' but it is not inevitable, and these descriptions are more about how the people were treated than about their innate capability.

I think these positive changes have had a greater impact on the lives of children and adults with Down syndrome than research on their intellectual and psychological abilities and remedies, therapies and treatments (Chapter 12). If I am correct, the message is that we can make a huge impact on their lives by sorting out our own and others' attitudes and beliefs, and then by creating a positive and expectant environment within which children with any disability are given opportunities to develop to the best of their ability.

In developed societies the change towards a much more positive outlook has resulted in the provision of support services and a policy of inclusion in the community. It is recognised that:

- People with Down syndrome do best when living in the community, rather than in large institutions, at first with their families and then more independently.
- Families cope better if they are supported and resourced, not stigmatised or isolated.

Consequently there is:

- Increasing guidance and support for parents, including education from birth and help with child management, which should:
  - Help the children to become more skilled and independent, and reduce behaviour problems
  - Help parents avoid becoming isolated and making the child too dependent on them.
- An increasing willingness to include children with Down syndrome in everyday activities such as gym clubs, cubs, scouts, swimming, horse riding and, for many, enabling education in mainstream schools.
- In later childhood and adulthood, there is access to college education, skill training or work preparation workshops, organized sports and recreational activities. More and more adults with Down syndrome are living in houses or

apartments in the community and provided with support (Chapters 10 and 13).

Parenting and telling others

Two issues that parents often ask about when I first meet them, are how they tell others the baby has Down syndrome, and what to do to start to help the baby.

Being the parent of a child with Down syndrome

As we saw earlier, being the parent of a child with Down syndrome does bring many challenges, and often demands much re-thinking about values and beliefs, and seeking out new knowledge and learning new skills (Chapter 2 and Section four). Here I want to reassure parents that they do not have to rush at it.

Take time and focus on parenting

As the child's parent, you are his or her best hope for the future. You are their main advocate and they will need and benefit from your support to a greater extent than other children, because of the Down syndrome. Don't lose sight of your fundamental parenting role. I believe that 70 − 80 % of your child's potential will be brought out simply by giving the same sort of parenting that you would give to any child. Try to treat the child, not as 'normal' − but as normally as possible.

Coping with your child's learning difficulty does not mean you have to become a highly qualified therapist or a specialist teacher. Specific skills can be developed when and if they are needed. Don't rush out to find treatments for the Down syndrome even if the urge to do something is very strong. Trying to correct or 'remedy' what has happened may get in the way of coming to terms with the situation and finding a balanced way of moving forward with all the family.

Some children will have additional complications such as a heart problem, or a feeding problem that is an immediate priority for parents. But for most new parents, there is time to focus on the tasks noted earlier, and just get to know the baby.

Most parents do want to feel confident about how to engage and help the baby. Here I describe what I tell them. Parents will find other professionals may have different views and may advise on more intensive or specific programmes of activity. This is discussed in later chapters, and it is for parents to decide what they feel is right for them.

Interacting, teaching and managing

Because children with Down syndrome have intellectual disability, parents do need to learn ways of engaging with them that are not usually necessary with typical children. These are not complicated approaches that require professional training. I emphasise that it is similar to any child but you need more **patience** and **perseverance,** and you will learn to get **pleasure** from the smallest gains, and show this to the child. I have three rules of thumb:

1   Put yourself into first or second gear and work at the child's speed (Chapter 8). The nervous system of people with Down syndrome works at a slower pace than typical people (Chapter 7).

2   Learning difficulties mean children have problems seeing the different aspects of things (analysing tasks and information), and spotting the key aspect in what they see or hear. They also have difficulty putting things together (synthesising), to form chunks of skill or knowledge; they need more practice to consolidate their learning. We need to learn how to break tasks into small chunks; to sensitively direct their attention to the key aspects and then help them put things together (Chapter 11),

3   Don't jump in too soon to help them or make them do something. This will just teach them to wait for you and stifle their initiative and confidence (Chapter 8).

I will illustrate these rules with some examples, which hopefully show it is not that complicated. There is a natural rhythm when we talk with other people. You say or do something and wait for a response. If it does not come within a short period of time you try again or think something is wrong. We all learn these natural rhythms in the first weeks of life. But this normal timing is too quick for a baby or child with Down syndrome, they take longer to process the incoming information and longer still to send out a response. Unless we work at their speed, we are likely to try again just as the baby is about to respond. This stops the response and they have to start all over again. If you wait for the baby the baby is in control of the exchange.

We did research looking at how mothers interacted with their babies in the first weeks of life, comparing those with babies with Down syndrome to those with typical babies. We found the mothers of the babies with Down syndrome tended to have more 'inputs' than the mothers of the typical babies. We interpreted this as due to worries and low expectations that the baby might not 'perform' without help. When we told the mothers to slow down and wait, or just to imitate what the baby did:

- The mothers of the babies with Down syndrome decreased the amount of 'input' to the baby, to levels similar to those of the mothers with typical babies.
- The babies with Down syndrome smiled and vocalised more.

Imitating is a very good technique for giving control to the other person and reflecting back the behaviour. This can help children to think about the meaning of their actions. I have often found it useful with children who are very intellectually disabled and have little communication. Many have spent years passively being 'seen to' by others. When they find they are controlling others it can bring much excitement and fun.

The message is simple. Instead of always trying to make the child do something, give them more control over the engagement. That way, they are more likely to learn to be active and to initiate things than become passive.

Here is a father of a 13-year-old boy with Down syndrome:

'When we go swimming I have to make sure I give him an extra five minutes to get out and get dressed – with his brothers I just say O.K., let's go, but I say to David, dry yourself, then I check him, then I say put on your shirt . . . sort of prompting and checking each step . . . it takes longer but it's worth making him do it himself.'

Most of us have experienced the frustration of watching someone struggling to do something. It is tempting to jump in saying, 'let me show you.' This does not help the person develop self-confidence. It is more likely to teach them to be dependent on others. I tell parents, and myself, to 'sit on your hands.' The best teachers (and I mean people who are good at helping others to learn – not just trained professionals) are patient and use subtle suggestions that are not critical and judgemental. They don't dominate, and they try to work out ways of making it easier for the person to understand the problem and to feel they have achieved it by themselves. There are lots programmes that describe how different tasks can be broken down in small steps (see Resources). Once parents understand the principles, they usually use them as opportunities arise. The main problem is finding the time.

I believe that a lot of the passivity and dependence on others reported as characteristic of individuals with Down syndrome is due to how we interact with them and our expectations of them, rather than faults in their neurological system.

How do we tell others?

Sooner, rather than later

Most parents face the difficult task of telling others about the baby, and usually quite soon after they have been given the diagnosis. It is not easy to say 'my baby has Down syndrome', especially if you are in a state of shock yourself. Putting off telling people usually happens because it is painful for the parent to go through it all again and to cope with all the issues and tensions. Putting it off also happens when the parent does not want to cause pain for someone else. This seldom works.

All of us, including medical professionals, can find reasons for putting it off. Yet most parents complain if they are not given the diagnosis fairly quickly (Chapter 2). It suggests there is something to hide, to avoid, or be frightened or ashamed of. People may interpret not being told as you thinking they cannot be trusted with the information, or in the case of young children, that they are too young, or in their words 'too stupid', to understand.

Relatives, friends and neighbours will use how you tell them as their cue to how they talk about and share the experience with you. Putting it off may not work.

Parents and family members often guess that something is wrong in hospital because they notice that routines for their baby are different to other babies. The same can happen at home. Children are sensitive to disturbance in the household. Conversations suddenly stop when they are around; there is tension in the family; the new baby stays in hospital longer, or goes to the doctor more often than babies of friends. Similarly, it can be difficult to hide from relatives, friends and neighbours that the baby has additional needs.

A bonus of telling others is not just the relief, but that you are more likely to tap into support when everyone is reasonably open and willing to talk. Even if you strongly suspect a negative reaction by the other person, such as a grandparent, it is better to tell them, rather than to use up energy worrying about it and avoiding the issue. Most parents find it a great relief when they have told others.

Delaying the telling

Most parents say they want to be told as soon as is reasonably possible, and especially when the doctor has strong suspicions and is ordering further checks. They become concerned if they do not know why. But some parents have told me that the delay was good, because they enjoyed the first days with the baby without the shock and concern of knowing they had Down syndrome.

'I think I recognised it *(the Down syndrome)* as soon as I saw her but shut it out. It was two days later when they told me. I am glad I had those two days . . . it may have been more correct to tell me as soon as the doctor had suspicions, but it would have stolen those first hours of happiness.'

Such feelings have also influenced telling the brothers and sisters:

> 'They were 5 and 7 years old when Jenny was born. I didn't tell
> them straight away. I was grappling with my feelings and didn't
> tell them for a few months. I didn't want to destroy their enjoy-
> ment of the new baby . . . like happened to me . . . I wanted the
> bonding to take place first.'

Some doctors, like this mother, also feel that one should wait until
the mother and child have bonded. However, there is no evidence
from our studies that being told about the baby having Down syndrome in the first hours or days after the birth has any long term
effects on bonding and attachment (Chapter 2). Nor does telling
the siblings sooner or later, appear to affect their relationships with
the baby – as long as there is a reasonable explanation for the delay.
This makes the timing of 'telling' a difficult job for doctors; as yet
we don't know how to decide which parents would prefer some
delay.

Sometimes if the relative is unwell or very old, parents decide not
to tell them. I have not heard of any instances where this has caused
a problem. I think because there is an acceptable reason for not
telling, and therefore no implications for trust or shame.

Reactions of relatives and friends

The initial telling often falls to the father as the mother is in hospital. Relatives and friends are usually waiting to hear about how it all
went. Fathers often have to leave the hospital having just heard, and
then tell the others. It is not easy when you are in a state of shock
yourself. Often when the others hear the news, they ask the same
questions that parents are still fighting with, 'Are you sure?', 'Has
there been some mistake?' Some react with optimistic reassurance
that many parents do not feel at that time. Others ask what you will
do, or give advice on how to cope. This is not helpful when parents
are grappling with similar questions and confused feelings.
Unfortunately some relatives and friends also share their shock,
upset and pain, and the parents find themselves having to support

them instead of receiving the support they need. Fortunately this happens less often, and parents usually find others are supportive.

The grandparents

Grandparents are important at this time and need to be told (Chapter 3). Like the parents, they will experience a range of feelings and reactions as described in Chapter 2. Understanding how you would want to be told can help how to tell them. A father told me that when he and his wife were being told he suddenly realised he would have to go and tell his mother and father and the family:

'It was their first granddaughter . . . they had always wanted a girl. They had been getting really excited. Mum had been knitting and Dad had helped me wallpaper the bedroom. Well, the doctor who told us was so good I thought it best to do as he did. I went to their house and sat them down together and said straight out, 'I've got some bad news, the little girl has got Down syndrome – she's a Down's baby.' They reacted just like we did. Mum cried and Dad said are you sure; there must be a mistake. I wanted to shout – How do I know if they're sure? I could feel my temper rising just like it had when I left the hospital. I told him that the doctor said he was 99.9% certain but would do a chromosome test and we would know the results in a couple of weeks. I told them that the doctor said it wasn't like it used to be . . . there was lots of things one could do to help . . . schools and exercises for the baby. But I can see them now; they were so sad and helpless . . . Mum asked how was J . . . taking it and I said, not too bad. Then I looked at her and said we'll need your help Mum, if we are going to get through. Well that was it. She just came over and hugged me and said of course we'll help, won't we Dad? We'll manage and don't you worry about the baby she's still one of the family. Well somehow after that things looked better . I found it easier to tell friends and my brother. It was best just to say, 'She's got Down syndrome.' Once I had said it everything was usually okay and every time I said it, it got easier. But you soon find out who your friends are. I was surprised just how kind people were – even people in our street who we only ever said Hello to . . . I was also surprised to find out just how many

people in our street had a relative or a friend with Down
syndrome . . .'

During the same home visit, the mother told me that it was such a
relief to come out of hospital with the baby knowing that her husband had told most of their friends and relatives.

Another parent told me,

'We found a fund of goodwill in our friends and relatives. We
needed to harness it and direct it.'

Telling the other children

If you have no other children you may prefer to skip this section.

Parents say that from about 4 years the siblings of a child with
Down syndrome begin asking questions: 'Why can't he talk like
me?' 'Why does she look different?', 'Why is she not jumping?'
Often it is social things that trigger the question: 'Why does she go
to a different school? . . . to hospital?' 'Why do people keep coming
to see him?'

A child who has a sibling with a disability, or who has a classmate
with a disability, is more likely to notice differences and ask questions sooner. These same things can trigger questions in a child with
Down syndrome. They see someone with Down syndrome on television and point out they look the same, or they ask why they go
to a different school. I discuss their understanding and awareness of
their own disability in Chapter 8.

The child's age and level of intellectual development will govern
how much sense they make of their observations or what you tell
them. If the other children in the family are quite young (under
three), they are unlikely to understand the idea of different. But they
will be sensitive to any distress and tension in the family and need
some explanation. It is important to help them to understand that
they have not *caused* any upset, and try to avoid indicating that their
new brother or sister is causing the distress. The older the child, the
more information he or she will understand. If they are 8 years or
older, they will already have some idea of intellectual disability.

HOW DO CHILDREN UNDERSTAND DIFFERENCES
IN OTHERS AND DISABILITY?

This developmental sequence is based on average ages –
some children will show the behaviour earlier and others later.

12-18 months – can recognise themselves and know if
   something has changed, for example a mark on the face.
   They can recognize others and begin to 'see' what is the
   same or different.

2-3 years – they understand that they are a boy or a girl and
   other characteristics about themselves such as hair colour.

3-4 years – they become very aware of physical and
   observable differences in others such as age, size, hair and
   skin colour. They begin to understand social groups such
   as relatives and friends. They talk about me and mine, their
   belongings and their mother, father, sister etc.

5-8 years –they begin to form social categories, grouping
   others using physical characteristics such as having blond
   hair, being taller, dark or light skinned, and observable
   behaviours such as being a fast runner, or a good reader.
   They begin to recognise and understand disability – some
   people can't walk, speak or see. An important change is
   that they begin to understand some characteristics are
   permanent such as ethnicity and gender. Most 6-7 years
   olds understand not being able to walk can be permanent,
   but three quarters still think intellectual disability is like
   being ill and you can get better.

7-8 – they begin to compare themselves with others and
   make judgements about desirable and undesirable
   characteristics. These comparisons begin to influence their
   self evaluation and their self esteem and reflect social
   beliefs and values.

8-9 years – they begin to make more abstract comparisons
   and more understanding of learning and intelligence. They
   are aware that intellectual ability and disability can be
   permanent.

There is a development sequence relating to how typical children understand themselves, other people and disability. Studies have also shown that it is similar in children with intellectual disability. I think is offers a good guideline about telling and explaining disability.

> 'When Alison was about three months old I felt ready to tell her brother. He was just over six. I started by pointing out the shape of her eyes . . . I said it was called Down syndrome. I got him to help with the exercises I had started doing. I explained she needed it to help her learn to walk sooner because she learned things a bit slower. He was fascinated. He told his friends that his sister was special and had Down syndrome. I remember one day when I found him showing three of his friends how to do the exercises and they were fascinated and all wanted a turn!'

How and what do I say to the children?

Some parents prefer to be reactive:

> 'I think it's a bit artificial to suddenly start to tell them – it makes an issue of it and there really is no issue. We didn't hide anything and when they started asking questions we answered them.'

Others are more proactive:

> 'I told her brother when he was five and about to start at school. I thought others might ask questions or say things and so it was best if I prepared him . . . it seems to have worked well because we have not had any problems.'

Many look for opportunities, and fit their explanations to what they feel the child will understand:

> 'When they were doing genetics at school, I took the opportunity of explaining about the extra chromosomes that caused the Down syndrome in Michael.'

I think telling them about disability is a bit like telling children about sex. If they ask a question or offer an opportunity we either ignore it, which helps no one, or often in our anxiety we 'grab the moment' and to make sure they understand, end up delivering a complex lecture with far more information than they want.

TELLING TOGETHER

Do the telling together as a family and with the baby present. I have no strong evidence for how important this is, but an 18-year-old brother of a girl with Down syndrome told me how, when she was born and he was twelve, his mother told him about his sister. He knew his father was out in the garden and, at the time, could not think why he did not tell him as well. It was a year or two before he discussed the Down syndrome with his father and they were both profoundly relieved. At eighteen, he said he understood why his father had not been able to tell him, but felt sad that there had been some tension, something to be avoided, in what otherwise was a very close relationship. Incidentally, most parents like to have the baby present when the doctor tells them about the Down syndrome – it shows it is not something to hide away.

So what do we tell the other children? I agree with most parents that you should say the baby has Down syndrome because this word will be around a lot and they need to feel secure in using it. But what does it mean? Children need some explanation that they understand and, and importantly, **words they can use to explain to others.** This level of understanding is seen in the questions they ask: Will he learn to walk? Will she come to my school? Why do you do those exercises with her? With younger children I prefer the word 'different', because I believe they understand this better than 'disability' or 'handicap.' I think you should avoid explanations like 'something wrong', or 'the brain doesn't work properly.' because this can be misunderstood. However, some people feel the word 'different' is not useful, because we are all different, and we may be avoiding the correct words 'disabled' or 'handicapped.' We may be in danger of over-emphasising the difference rather than the sameness.

Whatever words we choose, we must not suggest that Down syndrome is an illness or disease. As noted above, this is how young children usually try to make sense of what they are being told; they will have experienced being ill and feeling sick or in pain, and associate this with doctors and being physically examined and taking medicine and getting better. I think it is quite a good idea to point out that Down syndrome is not being ill and the baby is not sick, suffering or in pain. Of course, if the baby has other problems, like a heart condition, this can complicate things.

When I have asked parents how they explained it, most said they emphasised that the baby or child would be 'slower to learn things', or needed 'more time to learn things.' Most illustrated this by focusing on concrete things like sitting, walking, running, drawing, or doing puzzles. Using an activity that the child is into at the time is useful. For example, 'you can draw a man very well, but the new baby will need you to show him or her and will take longer.' Many parents also pointed out the physical features such as the shape of the eyes, when telling the child about the Down syndrome.

There are some excellent books for children at different ages (see Resources Section) and I have known several teenage siblings dip into this book.

How do siblings react to finding out about the Down syndrome?

If the family talks openly about the syndrome and the child, then the other children will take this in and use it as the basis for their understanding and feelings. The majority of six to ten year olds seem to take the news in their stride and carry on as before. If new information is available, they will seek it when they want it. At this age, many parents said the siblings thought the child with Down syndrome would grow out of it or get better; the 'illness' idea noted earlier. Explaining the difference between illness and disability, and its implications, is worthwhile.

Parents describe how children over ten, and particularly teenagers, reacted to the news much as they had themselves. Some protest that it cannot be true because the baby looks fine and is very happy and alert. This can hurt, as it is what parents want to believe, despite the evidence. Like their parents, they need to express their shock and grief and come to terms with what it means. Some need time on their own to think it through. Others need things to do. Many mothers talk about the support they got from older children, particularly daughters.

We found that less than 5% of parents felt their child reacted in a particularly negative way to the news. One 5 year old asked if it was his fault and became withdrawn for several weeks; a 9 year old became very aggressive and resentful and would not go near the new baby for some time; and a 15 year old girl developed behaviour problems, but she was already experiencing difficulties within the family. I think the younger children were caught up in the general feelings in the family at this time. With older children the diagnosis will interact with their own feelings of security and relationships within the family (Chapter 3).

We can underestimate our children at such times. A friend who has a child with severe and profound disabilities told this story. When the baby was a few weeks old, and shortly after he had told his son about his sister, a sympathetic neighbour, had gone through the rather harrowing 'How are you?', 'How is the poor little girl?', 'What a shame, but these things happen', set of questions and reassuring statements, when the three-and-a-half year-old brother looked up and said ' but we still love her, you know.'

How do the siblings tell their friends?

At some time, brothers and sisters have to tell others. They can find this difficult, and need help from their parents. An adult sister who had a younger brother with intellectual disability told me:

'I was always embarrassed about informing people about Peter's mental handicap. Explaining mental handicap to people when you are only young can be overwhelmingly difficult – even if you understand it yourself. It was also difficult coping with questions like – What does your brother do? Where does he go to school? etc. It was only as I became older that I ceased to use 'mental handicap' as an excuse for Peter's behaviour and was able to explain that he hasn't learnt to do it yet.'

Even parents get tired of having to explain their child to others. Sometimes a brother or sister will not admit or mention their sibling with Down syndrome to friends, because of the difficulty of explanations. Parents need to tell siblings in a way they can then tell others and possibly even give them some practice in telling others. I discuss using role-playing and drama in Section Four. The words need to be carefully selected, because labels can give out the wrong message (see Chapter 10). Using the correct term Down syndrome with the explanation that it 'takes him or her longer to learn things' and 'he has not learnt to do something yet', are useful.

TALKING OPENLY ABOUT DOWN SYNDROME

Parents often emphasise the importance of talking openly about the Down syndrome as soon as they feel reasonably all right. This shows they feel OK about their child with Down syndrome, which helps the other children, relatives, neighbours and friends, to feel comfortable asking questions and talking about it. Natural and everyday opportunities should be used for the family to voice ideas and raise topics for discussion. This is far better than reacting to a crisis or creating an artificial discussion along the lines of 'now it is time we had that chat.' It is certainly better than avoiding issues and implying there is something best kept hidden. Worries or issues should be raised openly. If family members, including the children, have aired their views, they are more likely to feel some ownership over decisions and become involved. If they disagree then at least this is out in the open.

What if I can't take the baby home?

From my experience, between 20 to 30% of parents in the UK find they cannot face taking the baby home from hospital. In other countries some have no option; parents may be encouraged to place the baby in an institution based on the false assumption that the baby may harm the family and it was best for the baby (Chapter 3).

Parents can agonise for days or weeks trying to decide what is best. They need to get an accurate picture of Down syndrome and reassess their feelings. But the decision is not just taken coldly and objectively based on facts; it has to come from the heart. The problem is made more difficult if the mother and father have different attitudes and reactions. They may have a very different understanding about Down syndrome and its' implications. They may have different aspirations for the future and fears of how a child with a disability will affect this.

About half the parents I have met found it helpful to visit a family who had a young child with Down syndrome. Half did not want to until several months after the birth. Some felt no need, but others feared they would be pressurised into making a decision by meeting a family who had taken the child home and was coping.

When parents are undecided, the situation tends to resolve itself in one of three ways:

1   The parents are reassured by getting information about Down syndrome and help and support (family and services); they breathe a sigh of relief and go and get the baby. In my experience nearly all these parents never look back.

2   The parents realise they cannot cope at that moment. They decide not to take the baby home, perhaps to have a break and stop talking about the problems for a few days.

> 'We were told we could leave the baby in the hospital and go home to give ourselves time to think . It did me good as I had a chance to get over the birth. We also talked and talked and got some information from someone who knew a lot about these babies.'

> 'Getting home where I felt safe and could take my own time was so helpful.'

> 'We decided not to talk about it for a few days. Then when we sat down we both knew we wanted to bring the baby home.'

3   Some parents do not resolve the problems but they take the baby home anyway. This seems to put an end to the emotional

stress of trying to make the decision. Sometimes it is one parent saying we will take the baby home and the other just complying. From my experience, about half find coping easy and enjoy the baby. In the other cases it causes friction and was never resolved (Chapter 3).

Sometimes the parents get so worn out dealing with contradictory information and feelings they cannot make a decision one way or the other. In these cases the family should seek help from an experienced and non-judgemental professional, usually a social worker or psychologist.

Parents who don't keep the baby

Accurate numbers of the parents who don't keep the baby are difficult to find and vary between countries. I estimated about one in ten in the UK during the 1980's, but this will have changed with the increase in screening and elective termination of pregnancy (Chapter 6). I do not believe that placing the baby for fostering or adoption is a cold decision. These parents just cannot face the prospect of having a child with Down syndrome. It is an awesome decision to make, and I firmly believe most parents do make the right decision for themselves, providing they are not pressurised by outside influences. To take home a child whom you know you can never love or care for, that you might find repulsive (Chapter 2), will not help the child or the family. To give up one's child is not easy, and those parents who do, need our understanding, not our criticism.

Just after the first edition of this book was published a mother telephoned me to thank me. I was at first surprised, because she said that reading the book had helped her and her husband decide to put the baby up for adoption. After some reflection, I realised that this confirmed my hope that the book would be an accurate review of information to help all parents, or would-be parents, of a child with Down syndrome, to make their own decisions with confidence.

I have been involved with a small number of parents who decided not to keep the child with Down syndrome. In two cases

I felt they could not come to terms with the idea of having had a child with a disability. Another parent had a brother with multiple health and behaviour problems (not Down syndrome), which had caused considerable difficulties within his family when growing up. He felt he had had enough of that sort of coping and could not take the risk. In another family, both parents were highly qualified and career oriented and came from families that expected and prized excellence. There was no room in their plans for a child that would not excel. This is one of the few times I felt the decision was very objective with little emotion.

There were also times when I felt the parents had not actually wanted a child for the child's sake. One couple were experiencing problems with their relationship and whilst initially they had not wanted children, thought it might help. When the baby turn out to have Down syndrome, it forced them to look at their relation-ship in more depth. Not only did they place the baby for adoption, but they separated. There was also a couple that had two children each from previous marriages and one from their present marriage. They were very happy and partly decided to have one more child so that their other child would, like the others in this extended family, have a brother or sister. They also had a family plan that all the children would grow up and be independent and so give them time for their many interests. Arriving at the decision to place the baby for adoption was long and painful, but when I last spoke with them they were even more convinced it had been the right deci-sion for them.

One mother came to the decision that her husband, who had a history of mental health problems, would not cope with having a child with Down syndrome. She had already acknowledged that he might have problems sharing her with any child. She also told me that I was wrong in saying that the decision to keep the child or not was from the heart. Clearly in some cases it is very reasoned, but still very difficult.

In several cases, a young couple found themselves pregnant and decided to marry, but when the baby arrived with Down syndrome this added to the problems and they separated. The mother then decided she could not cope on her own.

Adoption and fostering

Fortunately there are families who are willing to foster or adopt children with Down syndrome. These are often very committed families and some particularly ask for children with Down syndrome. From my experience the vast majority of these foster placements and adoptions are very successful. I know of legal cases when biological parents decide some years later they want their child with Down syndrome back, and foster parents fight for all they are worth to keep the child.

A few studies have compared families who adopt or foster a child with Down syndrome with biological families. Apart from the initial problems of coming to terms with the diagnosis for biological parents, there was no difference in the family's levels of adjustment, aspirations for the child or the attainments of the child.

Summary

Advice from parents is summarised in the following coping strategies:

1 Try to take each day as it comes – don't dwell too much on the future
2 Remember that all the family will feel upset and possibly stressed and irritable. Try to be calm and tolerant with each other
3 Don't be afraid to express you feelings, talking helps (Chapter 2)
4 Get to know your child – look for their uniqueness, not the Down syndrome
5 Tackle the situation together with the family
6 Avoid letting the child's disability become the focus of family life – keep your social lives as normal as possible
7 Take the initiative and tell your friends, relatives and neighbours about the child as soon as possible. The longer you leave it, the harder it becomes.
8 Do not hide the facts from other children in the family – explain simply that the baby is different and

will be slower in growing up. If the children are too young to understand, talk about it in front of them, and when they ask questions, answer them honestly.

9　Other people will take their cue from you – if you are embarrassed or avoid talking about the baby or the Down syndrome, they will act accordingly and you can lose a great deal of support

10　Take your baby out and do not be afraid of people seeing him or her – on most occasions people are supportive. But, develop a thick skin and be ready for tactless and hurtful remarks – teach people the truth about Down syndrome if you feel able.

11　Search out accurate information from different sources – beware the many myths and superstitions and be cautious about 'cures' or exciting new treatments (Chapter 11)

12　Talk to people with experience, especially other parents of children with Down syndrome

13　Start to learn how to help the baby, and begin to stimulate and play with him or her as soon as you feel able – but don't rush into things. Taking your time in the first months will not harm the baby's development

14　When you feel able, analyse your situation, work out your immediate and longer-term needs and then plan how to meet them.

2

Coming to terms with the diagnosis – feelings, reactions and adapting

- Am I the only one who feels like this?
- Are these feelings and reactions normal?
- Will we ever come to terms with the Down syndrome?
- How long will I feel like this and what can I do about it?

The first part of this chapter is about coming to terms with knowing your baby has Down syndrome, and trying to understand the complex feelings and reactions you may have at this time. With the increase in prenatal screening, many parents will have received this news much earlier; some of the descriptions below may be not be useful to them. The second part of the chapter describes the continuing journey of adaptation, and some of the problems that parents can experience.

'The baby has Down syndrome'

If you have recently been told your baby has Down syndrome you probably have many painful feelings, and feel overwhelmed:

'I heard the Down syndrome bit and then for the next hours I don't where I was, just bouncing about in this strange space like a zombie.'

'I felt so alone. Was it my fault? What did I do to deserve this?'

'I wanted to die and take the baby with me.'

'I've had difficult experiences in the past and always thought of myself as a coper, but this knocked me for six.'

Parents say it helps to know that others often share these feelings and reactions:

'Sometimes you feel like you're the only one going through this. It is such a relief when you find other parents are the same.'

Most parents, especially if it is the first baby, are optimistic. At the risk of exaggerating, they dream that the baby will be the best ever – dreams that often reflect the parents' own values, ambitions or lost opportunities. The child is imaginary, but parents are very attached to the image. A diagnosis of Down syndrome can shatter parents' dreams in an instant. A father (an academic psychologist) of an eight-year girl with Down syndrome wrote to me about this:

'. . . the cosy picture of stages of development of my little girl. I had never questioned that she would be intelligent and pretty, with a sweet nature and the object of universal admiration. These mental pictures now lay shattered at my feet. I was yet to learn that Louise would fulfil all these aspirations but in ways different and more wonderful than anything that my tormented mind, at that moment, could envisage.'

A young mother said:

'My dreams of my baby were shattered . . . in their place came nightmares . . . but as we got to know each other, I had new dreams of my new baby. They were different, but they were no less joyful and full of hope.'

Parents who are told about the Down syndrome in a caring way, who are given accurate information and who feel supported in the early days, may find it easier to accept the diagnosis. Parents are very sensitive at this time, and the right words can make a huge impact.

> 'The doctor said, "Enjoy her for who and what she is, because worrying about it is not going to change her." I found that very comforting and say it aloud to myself when things are difficult.'

Many studies have shown that large numbers of parents say they are not told in a caring way, or offered appropriate support and information. Some health professionals believe that there is no good way to break bad news, and that parents will inevitably react angrily to the teller. While this can happen, most parents voice their gratitude when it is done well. Some parents feel they were given too much information and reassurance at this time, especially if they had doubts about coping or taking the baby home. If you were told badly, you have a right to feel angry, and should not feel guilty if you express your feelings.

Coming to terms with the Diagnosis

The news takes away hopes for the future. It wipes out much of the knowledge gained over years of how to look after a baby and be a parent. There is now an empty space or a gap, in how the parent makes sense of the world. Our bodies react with increased arousal; this aroused state is why many of us find sleeping difficult when we have things on our minds. The instinctive reaction is to want to restore balance and wholeness in our understanding. It is a process of adaptation, of re-constructing our ideas and knowledge, and resolving our feelings as best we can. This is how I understand coming to terms with the diagnosis.

The journey of adaptation starts with the news. This can shatter our understanding at the time. It ends with the parent accepting the news sufficiently so they can get on with their life.

Acceptance

'Acceptance' has different meanings for different people. At one level it is accepting the diagnosis. But I see it as when the parent is able to think about the future, understanding it will be a challenge, but feel reasonably confident that they will cope. They begin to accept and help the baby develop, to realise they are unique, not that strange, and more normal than abnormal.

For some parents, it comes with little effort:

'We didn't need much information for us to accept her, other than she was a Down's baby and how it came about.'

'It didn't occur to us that we shouldn't take him home. He was ours no matter what he had got.'

Others take longer and make a conscious effort:

'About the second week after having him home I told myself to forget all about the Down syndrome and treat him like any child. I sort of shrugged my shoulders and took each day as it came. If a problem arose, I sorted it out, but I thought there was no point sitting and worrying about problems that might never happen.'

'It's really about getting things under control again. It's much better when you feel you have got some direction back in your life.'

For some, time was needed for healing:

'I joined the human race again when she was four months old.'

'It's difficult to say how long it took for the hurting to stop, but in its place has come a great feeling of strength.'

For others it is not about conscious effort but more about just carrying on with life and getting to know the child:

'I am not sure how it happened. One day I just looked at him and knew I loved him and that we would survive. I think it was then the pain went away.'

Some parents talk about accepting the child but rejecting the disability:

'I don't resent the baby. I resent the Down syndrome.'

Some parents feel they have to reject the disability or keep fighting against it for the sake of the child:

'I thought to myself, he may be a Down syndrome baby but he'll be the brightest one anyone around here has seen.'

'No, I didn't tell the neighbours she had Down syndrome. I felt they would treat her more normally if they didn't know.'

The babies were only a few months old when I collected these last two quotes. I talked to the parents again when the children were five years old. The first couple said it took them at least two years to come to terms with the disability. The other couple still felt that they had not come terms with the disability. They tended to avoid situations like school meetings, holidays and family occasions that made them aware of their child's disability.

I think coming to terms means seeing the child for him or herself – it is an unconditional acceptance that he or she has Down syndrome but is a unique person, with his or her own special qualities and particular problems.

'I hardly know what to wish for Thomas. It makes no sense to wish he was well, without problems or like the other children. I love Thomas the way he is.'

'He wouldn't be himself without the Down syndrome. He'd be a different person. I love him and want him as he is. Of course I wish he could speak more clearly and I would love to find him a girl friend.'

Individual pathways

We all have different ways of coming to terms. Some people want to talk with those they trust, some need space away from others in order to reflect quietly and express their feelings privately. Some find it best to get on with normal routines, others have a strong urge to make new plans or seek out solutions such as second opinions, cures or treatments. It is often a case of two steps forward and one step backwards. Some days you feel fine, and the next day you feel dark despair.

How we feel and react depends upon our past experience and knowledge, our hopes and plans for the future, our dreams of the children we want, and the things we value in life. The sheer range and depth of the feelings we experience can be surprising and frightening. The diagnosis has thrust a new identity on the parents – a parent of a baby with Down syndrome. For many it challenges who they thought they were. Parents have told me how shocked they were at the intensity of their feelings towards the baby, their partner and others at this time. Some never imagined they could ever reject their baby, let alone wish it was dead. Others never imagined they could feel such love for a baby with Down syndrome.

It is not surprising that members of the same family often react differently and come to terms in different ways and at different times. Grandparents sometimes predict a grim future based on their knowledge and experience of people with Down syndrome from the past. I am aware of several grandparents who obtained information on fostering and adoption, and one who actually arranged residential care, within days of hearing the diagnosis and before the parents had got over their initial shock (see Grandparents, Chapter 3).

How we adapt depends not just on the intensity and range of the feelings, but on external things like support and other resources (Chapter 1). For example, research has found that fathers who felt supported by their fathers find the adaptation less stressful, and that some fathers may have more difficulty adapting if the child is a boy than a girl. People have to find their own path and no one can really predict how he or she will feel and react until it happens. At such times we all become vulnerable and very sensitive and we need to be more tolerant of others and ourselves.

My hope is that understanding feelings and processes will help this, and with patience and understanding, all members of the family make the journey in the least painful and stressful way possible.

BONDING AND ATTACHMENT

Many people think all mothers have an instant surge of maternal love and attachment for a newborn baby – called 'bonding'. But this is not the case. Feelings can be disrupted because of tiredness after a difficult birth, separation from the baby, or even fears about being a parent. There is little evidence to show this damages a parent's future relationship with their baby. Many mothers just feel a sense of relief, some are so tired they simply need to recover. Being told the baby has Down syndrome can affect bonding. This has been used as a reason not to tell mothers about the diagnosis soon after the birth. But there is no evidence that being told sooner or later affects whether parents reject the baby or their later attachment to the child. We found positive and warm attachment to the children in over 70% of the parents, much the same as in typical families.

The idea of bonding at birth is too simple. Attachment has three phases:

1 Attachment to the dreamed-of child before or during pregnancy
2 The upsurge of feelings at the birth
3 Attachment that grows with the emerging new person. This starts with the first communication – eye-gaze, smiling and vocalising – and grows as the two people become more engaged.

This last phase is the most important and enduring.

Feelings and Reactions*

shock, numbness, disbelief, confusion, fear, grief, loss, panic, anger, guilt, distanced, protective, revolted, inadequate, hopelessness, resentment, bitterness, pain . . .

These are some of the many words used by parents, grandparents, siblings, relatives and friends when they first learn the baby has Down syndrome.

Feelings of shock

When first told their baby has Down syndrome most parents are deeply shocked. Many talk of 'going numb' and 'being unable to think straight':

> 'I heard the words 'Down syndrome' and from then on I just remember his [*the doctor's*] mouth moving. I think I asked if he was sure.'

Shock is felt in many ways – trembling or feeling very cold, sick or faint. It is a natural, biological reaction to something threatening. Our natural survival instinct means that when faced with a physical danger, the blood is taken to the muscles to help you run away faster. In such a state, it is not surprising that we find it difficult to take in information, or to think about what questions to ask.

Parents describe wanting to get away – out of the doctor's office and back to a safe place. Shock can be seen as nature's way of creating space by initially avoiding the threat and then approaching it when we feel ready. Parents recognise that what they have been told will have an enormous impact on their lives, but they need time, space and information, to make sense of the implications:

> 'I needed time for my mind to accept what I had been told.'

---

*My understanding of the feelings and reactions of parents at this time is strongly influenced by the model described by the eminent paediatrician, R Mackieth after many years experience of working with parents who had just discovered their baby or child had a severe disability. Mackeith R (1973), 'The feelings and behaviour of parents of handicapped children'. *Developmental Medicine and Child Neurology, 15,* 24–7.

Another physical reaction is to increase adrenaline and heighten alertness – originally to protect against danger. Many parents remember everything as 'crystal clear', but as if it were happening to someone else:

> 'I was up in the corner watching it all but it was me he was talking to.'

> 'I went very calm and asked lots of questions. I don't know what the doctor thought of me. When I got out I just went to pieces.'

In physical accidents, people often stay calm until the danger is over. Then they go into shock. This way of coping is like **distancing** oneself from the threat and is a common reaction. The mind knows it can't cope with the threat immediately and retreats, usually to return at its own pace and in a less threatening situation.

> 'He was telling me that Matthew had Down syndrome and I remember thinking about what I needed from the shops that afternoon.'

> 'I can remember carrying him around the hospital and feeling as if my body had no substance, as if it was cotton wool.'

Feelings of disbelief

It is not uncommon for parents to become irrational and confused, and to find it hard to believe what they have been told:

> 'I told him there must be a mistake. I've just been feeding the baby and she's all right.'

> 'I thought he must have mixed my baby up with someone else's – I was too young to have a Down's baby.'

> 'He was my baby and as far as I was concerned, he was perfect.'

This is often labelled as denial, but I prefer to call it disbelief or deferment. Your mind registers the news as a threat with huge implications for your future life. You need to be sure that the information given is valid before you start the major task of re-organising your understanding and your life. It makes sense to hold the threat at bay and approach it in your own time and when you feel ready. It is sensible to ask for a second opinion, if you feel unsure. These are all natural ways of coping and should not be seen as weakness or bizarre behaviour.

A minority of parents deny that the child has a disability, and may need special help. Denial is when somebody cannot accept the information, despite being given considerable evidence.

Some parents appear to accept the diagnosis, but not the potential implications or severity. They may have expectations that the child will be very able, or that a cure will be found. This can be a great strain, and can prevent the parent from adjusting to the needs of the child and finding appropriate help:

'I didn't want them [professional early support people] to come to the house, as that would show there really was problem.'

'I spent at lot of time in the first year avoiding anything to do with Down syndrome – especially services that offered therapy and things – and kept looking for information on what might stop it . . . like a cure.'

These situations are difficult and take a while to work through. However, parents do need to be optimistic, and what might be realistic acceptance to one is negative and pessimistic to another. I will come back to this in later sections

Feelings of Loss and Grief

Most parents experience a sense of grief and loss when they are told the baby has Down syndrome. As noted above, it is as if the child of their imagination is dead, and their hopes and dreams are taken away in an instant.

'I was just shattered when he told me. I could feel this great emptiness inside me. A great feeling of having lost something. It was like when my mother died.'

'Knowing that she would never be a normal child was like a bereavement.'

The fact that the child was imaginary does not lessen feelings of grief and loss. Some parents need to recognise and express their sense of bereavement and mourn their loss. Many parents never really get over their feelings of loss, and combined with other feelings, they experience what is called chronic sorrow. This is much the same as when a loved person in our lives dies. They can never be replaced.

Other parents experience more of a deep disappointment. For many it is a confused feeling. They feel the grief and loss, but have a baby to care for:

'For three or four weeks I didn't do anything with the baby except wash her, change her and feed her. I kept finding myself thinking about all the things I had hoped she would do . . . I would pick up the little cardigan I had knitted when I was expecting and remember all the thoughts that I had had when I was knitting it. After a while I started to tell myself to stop thinking about it. I made myself think about doings things with her. The exercises and games to help her develop were very good as they kept me busy.'

'It was really funny – you know strange – there I was washing the baby but somehow feeling it was unreal.'

Feelings of protection, revulsion, rejection

Many parents say that they have experienced these feelings in varying degrees. They are instinctive and fundamental. Parents feel protective toward the helpless child, and often at the same time, they feel revulsion towards, and a rejection of, the disability:

'. . . as he started to tell us all the facts about Down syndrome and problems that might happen, I felt this huge desire to grab the baby and run away . . . I saw it all as a threat to an innocent baby . . . my precious baby . . .'

'I felt sick when he told me. I looked at the baby and I could see it . . . I could see the Down's look . . . I didn't even want to touch him . . . not then. I sat looking at him for hours in the hospital, there was no one to talk to because my husband wasn't coming in till later. How could I tell him? How do you tell anyone you feel like that about your own child? Slowly I pulled myself together and changed him and then I started to feed him. It didn't feel so bad then, but I still don't like to think about it – him being a Down's, I mean.'

This mother made these comments when her baby was a month old. By six months she was very happy with him.

'We both looked at the baby and instinctively I was aware that we were thinking the same thing – poor little thing lying so peacefully, causing no trouble for anyone, through all the dramatics of the last few days – totally unaware of the explosive effects of your birth. I think both my wife and I felt a surge of love for her at that moment. Sarah, as a unique person, had entered our lives."

A letter from a father

These are all natural, biological reactions. If we did not feel protective of the helpless child, children would not survive. Feelings of revulsion at something unusual and different are a natural, if primitive, way of protecting the species. Rejecting the child avoids many threats to the future. Recognising these two instinctive, biological and quite normal feelings of protection and rejection or revulsion, can help us understand how we can love and care for the child on the one hand, and reject, or feel revolted by the characteristics of the disability on the other. This can seem strange, as the child cannot be separated from the disability. As most parents testify, they eventually realise the child would not be who they are without the Down syndrome.

Many people find it difficult to talk about their feelings of revulsion. In our society we are not supposed to have, or admit to, such feelings, but they are quite common. Revulsion may be too strong a word for these feelings and reactions, but certainly wanting to reject the baby is common.

Three out of four mothers in our research admitted to some feelings of rejection in the first months. Many have told me how they wished for the baby to die, and in some cases thought about ways this could happen. This can be no more than wishing the problem away, and with it the pain and hurt. It can also be a way of imagining what life would be like without the baby or disability, which can help put things in perspective and help you to cope. For example, by showing it might not be that different. Planning how to kill the baby is probably quite common, and can be very upsetting:

'My wife and I wished that Michael had a heart disease that would lead to his death. What I found very disturbing was that I actually entertained notions of murdering him in some way. The thing that made me most wretched of all was that I could actually entertain such notions about my own son.'

Michael is now 18, has just left a mainstream school and goes to college were he hopes to complete his third, foundation level GNVQ. He left Scouts to attend the Lads and Girls Club, is looking for a girlfriend and wants to improve his stage singing and dance routine. He skis and swims and is loved very dearly by his parents and two sisters.

Feelings of Guilt

Many parents feel guilty about their feelings of revulsion or wanting to reject the child. Some just feel resentful about the impact of child and the disability on their lives.

'. . . deep down I have never been able to forgive him for that genetic confusion that produced him. The contradiction haunts me – here I am advocating the rights of every human being, a belief in the educability of all and a dislike of elitism, but when it happens to me I fail to cope adequately.'

(Charles Hannam, Manchester Guardian. 14.10.1979)

Guilty feelings about causing the disability are also common and, although irrational, they may be very strong for some parents. Feelings of guilt, revulsion and protection can lead parents to over-compensate or overprotect the child:

'I just can't stop thinking I did something to make all this happen . . . and I never feel I am doing enough to put it right and make it up to him [the child].'

Many parents have worries during pregnancy and after the birth many feel such worries were premonitions. Some parents think that events during pregnancy caused the Down syndrome. This is all part of trying to make sense of why it happened. As yet, there is no evidence to link particular premonitions, or events during pregnancy, to the incidence of Down syndrome births (Chapters 4 and 5).

Feelings of over-protectiveness

I think this is an overused word often thrown at parents with little thought. But it is an issue we all face with our children. Feeling protective towards a baby will usually lead to warm loving care. But it can make us very sensitive. Any remark about the child or the disability can be seen out of all proportion. Sometimes, the feelings can be so strong that we protect the baby, and ourselves, from normal everyday experiences.

'Looking back I was so sensitive and touchy in those first weeks . . . my brother-in-law said in fun [to the baby], "What a little button nose you've got" – and I felt myself get red hot – every time someone said things like "he'll be a bit slower" or " he'll need special help", I kept thinking they were being critical and somehow getting at him.'

A mother of a three year old.

These feelings and their consequences, can persist into later life, or return if the child has a medical problem or becomes ill. If parents are overly protective and indulgent with the child with Down syndrome it can create an imbalance in the family – especially for the other children. It can result in poor management of behaviour problems, and slower attainment of independence for the child with Down syndrome.

Feeling protective towards those we feel are ill or less able is almost universal, and when combined with frustration watching others trying to do something we find easy (Chapter 1), it can become a powerful force to train dependency:

> 'His brothers and sisters tend to do things for him . . . he can get crisps out of a machine but if they are around they do it, and he lets them. I suppose it's some kind of instinctive protection, but it stops him doing it.'
>
> Father of a 13 year old.

When children with Down syndrome attend mainstream school, it can be difficult preventing the other children from being overly protective, or helping them to the point they do little for themselves.

Sometimes one parent feels very protective of the baby – usually the mother –and the other feels revulsion, resentment or fear of what it means for the family. This can get complicated when family members start to take sides, reacting to their own feelings of protection or rejection.

Feelings of Unfairness, Resentment and Anger

Not surprisingly, a lot of parents experience feelings of unfairness and resentment. The questions, 'why me?' and 'what did I do to deserve this?' are often heard by the doctor telling the parents about the condition. They are normal and honest reactions. The strength of our hopes and ambitions, and how much we have invested in the idea of the new baby – the perfect baby – will influence how much we feel we have been cheated by the baby having Down syndrome.

Angry feelings are sometimes directed at the nearest people to us. This can lead to parents becoming isolated, because people may

THE PROTECTION AND REJECTION TUG-OF-WAR

A somewhat extreme example of this situation was a young couple whose first baby had Down syndrome and was about two or three weeks old. The baby was in hospital while the parents decided what to do (chapter 1). The mother had left her husband and moved in with her mother. She felt very protective of the baby and would react against any 'negative' comments. She also needed the baby. She said she could not believe how unloving and selfish the father was. The father told me that she did not understand how disabled these children could be, and that they could destroy the family. He said her problem was that she was not very intelligent, didn't listen and always reacted too emotionally to things and was *"putting her head in the sand"*. By this stage the grandparents and relatives had taken sides and had reinforced the beliefs that the couple had about each other. The two camps had arrived at different ends of the revulsion-protection dimension and were angry and distraught. We had several discussions over a two or three day period. At first the couple focussed on their own feelings, then each other's and the rest of the family. The mother remained determined to bring the baby home regardless of how disabled she might be. But she agreed that she had to face up to the implications of the child's disability, and to try and understand that the father was trying to protect their future family. The father acknowledged that he was revolted by the idea of having a child with a disability, but had never met any, and was willing to visit a nursery and school with several young children with Down syndrome. He did not want to talk to other parents because they might try to persuade him. The day after the visit, the couple got together and talked, and later brought the child home for a trial period. When I last heard from them they had two other children and the eldest had just started secondary school.

avoid them, or avoid talking about things likely to upset them. Sometimes parents become angry with anyone who crosses their path. One father recalled being very angry with a plumber working on his house:

> 'It wasn't his fault. He was just the first person I met after leaving the hospital.'

Afterwards, this father felt badly about his anger, which was unlike him. This can have an effect on our sense of who we are, and undermine feelings of competence. Family, friends and professionals can be very helpful, either practically or as a listening ear. Attention can get focussed on the baby with Down syndrome to the detriment of other family members. Older brothers and sisters can feel left out; parents can neglect their own needs in their struggle to help the baby. Taking time for everybody is important.

> 'It was really helpful to talk to someone outside the family – someone who came to see me, not Christopher.'

For most parents, angry feelings get less with time. But they can resurface unexpectedly at a later date, for example when a friend or relative has a baby, or when they see other families doing things they cannot do.

Feelings of Inadequacy

Some parents have an overwhelming feeling of inadequacy that can undermine their self-esteem. It is as though their ability to reproduce is in question.

> 'I felt I had failed as a human being. I got so angry that all these young girls in the ward could produce healthy babies and I couldn't even do that.'

Even when they know that there was nothing they could have done to prevent the disability (Chapter 4), such feelings can remain and last a long time. The father of an eleven-year old boy with Down syndrome, whom I had known since shortly after the birth,

BLAMING OTHERS

Some parents will have had prenatal screening (blood tests and ultrasound, see Chapter 6) which failed to detect the Down syndrome. These tests do not detect 100% of Down syndrome pregnancies. Parents who think these tests are 100% accurate, are not only likely to feel shocked, but may be more likely to experience disbelief, anger, resentment and rejection of the baby. The same seems to be true for some parents not offered the tests but who feel they should have been. Feeling angry about someone else's mistake can cause greater problems in coming to terms with the diagnosis.

Research involving people who have suffered from a negative event such as an accident or loss, have found that blaming others is linked to poorer adjustment. The very few studies of parents with a baby with a disability support this. It seems to be about feeling in control and unable to do anything about what has happened. My experience is that until parents let go of their resentment and anger about what they see as someone else's mistake, they are less able to address their own feelings and learn how to live with their child.

The most difficult situation is when the father blames the mother, or vice versa. It is particularly difficult if one parent took the decision to have a child and the other agreed reluctantly, or was not involved in the decision. Sometimes a grandparent blames their son or daughter in law, with comments such as 'we never had anything like that in our family.' It is essential that everybody understands the causes of Down syndrome (Chapter 4).

and who had always seemed to have come to terms, surprised me when I asked (a few months after his elder sons had left home) if he would change anything:

'I wish we had had another child after Steven [*who has Down syndrome*]. Now when we go out, I feel that people are looking at us and wondering if we can have normal children.'

My impression is that these feelings are more likely with a first-born baby. It is often later, when parents have another baby, that they realise just how strong these feelings were:

> 'It suddenly struck me after John was born. We both said something like, "Well we did it this time" meaning we could produce a normal baby. It was only then that we talked about how we both had this feeling of not being normal ourselves. It had been there at the back of our minds, but we had never talked about it. It was such a relief to be able to talk about it and to find that Tony had the same thoughts.'

SEXUAL RELATIONSHIPS

The sexual relationships between partners can also be affected. This is not uncommon after the birth of any child. But when the child has a disability, the additional stress and worry about any future children can make it more difficult. This is not something parents easily talk about. When I have raised it parents are often relieved that others have felt the same. Talking about it – together, or with someone else – can help. The longer it is left, the more difficult it can become to return to a loving relationship, which all the family needs.

Feelings of Depression

Feelings of inadequacy and loss of self-esteem can strike deep, especially if you already feel insecure. For some parents, the birth will trigger depression. Many people believe that depressed feelings will resolve given time, and that professional help is not needed because they know their depression was caused by having a baby with Down syndrome. This may be true, but severe depression is seldom caused by one event. Other factors can make the person vulnerable. If the depression persists, if they cannot find any joy in their life and if they suffer from chronic fatigue, they should seek professional help. Depression can be treated.

TALKING TO A STRANGER

Sometimes, it can be very difficult to talk to your partner, especially in an atmosphere of uncertainty and anxiety, and with such a mix of deep and complex feelings. Emotions are often running high. Fear of upsetting them when they are trying to cope is common. This is often part of protecting those we care for. Many of us find it easier to confide in a 'stranger': it can help to talk to someone else who is more detached from the situation. If our partner does this we should try not to feel it is a criticism of ourselves, nor an indication that the relationship has problems. We need to feel there will be no repercussions from what we say. We can voice our fears without feeling judged or threatened.

Feelings of Embarrassment

Having a child who looks different, who can behave differently, and who sometimes needs to be treated differently in public, can be embarrassing. If family members feel it strongly and fail to deal with it, there is a danger of social withdrawal and isolation. Feeling different and isolated are common reactions for many family members.

In the first weeks parents may need to get over the initial shock and adjustment in the company of close friends and supportive relatives. But later on it is important to take your courage in both hands and go out with the baby and let people see there is nothing to fear or feel ashamed of (see stigma – Chapter 8). Siblings will also need to learn how to deal with people staring or making silly comments, and they may need help explaining to others (Chapters 1 and 3). It is irritating but needs to be faced. Most families become immune to such things.

Feelings of Uncertainty and Anxiety

These feelings and their implications were partly discussed earlier. They are probably the most common reaction and every parent experiences them to a greater or lesser degree.

'When he told me – somehow she wasn't a person anymore – just a big question mark'

'Questions kept going round inside my head – I got in such a state I couldn't even sort them out, let alone look for answers.'

'We didn't get told much in hospital at all, and especially with him being our first, we don't know whether something is a normal reaction or is typical of the Down's group of children.'

'I just couldn't think what was best. I felt useless . . . I would try to do something with him but I usually gave up because I wasn't sure what to do.'

Babies with Down syndrome generally do what babies do. Many parents whose baby with Down syndrome was their second, third or later, say that they quickly realised, with relief, that the new baby was just like their others.

The continuing journey of adaptation

Two or three months after the birth, many parents are feeling quite positive. The baby is not as bad as they thought; they have got over the shock and are feeling hopeful and optimistic. Most can now see beyond the 'Down syndrome', to the baby. The baby's personality is emerging, he or she is making eye contact, smiling, and responding to being tickled and seeing the parent's face.

I do not think it is accidental that this stage coincides with many parents feeling they are through the worst. Around this time parents often tell us that the baby seems 'quite normal.' Some feel they are 'even quicker at doing things than their other children.' In a sense, the parent is comparing the actual baby to the imaginary one they created from what they know about Down syndrome. They are looking for proof of the disability or how much the child might be affected. This can be a quite euphoric period for many parents. They have come through the first difficult weeks, and many of their fears about the baby have not materialised.

Between six and twelve months, the first signs of slow development become more noticeable for the majority of babies with Down syndrome. For some parents, this is the first real sign of the disability. It can happen quite suddenly, perhaps when they are at the clinic or at a friend's house, and there is a baby of similar age. When this happens, parents can experience many of feelings they had just after the birth; they may have to work through them again and construct new understandings.

In an extreme example we had a boy in our research who did not have very strong features of Down syndrome and whose early development was not obviously slow or different. When he was about three years old, his mother – who had accepted he had Down syndrome and carried out all the early stimulation work and learnt all she could – began to doubt the diagnosis. He was not what the books described. She experienced a period of very mixed feelings until he finally went to mainstream school and she began to see differences with the other children.

The period following the diagnosis is usually the worst for most parents. But later on there may be more emotional upheavals and a need to re-think things. With any family, the journey of adaptation is a continual one. Each day we change and learn more about one another. The typical family life cycle is full of events that bring change – births, marriages, deaths, illness, starting school, leaving school, coming of age, first job, first love, changing jobs, moving house, and so on. Each event can trigger feelings and reactions, and some will bring back feelings you had when you first heard your child had Down syndrome. These feelings can bring back reflections on what might have been.

Parents can experience a 'crisis' if the child is diagnosed with further problems, such as severe heart defect, hearing or visual impairment or later on, severe behavioural disorders (Chapter 9). Professionals can make the mistake of feeling that because parents have survived an initial diagnosis of Down syndrome, further problems will be easier to cope with. This is not true; they can be even more difficult. The way professionals work can also add to these difficulties:

'In the first years everybody told me how wonderfully he was doing. The home intervention visitor was really lovely and so positive. Then I went to the meeting with a range of professionals to sort out his statement of special education needs. Each took their turn to speak and each emphasised his needs. It was not what I was expecting. It was a shock and I had to go home and think about him in a new light.'

Parents who have coped by wishful thinking or by denying the disability, often constructing an unrealistic and overly optimistic view of the child and their future attainments are most vulnerable at these times. Those parents who have organised their resources and used active coping (Chapter 1) appear to experience less emotional upheaval later on. This is why I stress the importance of recognising the very wide range of abilities and personalities of people with Down syndrome (Chapters 8 and 10).

I am not sure what marks the final point in the journey of adaptation or coming to terms, or even if it ever really happens. I think it means seeing and loving the child for him or herself.

Positive parenting

Parents often say that well-meaning professionals and relatives insist on them accepting their child with Down syndrome in a 'nothing can be done about it' sort of way. This can add to their depression. It is sad that if a parent is optimistic and hopeful, relatives and professionals may conclude that they have not really accepted the diagnosis. It can feel as if you have to concentrate on the negative aspects of the condition in order to convince others that you are not being unrealistic.

In the first months many parents are frightened to be hopeful. They are trying to find a balance between their fears of the worst and their dreams of the best. It is important to realise that the child will have limitations as well as strengths. We can't all have brilliant, sweet natured children. What we can have is *our* child. They are themselves, and all we can do is provide them with the best opportunities to help them develop as best they can.

Many parents know instinctively that they need to feel hopeful and optimistic about the future of their children.

'You have to believe she has a future. Without hope there would be no reason to get up each morning.'

The parent or grandparent who has few expectations or hopes for the future runs the risk of increasing the child's difficulties by not providing an environment of opportunity. As one of our parents wrote:

'We need to learn to build on things they can do instead of perhaps dwelling on the things they might never do.'

Children with Down syndrome achieve more when their parents take a positive, hopeful, problem-solving approach and expect progress and achievement. If you assume your child cannot do something, you may not give the necessary help and encouragement. When the child does not manage to do it, it can be seen as proof that they were incapable.

Getting and coping with information

Many anxieties and uncertainties can be reduced with accurate information. More and more hospitals do provide information, and hopefully link the new parent to help when they take the baby home. Many have special leaflets – either their own or from national bodies. We found that while most parents want these information leaflets, about half cannot face them for some time after being told the diagnosis. Some describe holding them, but not being able to open them up. This is natural, and as I said earlier, distancing yourself until you feel ready is a positive coping strategy.

Some parents find these leaflets overly reassuring (possibly like parts of this book), with positive parent quotes and pictures of happy families. They also felt less happy if they could not identify with the families in the pictures or the quotes. You may have similar thoughts about the quotes and photographs in this book – they are mostly from English families and parents I have met.

There are many sources of information available to parents when they feel ready (see Resources). In most developed countries there are National Associations for Down syndrome and there is a European and an International Association. Some countries have telephone helplines. The Internet can be used for finding up-to-date research or chat-rooms with other parents. Your doctor or local hospital should put you in touch with local groups and parent support groups. If not, contact the Associations for Down syndrome.

Other parents are often a major source of information and support. But just because they have had similar experiences does not automatically mean you will get on with them, and find them supportive. If the other person or family is very different, you may not see the comparison as valid or that what they say and think does not fit well into your understanding.

CHALLENGES TO OUR VIEWS

Information is not always reassuring; it often challenges how we understand our world. We all tend to hear what we want to hear, and often reject anything that is too great a challenge. Parents of a new baby with Down syndrome will get what seems to be contradictory information, which increases anxiety and causes stress. A natural reaction to feeling under threat is to seek out a safe place. Parents who perceive society as hostile often avoid engaging with others, and become isolated. Others form small social networks of like-minded people. This is supportive, but not challenging. Healthy support groups feel safe, but offer new information and challenges that can be explored within the safety of the group.

Activities and early intervention programmes

Activities which stimulate the child's development can sometimes be very helpful. See Chapter 11 for details of these. Here are some quotes from parents in our early support programme. I asked them what had been helpful:

'My husband and I felt that we were doing something, we didn't feel so inadequate.'

'Just knowing that other people, experts and even other parents, found it useful to do something, gave me all the confidence I needed to keep going.'

'They [*the research team*] never really told me anything new . . . it was often common sense . . . but it was very important because I just dithered around at first . . . I didn't feel confident in myself.'

'My husband was a lot better than me at helping Jamie at first. He enjoyed being able to contribute something positive. That's why working out a set of activities to do kept us both busy . . . we did it together and it was nice'

For other parents, these activities are seen as a constant reminder and can cause problems; they feel guilty about not doing them, or simply do not want to do them. There is no strong evidence for the benefits of starting exercises or stimulation activities in the first weeks or months (see Chapter 11). The sort of everyday handling any baby should receive is enough for the majority of babies with Down syndrome. It is better for the baby and the family to take time to get to know each other, rather than the parents get side tracked into the role of therapist.

A few parents find it difficult to accept that it is worthwhile to do anything. After every possible stimulation, their baby will still have Down syndrome and intellectual disability. Such conflict requires a long hard look at our values and what we think life is about. We might start by asking another almost impossible question. Why do we have children? Our answer will partly reflect the extent to which we can accept the child's disability. Most societies today value intelligence, physical ability and appearance and seek after material benefits. Such aspirations are not likely for a child with Down syndrome. We need to know that there are other goals and other ways of life that bring fulfilment.

Getting financial and practical support

Many countries offer financial and other types of support for families who have a child with a disability. Parents need to contact the appropriate social service department to find out more about what is available. Some parents don't like to do this. Some feel that taking the help is stigmatising, or is too public a recognition of the child's disability. Others can feel that seeking help – such as respite care – reflects on their competence. From my experience parents who feel like this are more likely to experience stress.

This is unfortunate and reflects how we view such benefits. I want to live in a society that does its best for all people, and provides help when some find they have greater needs at some time than others. Most of us will need help at sometime, whether it is social benefits or health care. Nearly all adults with Down syndrome will need support to obtain the necessary resources (benefits). Parents must take an outward-looking approach, engage with society and access the help and services they are entitled to. The overall goal of this is help for the child.

Often the support provided – financial, respite, home care – is based on an assessment of the severity of the disability and family circumstances. More enlightened systems are based on the needs of the child and family. When we first started to work with parents we made an error in terms of these assessments. Our emphasis was so much on being positive and optimistic that parents expressed just how well the child was doing and how well they were coping. The assessors naturally felt the need was low and parents were denied benefits and support. By itself, Down syndrome is not sufficient to expect to receive help; and in my view this is correct. However, many children with Down syndrome have additional health problems, including hearing and visual problems, They can be seen as having some form of physical disability. We had to learn to itemise these problems as objectively as possible, without losing our positive view.

Working with professionals and the services

In terms of Down syndrome, I am a professional when I deal with other people's children. I try to be reasonably objective and objectively reasonable in my dealings with them. From a professional perspective children can (and do) make unreasonable demands on their parents – and from a child's perspective parents make unreasonable demands on them. Some years ago my son asked (actually, he told me) to fix his bicycle. I said 'I'm busy; why should I?' He replied, 'because you're *my* dad.' This is the nature of the special parent-child relationship. Being a child's parent means you are their advocate. As their advocates you must favour them, and may make demands that appear unreasonable to the professional.

I think parents and professionals should think very carefully about their differences and roles in the child's life.

Parent-professional differences

- The role of parents is broad and diffuse, they are responsible for all aspects of their child's life – they need to see the whole child.
  The role of professionals is set within defined limits with specific aims. They bring expertise to that aspect, but may not see the whole picture.

- Parents have more interactions over a wider range of contexts – therefore have a broader picture of the child.
  Professionals have fewer interactions and within restricted contexts – they need the parent to give them the broader understanding.

- Parents are more emotionally involved; they may be less able to deal with treatment failure and slow progress; they may be more impatient and less objective.
  Professionals are less attached to the child; they may be more patient and less stressed by any lack of progress; they should bring detached objectivity to the partnership but understand that the parent may feel more upset when things don't work or don't work quickly.

- The interactions of parents with their child is usually spontaneous, unselfconscious and less directed than a professional. They enjoy the interaction for it's own sake. They are more opportunistic. The child therefore has a different and hopefully more relaxed social experience.
  Professionals try to make their interactions as purposeful as possible within a set of job expectations. They work for, and try to make the child reach some goal.

- Parents should be highly partial to their child; they have the responsibility and are the main advocates.
  Professionals have responsibility for many children and must avoid favouritism.

- Parents do not usually choose to be involved in disability.
  Professionals usual choose this involvement and have high motivation.

These differences can cause conflict in the relationship. For example, a therapist gains job satisfaction from seeing the child make progress in her speciality. She or he defines an objective and treatment plan and advises parents how to help. But what if the parent does not have the resources to fit this into all her other roles? What if other family members are not supportive and do not believe that the effort is worthwhile, or if progress is very slow? Do the parents blame themselves and feel guilty? Do family members begin to argue? Do parents become professionalised and forget just to be parents?

From my experience, many parents get caught up in this 'professionalised' parent role. I have seen it most clearly in early intervention programmes, and parents have eloquently described it:

'Sometimes it seems that professionals can only deal with parents who become as professional as themselves. I believe this has its dangers in that a parent who has become more 'professional' is sometimes unable to become once again, a subjective loving and caring parent for their child. The pleasures of watching one's child develop become overtaken by the need to measure development as would the professional. I know this happened to me and I regret very much all those lost pleasures. After all a child has one mother – professionals come and go.'

Mrs. L Roberts, about her 3 year-old daughter with Down syndrome.
(Conference on Parent-professional Relationships, 1991.
Mid-Glamorgan, Wales)

'The prolific use of checklists often clouds the simple sweetness of success. No sooner is one skill mastered, than another skill from the checklist is presented leaving little time for basking in the glory of what was possibly a hard fought achievement.'

Mrs.D.Fulwood mother of a child with Down syndrome; article 'Mum or Supermum?' in *Australian Citizen Limited* (August 1981: p241–247).

Satisfaction for parents should be more than just the believing that they are doing the best for their child; it should be about enjoying their interactions with the child.

Not all parents want to take on the 'political' role of fighting for the rights of people with disability. They may not get the same feeling of satisfaction as the professional from working with people with a disability. The professional has spent time training for this, it is part of their identity and gives them status in society. In contrast, the parent may feel they have little status in their role as the parent of the child with disability; they may even feel stigmatised. I have seen this cause conflict most often in clashes about special or mainstream schools and the rights of adults with intellectual disability to make decisions for themselves (Section Four).

Unfortunately many parents of a child with disability share one common experience. They have had to battle with professional administrations and often family and friends, to secure a meaningful future for their child. I noted this from something I read many years ago, but have lost the reference. I still have no reason to doubt it is true. Problems arise because of a scarcity of resources and professional help, and complex administrations. They are also more likely when the parent's view of the child and his or her needs clashes with that of the professional (see Chapter 10 on different models of disability). Part of the process of adapting to the child and to the disability, is to develop skills to find ones way through the administrative system and how best to work with professionals. This is discussed in more detail in Chapter 12.

Summary

When parents, and close relatives or friends, find the baby has Down syndrome, they experience a wide and varied range of emotions and reactions. Nearly all experience shock and often feel numb, confused and disorganized and cannot believe it is true. This is the beginning of a process of adaptation in which they have to re-construct how they make sense of their lives. How parents react and adapt and the emotions they experience, depends on their life experiences, personality, attitudes to life and children, plans for the future and resources such as support and information.

These feelings come and go over the first weeks, and mostly diminish in time. The end of initial period of adaptation is when the parent accepts the child has Down syndrome, begins to make plans and is able to get on with their life. Parents continue to adapt as the child grows but feelings can return if more difficulties arise, and especially with normal life events that highlight the disability. Parents most able to cope are those who have developed appropriate skills and coping strategies and who have gathered information.

In their concern to do the best for the child, some parents lose sight of their parenting role. It is important to focus on being a parent and caring for the whole family.

3

What is the effect on the family?

- **What effect will the child with Down syndrome have on the parents' relationship?**
- **What effect will the child have on his or her siblings and on the grandparents?**
- **What might the effect be on the family as a whole?**

The pathological view of Down syndrome

For many years medical practitioners, and most other professionals, believed that a person with Down syndrome would be a major burden to the parent and the family, causing difficulties in the parents' relationship and problems for the other children. Many also believed that these babies were too damaged to benefit from living with a family, and being encouraged and stimulated like any child. This was also the common view of western society and so was usually shared by parents, grandparents, friends and relatives (Chapter 8). It is not surprising therefore, that many babies and young children with Down syndrome were placed in institutions. Such beliefs are still common in some countries, where many children and young people with Down syndrome still live in institutions. This is at a time when a large body of research shows that living in a caring and supportive family is of the utmost benefit to any child with Down syndrome (Chapters 8 and 10).

The same focus on impairments and problems – the pathological approach – was seen in research on families well into the 1980's. Questions were asked about stress, behaviour problems and marital difficulties, rather than parent satisfaction, family well-being and positive strategies for adapting and coping. Even today, very few studies ask families what they feel they have gained from having a member with Down syndrome. It seems most people assume that there can be no benefits, or if there are, they are unimportant. Even in this new millennium, many expectant parents say that health professionals involved in prenatal screening take a neutral view or emphasise the potential negative aspects of having a child with Down syndrome.

I have found Down syndrome being used as an example of a genetic mutation in the 'Health and Disease' section of current human biology textbooks for 14 –16 year olds. It is described as resulting in 'serious chest, heart and mental defects, often leading to death at an early age'. For most young people this biased and out-of-date information will be all they have to form their understanding of Down syndrome. It is not difficult to see how they confuse Down syndrome with serious illness.

Fortunately this image is being changed by publicity from voluntary organisations, parents taking their children out, children and young people with Down syndrome being included in mainstream life and acting in film and TV, and standing up for their rights.

My own view switched from this 'pathological' model because the families in our early research began to describe lots of positive things in our conversations over cups of tea, after the formal bit of the research was over. We then started formally to ask questions about any positive changes in their lives. 70 to 80% of the time, their responses fell into the very positive to neutral categories. Similar results are being reported by studies from several different countries. The parents described changing their values and becoming more compassionate, stronger marriages, making more friends and extending their life, and making the most of each day.

I can say with quite a lot of confidence, that the probability of a child with Down syndrome damaging the family is far less than the probability that the family is enhanced and benefits from having a member with Down syndrome.

This should be kept in mind if you decide to read this chapter, as I will be describing possible problems and how they can occur. I believe that if we have some idea of what can go wrong, it helps to reduce the risks and increases the chances of things going right. I hope it will get rid of some unnecessary worries and suggest strategies to deal with potential problems.

What is the effect on the parent's relationship?

Whether you have a child with disability or not, most parents get into conflict at some time about how to treat the children. The other major source of conflict is about finances. Such conflict can be healthy, as we need different views to make us think and move forward. But, especially at the early stages, the potential for conflict can be greater if the child has a disability. Complex feelings about the child, oneself and others, can result in anxiety beneath the surface.

Studies of families who have a child with Down syndrome show that there is no evidence of more difficulties between partners than in similar groups of families with typical children. The families in our research have, in fact, a lower rate of relationship breakdown than one would expect from national figures. We also found that measures of marital relationship problems were lower than that found for families with typical children. Most of the mothers we spoke to felt the relationship had remained the same or improved. Many parents say that having a child with Down syndrome has brought them closer together, and that facing the challenge has made them stronger as people and as a couple.

An old college tutor of mine once told me that marriages stay together because the partners learn to trust each other and respect each other. I think this is what happens when a couple find themselves with a baby with Down syndrome. It provides an opportunity to demonstrate each other's strengths, and their love and concern, as never before.

> 'The doctor told me he was a Down syndrome . . . I had to tell Frank, I was dreading it. I thought he would blame me and not want anything to do with the baby. Well, for the first few days after I told him he didn't say anything about the baby. I was still in hospital. He came in with some flowers and said "Sorry," that's all – just sorry. After a minute he looked at me and said, "I haven't been much help, but it's over. He's our baby and I think we will cope. We'll have a damn good try." You know, we had been married for five years and I didn't think he had it in him . . . but we never looked back from that day. This little one really brought us together . . .she's brought a lot of love into this family'.

Relationship Breakdown

It would be nice if all couples had a positive experience, but for some, the birth of a baby with Down syndrome can be a catastrophe. If you don't have emotional or practical support you are more likely to experience stress. If your relationship with your partner is poor, this is not only a lack of support, but is an added source of stress. These families have a higher chance of poor family relationships and behaviour problems in the children.

Couples separate for many reasons. Unfortunately, it is common to hear people lay the blame for family stress or a relationship breakdown on the fact that a child in the family has Down syndrome. Perhaps this is because the condition is so obvious and people fail to look beyond it. This can happen if all the attention is on the Down syndrome. Stepping back can give a broader perspective and allow parents to examine the different factors causing them stress.

If the parents have a good relationship, the birth of their baby can bring them even closer, but if the relationship is poor, then the birth can cause considerable disruption. Several studies, including ours, have reported that when partners split up because of the birth, there were difficulties *before* birth. Some couples, despite problems, stay together because of the children, possibly more so if the child has a disability.

WHAT ABOUT SINGLE PARENTS?

I talk about mothers and fathers and families in a traditional way. But families take many forms. Research on single parent families has found no differences in the effects on the children, provided the parent had the resources to cope. They did not find slower progress or more behavioural problems in these families. The support may come from different people in the household or close by – these people can be as much 'family' as relatives living at a distance.

The available research also shows that many single parents who are caring for the child with Down syndrome form new relationships. They are no more likely or unlikely to do this compared with the general population, but the time between the separation and the next relationship is longer when there is a child with a disability. My view, endorsed by some of the mothers in new relationships, is that they make sure the new partner understands the disability and shares their views of the child.

What sort of problems can parents have?

I have hesitated about writing this section. Relationships between spouses and partners are complex, and I do not feel at all competent or confident in talking about them. However, I made a promise that this book should be as honest as I can make it and I have tried not to avoid areas of difficulty.

Our observations are that about one in five couples do experience conflict. These observations are mainly based on what mothers tell us; it has been more difficult to meet the fathers, who tend to be out at work and men are less likely to discuss their problems.

Contradictory and changing feelings

As described in Chapter 2 there are many complex feelings and reactions to having a baby with Down syndrome. If the parents have contradictory feelings towards their child with Down syndrome, such as resentment or protection, they may treat the child inconsistently or differently. Their view or understanding about the disability can result in quite different approaches to parenting and valuing the child. In turn, this causes conflict between the parents and confusion for the child. Such feelings and views interact with other ideas about discipline, the child's level of understanding and the parents' aspirations for the child. In the extreme, it can be about how much time or even money to invest in helping the child. All couples have topics that are not openly explored and areas around which they tread carefully, but in this case talking is important if the parents are going to develop a shared understanding and support each other and help the child together.

Expressing feelings

Mothers seem more willing than fathers to discuss problems and join support groups – usually of other mothers. This may simply be a case of having more opportunity, but I know many fathers, like myself, who recoil from the idea of meeting with a group. As one father told me, 'My wife likes nothing better than to talk a problem to death. She keeps on and on – it drives me round the bend'.

On the other hand I know many men who talk about their feelings, but often to another person in an informal setting:

> 'He never really talked to me about his feelings. I thought why does he bottle them up . . . doesn't he trust me to understand . . . then I started to think he was cold and didn't have any feelings like that. Later my friend told me that he used to talk about things and worries about the baby with her husband for hours. He should have talked to me . . . I felt lonely and needed to talk'.

At this time this couple's child was 18 months old. Five years later I asked the mother about this again. She said her husband still did not talk about it, but that the way he is with their daughter was wonderful. She felt he had been trying to protect her, but hoped that one day they would be able to talk about those first months. I was never able to talk to him, but they are still together, their eldest child is married and their daughter with Down syndrome is now in her early 20's, and very happy. All three are always doing things together.

Reactions to the disability

Parents can differ in their reactions to their child's disability. Fathers are more likely to ask questions about the effect on the family, on the mother and about residential care. I do not think this is because they are less humane. I think that it is 'instinctive' for the father to try to protect his family, whereas the mother is more likely to feel protective towards the new baby (Chapter 2).

Mothers may take on the main responsibilities for the care and treatment of the child, while the fathers often direct their energies into their work and providing for the family. Like this mother, you may recognize that your partner has difficulty coming to terms with your child:

'I know he loves John but he just can't bring himself to do things with him. So I do all the work with schools and hospitals and look after John, and he [the husband] gets on with the business and the other children. We all understand the problems and it works all right for us. I did resent it at first but if you are going to keep your family together it is worthwhile – you have to make some compromises'.

The 'traditional family' model is rapidly changing in many societies. Some fathers are very involved with their babies and many mothers work or are the main breadwinners. In these families I think there is often more equality and partnership, more willingness to talk and less defensiveness.

Views about the child's achievement and progress

A common source of conflict is that mothers often feel the baby is achieving more than the fathers think. Many fathers believe that they are more objective and less emotional than mothers. These differences may be because new behaviours in a child develop unevenly. A behaviour will appear and you think it is learned, it disappears for a few days, before reappearing, lasting a bit longer, until it becomes well established (Chapter 10). Mothers are likely to see the behaviour first because they are with the baby more often. When I ask mothers and fathers to tick off what the baby can do on a developmental checklist, I usually find that mothers tick most, fathers a bit less, and I tick the least – because I have spent very little time with the baby. This difference lessens as the child grows older. Even so, one father, when filling in a checklist about his teenage daughter, remarked, 'I'm not at home enough to know about all those – the wife will know better'.

Future education of the child

Parents can get into conflict over the future education of their child. One parent may feel that the other has unrealistic expectations of the child's ability, or that the child would be better in a special school, rather than a mainstream school. One parent may be trying to protect the child or worried about the child being labelled or stigmatised. Such conflicts can be reduced if parents recognize that it is difficult to assess the child's abilities, and that they are quite likely to disagree. Get the best professional advice you can, then use this assessment to work out your joint position. These issues are described in Chapters 10 and 13.

Future children

Problems can arise if one partner wants to have another child and the other does not. Sometimes a parent is afraid that a subsequent child will have a disability or perhaps feel they need to concentrate on the child with Down syndrome. Some older parents with a child with Down syndrome may already have children from a previous marriage and may not want more children. Less commonly, the partner who has no other children may have strong feelings of inadequacy and guilt that they could not produce a 'normal' child, especially for the new relationship. In my limited experience, this puts the relationship at risk unless the parents can address the issues.

Talking together and with somebody else who is not emotionally involved, is usually helpful.

Overall, most couples do not find that having a child with Down syndrome damages their relationship, provided it is fairly strong before the birth, that they can arrive at a reasonably shared view of the child, and that they come to terms with the disability.

What is the effect on brothers and sisters?

There is surprisingly little research on this subject. Some early studies found older sisters at risk for disturbed behaviour but this was about them taking the responsibility for child-care in quite large families. Others studies include a range of conditions, not just Down syndrome. I have mainly used our work and describe it in some detail. I use 'sibling' to refer to brothers or sisters living at home, up to the late teenage years or early adulthood.

The Overall Picture

Like most other studies, we found that the relationship between all the children in families with a child with Down syndrome was similar to families without a member with Down syndrome. 80% of the siblings we spoke to felt that their relationships were good, not just with their brother or sister with Down syndrome, but also with their parents. We found no differences between boys or girls or whether the sibling was of the same or different gender to the one with Down syndrome. We did not find that the level of intellectual disability, by itself, made any difference.

In most families, children prefer different siblings and one parent or the other, at different times or for different things, depending on age, shared interests and personality. We found the same if a member had Down syndrome. Parents often commented on how helpful the siblings were in engaging with and helping the child with Down syndrome learn new skills. My view is that siblings are more relaxed than parents or professionals, and focus on the fun of interacting with the child with Down syndrome rather than trying to achieve a goal.

The main source of information for siblings on forming their understanding of Down syndrome is their parents. This is why we find siblings views reflect their parents. If the parents see their main role as providing therapy for the child with Down syndrome then the siblings appear to take on the role of therapists, and parents often comment how well they do the exercises and so on. If the parent constantly refers to the problems the child causes, the siblings are more likely to see their brother or sister as a problem. However, it can happen that they become more protective toward the sibling and their relationship with the parent is less easy.

Positive effects having a sibling with Down syndrome

When we asked older brothers and sisters how they felt about having a sibling with Down syndrome, 8 out of 10 talked about positive effects; over half of these seldom mentioned a negative effect. They talked about benefits such as not getting stuck on trivial things and feeling competent that they can cope. Teenage siblings mentioned understanding the responsibilities of being a parent, and how the society they live in affects their lives.

> 'Mary has taught me not to take things so seriously. She lets me know life is OK. If I've had a row with my friend, lost my books or been told off at school and am in a bad mood, she'll laugh and say " it's a nice day". I think if she can cope I can. She's so positive and gets fun out of the smallest thing. She also tries very hard to learn things and so I don't give up either. You learn to sort out problems. I'm glad she's my sister'.
>
> Teenage sister, 2 years older.

Not surprisingly, the positive siblings were more likely to come from families who got on well together. They rated their families high on questions involving family relationships – talking together, shared decision making, reasonable sharing of family resources, feeling emotionally and practically supported. Their sibling with Down syndrome was also more likely to have advanced self-help and social skills – they could do more things for themselves, communicate quite well and behave in a socially appropriate way – than those of siblings who were more negative. While some of this will be due to the positive family environment of the child with Down syndrome, some will come from inherent characteristics. A minority of children with Down syndrome do have difficult behaviours and make high demands on the family resources (Chapter 9).

The siblings who made no negative or mainly neutral comments, tended to be older. It is possible that they felt protective and defensive of their younger sibling. Those who were closer in age to the child with Down syndrome, were usually positive, but also made more critical comments. Their gripes were common to all siblings, and included interfering with games and belongings, arguments about TV programmes or music, and being noisy when they were doing homework, and parents commented more often about their children competing for their attention.

> Less than 1 in 8 siblings we spoke to made more negative comments than positive ones. Negative comments were more likely from siblings who felt they were not coping with the demands of school, or the demands of their parents, and if they felt their parents were showing favouritism towards the child with Down syndrome. This is not just about the Down syndrome, but also about the family situation and relationships. Negative comments were more likely if the child with Down syndrome had difficult behaviour and general low functioning.

Siblings reflect their parent's attitudes, beliefs and values about disability. If the parent signals that the child with Down syndrome is a burden, a drain on resources, a constant worry and so on, it is not surprising that the other children adopt this way of thinking. This is why I advise parents and carers to try to sort out their feelings and beliefs, and not just put all their energy into helping the baby with Down syndrome.

**WHAT ARE SIBLINGS OF CHILDREN WITH
DOWN SYNDROME LIKE AS PEOPLE?**

In my experience, siblings of children with Down syndrome
are often very tolerant young people, with remarkable
understanding and maturity in their dealings with others and
sense of self. Parents often described positive effects such as
the sibling voluntarily helping others, and showing sympathy,
understanding and altruism. Other frequent descriptions were
that they seemed more competent and self-sufficient than
their friends and achieved their goals. Teachers have reported
similar observations about compassion and moral
development when they have a child with Down syndrome in
their mainstream class. This positive effect is more likely when
the school's approach is about developing social behaviour
rather than competitive achievement. There are very few
studies about this, but I believe the child with Down
syndrome – unless they are one of the few with severe
difficulties – can be a catalyst to make other children reflect
upon issues like fairness, helping others and achievement for
its own sake.

What problems can siblings have?

Behaviour problems

We found that parents rated about one in five siblings as having significant behaviour problems, which is about the same as families
without a member with Down syndrome. So siblings of children with
Down syndrome are no more likely to have behaviour problems.

Poor family relationships are strongly associated with behaviour
problems for both the siblings and the child with Down syndrome.
If families are having problems getting on together, the child with
Down syndrome can add to their problems. For example, if the
child is less able and resources are limited, this strain is felt by all
members of the family.

How the father can help

We found that siblings were likely to have less behaviour problems in families where fathers' recognised when the family needed more support and organised it. This may seem strange, but some fathers are very self-reliant and may not be aware of the amount of effort the mother and children are making in coping with the child with Down syndrome. Some feel there is nothing they can do and rely on hope or wishful thinking. This can add to the problems. Ours was a small study and the results are tentative; but it does make sense that both parents should give time to family relationships and working out strategies to solve problems. If the child with Down syndrome is demanding a lot of mother's attention, she will have less time for the other siblings. Or the other children may be taking on more responsibility for themselves and their siblings. What the father does in these situations is important. As the traditional roles of mother and father change, research findings will change.

Siblings are as likely as anyone else to focus on the Down syndrome and blame it for all their problems, to feel that life is unfair or to feel 'put upon' – a not infrequent view of teenagers in many families, with or without a member with a disability. We found a small number of siblings who said their brother or sister with Down syndrome was a burden on the family, and that they had different responsibilities at home to their friends. But whilst a third of the siblings felt parents expected more of them than their friends, only half of these had behaviour problems. So it is only when this feeling is combined with other problems, especially in family relationships, that increased behaviour problems are found.

High expectations and pressure from parents

Some children think their parent(s) is disappointed because their sibling with Down syndrome will not achieve the things they want for their children. They may strive hard to make up for the parents' sense of loss. The research on this issue is patchy. When we asked siblings, one third said that parents expected more of them because of having a child with Down syndrome, and around two-thirds felt no higher expectation or pressure. About half those feeling under pressure said their parents expected greater achievement, and the other half said better behaviour and more responsibility in the home was expected. The latter were usually older siblings. A small number who felt their parents expected more from them, were also rated by their parents as having higher than average behaviour problems – again these families had more relationship problems as a whole.

Many of the siblings who felt more responsibility was expected from them had a more demanding sibling with Down syndrome who needed more supervision. However, in some cases our observations of the child's behaviour did not always coincide with the view of the family. I felt that some parents were disappointed about having a child with Down syndrome, and so felt any additional demands were excessive and this influenced the whole family view.

I have heard parents chastising a sibling by comparing them with the one with Down syndrome, or telling them to be grateful they are not like them and to behave better. It can't help when a child grows up feeling guilty or responsible for a sibling – especially when there is little they can do. In the past siblings were often burdened in a similar way if they believed it was for their protection that their brother or sister had been placed in an institution. When I hear such negative comments I wonder if the parent has still not fully come to terms with having a child with Down syndrome. Some parents never really do, but because they are aware of the pitfalls, they still make a good job of parenting their children.

Lower Self Esteem

Parents can experience lowered self-esteem, because their child is less valued by society. The same can be true for siblings. Although our research found that most of the siblings had high self-esteem and felt good about themselves, there were a small number with lower self esteem. Amongst these were several who had a brother or sister with Down syndrome who was less competent in skills like going out, using local amenities, and communicating. The siblings with lower self-esteem were also more likely to feel anxious and lacking in support from their parents. If the sibling feels insecure and different, and has a brother or sister who is less socially competent, it may affect their feelings about themselves. If they feel valued and supported by parents who are not anxious, they are able to cope better with difficulties.

Do siblings get involved in the helping role?

95% of siblings said they did help at home, and their parents confirmed this. This is much the same in families without a child with Down syndrome, but the comparison probably hides the sort of help, and the daily consistency and responsibilities in providing the help. The amount of help varies depending on family circumstances and resources such as finances, one or two parents, the mother's health, and helpful neighbours, relatives and friends. 60% felt they took on more household responsibilities than their friends; 20% felt they did less and 20% felt it was about the same. Siblings are likely to experience problems if they feel different to their friends, and especially if they feel unsupported or are experiencing problems in coping with other things as well. It is important to be sensitive to their complaints about having to do too much and to regularly review how the whole family is coping with what they do to help

What help do siblings give?

About a quarter of siblings mentioned minding/supervising. Three quarters mentioned teaching and helping their sibling learn new things. These ranged from play, sports, leisure, computers, to helping more formally with management and behaviour training programmes. A third specifically mentioned they helped in teaching reading, speech, arithmetic, money, drawing and writing. A few (7%) said they were involved in the physical caretaking tasks such as feeding, washing and dressing, and 5% in coping with emotional problems. The latter tended to have younger siblings with Down syndrome or those who were amongst the most disabled.

What problems can siblings experience?

Embarrassment and explaining to others

Most siblings will experience people staring at them when out with their brother or sister with Down syndrome, or having to explain about their sibling to others. Most appear to cope, especially if they have seen how the family cope. Parents, close relatives and friends can help reduce such problems. This includes inviting the siblings' friends home and being open about the Down syndrome, and helping them with how to tell others (Chapter 1).

Teasing and name-calling

At some stage most siblings say they have been teased or called names because of having a brother or sister with Down syndrome. For most it was not a big problem, but it is important that parents listen, and take the sibling's upset feelings seriously. Explain that some children don't understand, or that, like most bullies, the name-callers are unhappy about themselves and need to pick on others' differences to make themselves feel better. If it is a constant problem and the sibling does not feel supported or feels unable to talk about it with their parents, they can become resentful about their brother or sister with Down syndrome. If they have low self-esteem and confidence, this name-calling can become damaging and lead to withdrawal and isolation. This is not common.

The school and/or the parents should deal with bullying. Where the problem involves more than one child at school, it can help to offer to talk to the class or get someone from the voluntary society into the school to raise understanding about Down syndrome. Many parents that I know have raised money and bought books about Down syndrome for the school library. If there is a problem with children in the neighbourhood that cannot be reached through the school, some parents have gone out of their way to 'educate' them. For example, stopping them in the street and talking, or inviting them into their home. They have also taken opportunities to talk about and explain Down syndrome to other parents. Of course this is dependent on the neighbourhood and society you live in.

Some parents' worry that there may be problems if the sibling with Down syndrome attends the same school as his brother(s) or sister(s), for example giving protection against bullies or being teased. This is rare and most schools that integrate children with Down syndrome have a policy of explaining it and dealing with such issues. But it is something to check when selecting schools (Chapter 13). It is something that you can plan for and prepare your children for – without making it too much of an issue.

Restrictions on family life

Children grow up thinking their experiences are 'normal'. Most siblings do not think that having a brother or sister with Down syndrome has restricted their lives. But, parents are more likely to think it has. Many feel they have been unable to give the other children as much attention as they wanted and have had to restrict family events such as holidays and outings. Some mothers have been unable to work and help with the finances, and some fathers do not take some employment opportunities because it would change the services available to their child.

In our studies, younger siblings were more likely say there were no restrictive effects. They are unlikely to be aware of what they are missing until around eight years of age, when they make comparisons with their friends or what they read or see on TV. With older siblings, the bigger the age gap the more likely they are to describe some restrictions. When older siblings reflect back on their childhood, they are more likely to mention restrictions, but without resentment or bitterness. Those that do feel resentful do not usually relate this to the sibling with a disability, but to more general relationship problems in the family, or specific problems with their parents. The exception is for those with a very severely disable sibling and limited family resources.

Anxiety and uncertainty about the future

Siblings can feel anxious if they are not sure about what future role is expected of them. If the family has a clear plan for the future care of the child with Down syndrome this can help. A plan allows them to keep more control of their future lives. Even if they disagree with their parents, they at least have a base from which to develop their own solutions.

Some siblings are expected by their parents to take on the responsibility of their brother or sister:

> 'I grew up with this role of taking care of him. My mother told me when I was about 16 that I would have to look after him when she couldn't. She was very frightened he would be put in an institution and not be looked after. He isn't good with strangers because he has always been with us. A bit over-protected I suppose. At the time I didn't mind. I planned my life around him – didn't think I would marry – worked out my career and where to live, all around him. Looking back it was wrong of her to expect me to do that. I know it now, but I still feel guilty I made a life for myself'.
>
> An adult sister, 5 years older.

Fortunately most parents do not think like this. All parents worry about the future for their child with disability, and equally about their other children and the burden of responsibility. There are an increasing range of possibilities for young adults with Down syndrome to lead independent lives and so reduce the likelihood of making the sibling feel responsible (Chapter 13).

The views of mothers about problems for siblings.

I will end this section with an overview from our research, of mothers' views on possible problems for siblings of a child with Down syndrome. The overall picture is very positive.

We talked to mothers living in the North of England in the early 1990's about possible problems for siblings. All these mothers lived in their own houses, most had a husband and none was very poor. Given different circumstances the findings could change.

Table 1 shows the ten most common negative effects and the chances that it might be a problem. Only two issues raised more negative than positive comments. These were that the sibling had less time for him or herself and was less able to do hobbies and activities at home. The mothers who said this often had inadequate housing with little space or outdoor play areas, and the child with

---

DO SIBLINGS TAKE ON THE CARING ROLE IN ADULTHOOD?

There is not much research on adult siblings and less that is specific to Down syndrome. This information is taken from what we know about siblings of people with significant disability.

Most adult siblings feel some duty and responsibility toward their brother or sister with disability. Some recent studies suggest about a third of younger siblings plan to live together when they are adults. A lot of the sisters of the young people in our study are quite adamant that they will look after their brother or sister with Down syndrome when their parents cannot. This changes as they get older and more independent. How many actually do live together is not known, but it is quite rare.

Siblings who have partners and families of their own are less likely to say they will take on the day-to-day care for their sibling with disability. Most maintain regular contact and provide emotional support, but fewer have direct involvement and give practical support. Higher levels of involvement are likely if the sibling is older, a sister rather than a brother, if they live close by and have regular weekly contact.

Down syndrome was active, excitable or less able, and so got into things and demanded more attention.

Only a quarter of the mothers felt there was one negative effect or more, and only one sibling was thought to have experienced 9 negative effects.

What about the grandparents?

Not all parents will have grandparents, let alone supportive grandparents, to turn to. They are often a major resource for families; I know of several who have 'adopted' a grandparent, for example, an older neighbour who was pleased to be asked to help with the child with Down syndrome. Sometimes parents have to show others that such help is welcome.

Table 1 Effects on siblings of having a brother or sister with Down syndrome as reported by mothers

	No negative effects	Mixed effects	Negative effects
Less time for oneself	64%	24%	12%
Bad attitudes/behaviour of other children	76%	14%	10%
Relationship with mother	78%	21%	2%
Relationship with father	77%	18%	6%
Relationships with other siblings	80%	12%	8%
Able to do hobbies and activities at home	78%	16%	6%
Making friends	86%	14%	2%
Bringing friends home	86%	7%	7%
Going out with friends	91%	5%	4%
School work/attainments	84%	14%	2%

In Chapter 2, I discussed the feelings and reactions of grandparents to the diagnosis of Down syndrome and how to tell them. In the early days many grandparents are very bewildered and upset, and their feelings can be forgotten as people focus in on the immediate family. It is important to keep them involved and informed. For example, home visits by professionals could be arranged for times when the grandparent is there. Grandparents with little to do may be left to brood and worry:

'I worried about what was best for my new grandson, of course, but my real hear-ache was for my daughter and son-in-law. I could see their anguish and more than them perhaps, that they were not able to experience the joy of becoming a parent. I did feel angry at that. I remember my joy and felt so useless that I could not make it happen for them'.

Grandparents need to take their own journey to learn how to be a grandparent of a child with Down syndrome and a parent of a child who has a child with Down syndrome.

What can grandparents do?

Grandparents have a very special role to play when the baby is born. If they can come to terms with the diagnosis, they can be very supportive both practically and emotionally. Research has found that fathers who feel their fathers were supportive are more likely to adjust to the diagnosis more quickly, to experience less stress and anxiety and to feel that they could then support their partner and the family better:

> 'We would not have survived without Mum and Dad. From the beginning they loved him and could never do enough to help. They wanted to learn all about what the doctors told us and about how to do the exercises. Dad was great at them. We could call on them any time. I never felt they resented the baby'.

Grandparents like to feel they are needed and can help. But there seem to be two extremes – those who take over so the parent feels left out, and those who hover around the edge not wanting to interfere and not quite knowing what to do. As I discussed in Chapter 1, parents need think about the strengths and weaknesses of family resources and how best to use them. One grandparent may be a bit too old to lift and carry babies, or not too good playing with young children, but they might be good listeners or information seekers. Others may be a great help in caring for and stimulating child.

There is so much good and positive help that grandparents can give. As a grandparent myself, I feel we have to learn not to be too influential, too knowing, too protective. We should offer our help and understanding, and then let sons and daughters accept, reject and direct it according to their needs.

Compared to parents, grandparents can:

- Be more relaxed with the child – they are less concerned about discipline and spoiling the child, and feel less pressure about their development and attainments.
- Offer the gift of time- they are removed from the everyday care of the child and have time away from the child to reflect.

- Be patient – in playing with the child or teaching them new skills.

These strengths echo those I described earlier for siblings.

Possible Problems

Although most grandparents are supportive, we found that just over 40% of the families in our studies experienced some problems. If there are problems it can help if someone from outside the family can be found to talk with the grandparent(s).

Difficulty accepting the diagnosis and differing views of Down syndrome

Grandparents can find it difficult to accept or appreciate the consequences of the condition. They may take time to adjust and avoid making contact with the parent for a while. This can be mistaken for disinterest. Parents may need to make the contact and help the grandparent – often by asking for help.

Grandparents may question whether the doctors are sure of the diagnosis. Even when they accept it, some may talk of the child 'growing out of it,' or insist 'Just look at her, she can't be that bad, someone has got it wrong'. Even comments such as 'Just see how well he's doing, I'm sure he's going to be a bright boy even if he does have Down syndrome,' can upset parents who are trying to be realistic.

> 'My mother was not much help. She felt the baby was being messed around with by all the doctors. I know she was just trying to support me . . . but she would not let the baby do anything. She'd prefer her *(the baby)* to just sit there. She always asks – 'Why does she have to do these exercises, she'll do them in time herself'.

These pessimistic views and predictions of a grim future may be based on past knowledge and experiences of people with Down syndrome. The problem is similar that discussed earlier when the mother and father hold different views. The solutions are the same. Patient open discussions, and access to the books, information and support that the parents have.

Family resources work best when all the members share the same beliefs, values and hopes for the child with Down syndrome.

Blaming

More serious, and less common is when grandparents start hinting that they have never had anything like this before *in their* half of the family. These comments can be very hurtful to the son-in-law or daughter-in-law. Sometimes they are a quite blatant accusation. The grandparent is feeling defensive and trying to protect their child (Chapter 2). The grandparent should be directed to information about what causes Down syndrome (Chapter 4).

Such remarks can cause long-term damage in family relationships. The accused in-law is already likely to feel inadequate and perhaps that they have 'let down' their partner and the child. Such accusations can create tension between the parents. The son or daughter of the grandparent making the comments can be caught in the middle. Often, they will naturally feel protective of their parent and more accepting of such comments than their partner. Equally, they can feel very protective toward their partner and then become estranged from their parent, which can make the partner feel guilty and around it all goes. Given such tensions it is no wonder any feelings of resentment toward the baby can become difficult to resolve.

If you are a grandparent reading this, and find yourself inclined to make such remarks, please find out about the causes of Down syndrome, and please think about the consequences of whatever you say. If you are a parent on the receiving end of such remarks, try to understand that they usually reflect the grandparents' own difficulties in accepting that they have a grandson or granddaughter with Down syndrome, and their protectiveness towards you.

Conflict over keeping the baby

The last and most difficult problem arises when there is conflict between the parents over whether to care for the baby themselves or seek fostering (Chapter 1). This is not common, but when it happens it can produce much anguish. Grandparents need to tread very carefully and examine their feelings before giving advice. It is such a difficult time for parents that they can find themselves buckling under pressure. When parents and grandparents have confused or conflicting ideas it is helpful to find a non-emotionally involved person, usually a professional, who can talk with all the family.

The positive effects for grandparents

Like parents, many grandparents also experience benefits that the child with Down syndrome brings:

> 'My daughter and I have come much closer since he was born *(the child with Down syndrome)*. I seemed to have been more involved than with the other children and it has been so enlightening to find a different way of looking at things'.

> 'I don't think I will ever completely accept what has happened to my child, but it doesn't stop the way we love our granddaughter. She radiates happiness and joy and I feel privileged to know her. Sometimes I find myself feeling it was nice she had Down syndrome. But then tell myself off for being so selfish'.

What are the effects on the family?

This section is in three parts: What we know about health, stress and anxiety; about social life and employment, and finally some suggestions for coping with possible effects on the family.

Health and Stress

Do families with a child with Down syndrome suffer more ill health than other families?

There is no evidence that families of children with Down syndrome have more medical problems or catch more illnesses. A few children with Down syndrome also have an additional severe physical disability. Like other parents of children with physical disability this results in greater caretaking demands and parents and carers may have to do much more lifting and carrying with quite old and heavy children. These parents tend to be at risk for back and muscular strain problems. This can be helped if they learn how to lift safely and use special equipment.

Do families with a child with Down syndrome have more stress and strain than other families?

As described in Chapter 1, having a child with Down syndrome does not inevitably result in more stress and problems for families. Children with Down syndrome are all very different, and families differ in terms of resources and underlying levels of stress and health.

Deciding what affect the Down syndrome causes is difficult. Life events such as moving house, getting married, changing work, gaining a qualification, and getting ill can all cause us stress. Having a child with Down syndrome brings extra things to deal with, such as coming to terms with the diagnosis, coping with any medical problems, selecting schools and arranging future care. The child usually makes extra demands on time and supervision and so when other stressors arise they can interact with this and together increase the stress experienced. However, many of these life-events are temporary.

We found that in the early years, mothers of children with Down syndrome had slightly higher than average 'stress and strain' scores, but they did not have significant health problems. Only 20-30% fell into the category of major problems – about the same as mothers of typical children – and usually associated with things like unemployment, physical ill health, poor family relationships and stress at work. For most mothers, the issues are the same as with any young child. Stress scores increased as the child with Down syndrome got older and decreased in the teenage years and early adulthood. This is probably due to increased difficulties in managing and entertaining a larger and older child. It improves as the child becomes more self-sufficient and self-regulating.

Some more recent studies are suggesting higher average stress levels than those found for mothers of typical children. It is not clear why, but it may relate to the changing life-styles of current young families and the increased demands on mothers. My suspicion is that these demands and the increased demands of having a child with Down syndrome compound.

Life events such as relationship breakdown, long-term unemployment and chronic illness are more likely to cause sustained
stress. If several life events happen at the same time, then the strain
is greater. How much this affects us depends on the resources we
have to cope (Chapter 1).

A minority of families experienced high levels of stress throughout the child-rearing years, and this was not just about the problems
with the child. When we compared families whose children had
similar levels of needs and demands, we found that those who felt
less stressed and highly satisfied with life also had strong parental
relationships, reasonable finances, practical and social support from
others and practical coping skills (Chapter 1). These families had
reasonable support from the early years, and they made use of the
local services. Practical problems caused stress, such as having to take
time off work because the child had a medical problem and needed
to visit the hospital, or if the child was frequently off school because
of illness.

> Overall, parents of children with Down syndrome have lower
> levels of stress and loss of vitality than families with children
> with severe intellectual or physical disabilities. This is largely
> because the children with Down syndrome are easier to
> manage and make fewer demands on family resources.

Stress and changes in society

Compared to earlier studies, some recent studies are indicating that
parents of children with Down syndrome have higher ratings of
stress and anxiety compared to the averages for the general population. However the levels are not those requiring treatment. There
are parents who do need treatment, but they have other complex
problems. A recent study of Swedish families, for example, found
somewhat higher percentages of stress and strain than we did. This
might be due to the differences in Swedish and English people, differences in the questionnaires used, or changing pressures on
families in the ten years between the studies.

In the Swedish study, mothers of children with Down syndrome
rated themselves as having lower vitality and more feelings of

anxiety and depression than the general population. They were more likely to evaluate their health as poor, felt tired more often, and said that these feelings interfered with their daily life, work and social activities. The fathers also had higher average scores on anxiety and depression, and to a lesser degree, vitality. 67% of mothers and 57% of fathers said they felt 'stress' about the demands on their time made by their children, compared to 46% and 35% for mothers and fathers of typical children. 44% of mothers of children with Down syndrome felt worn out much of the time compared to 27% of the other mothers.

I want to emphasise again that such difficulties are not inevitable because the child has Down syndrome. They arise when the resources to cope are inadequate. The majority of the families who are well adjustment and having shared and positive views of the child, and also have reasonable support, do not experience higher levels of stress and fatigue than similar families without a child with Down syndrome.

Are there differences between mothers and fathers?
More mothers report feelings of stress and less vitality than fathers in all families – with or without a disabled member. This is not surprising as most mothers are more involved in the daily care of children and running the home. We found that fathers were the main source of help, but that they were more likely to play and entertain the children than do the housework. Although the majority of mothers were happy with the division of labour, many wanted more help.

The difference in stress scores between mothers and fathers of children with Down syndrome disappear as the child gets older, probably due to the father becoming more involved with the older child.

Do less able children with Down syndrome cause more stress and family problems?
No! It used to be believed, and still is in many places, that the level of intellectual or physical disability and the nature of the condition, could predict the level of strain on families. But this has not been found in research studies. This is not surprising, as children with the same condition vary greatly and families vary in how they cope. But

many people are surprised that the severity of intellectual or physical disability is not directly related to how much stress the family
experiences. There are many parents and families who have a
severely disabled child, and who are coping well and feel satisfied
with their lives. There are others, who have a child with a mild disability that is causing them all sorts of problems. However the more
complex the problems and especially behaviour problems, the more
at risk the families are to experience stress and anxiety.

Social Activities, Going Out and Employment

Does the presence of a child with Down syndrome restrict the families' social activities?

Studies that have compared families with a *young* child with Down
syndrome with families of typical children, do not find major differences in social aspects such as parents getting out together, family
outings and holidays. Two thirds of our parents were content with
their social activities when the child was young, and only 15% felt
the child with Down syndrome restricted their social life more than
a typical child would. In the early years, less than 10% of the parents
told us the child had actually spoilt family holidays, and even with
older children the figure never rose above 20%.

A few parents noted that a holiday can disturb a young child's
routine, and that it takes them a while to settle down afterwards.
But this may not be a bad thing for the child and can help them
become more adaptable.

Fortunately, only a minority of children with Down syndrome
have major medical and health problems. But they may be susceptible to illness particularly respiratory problems and parents may find
time is spent in surgeries and clinics (Chapter 7). We found that
some parents went out together less often when their child had
severe health problems, mainly because they didn't have experienced child-minders who they felt they could trust in a crisis.

> 'We have to watch her very closely because of her heart, so we
> tend to go out separately and probably less often'.

Other families with children who had health problems did not feel so restricted. They seemed more able to leave the child and trust someone else to look after them. This is about aspects of the parent such as willingness to take a risk, coping with their fears, feelings of protectiveness, as well as their access to resources.

BEHAVIOUR AND OUTINGS

Behaviour problems can disrupt family outings and everyday tasks like shopping. Some families gave up going on family outings and holidays because of the child's behaviour, but many carefully selected the holiday because of problems with sleeping, running away, and temper tantrums.

'I like B__ (a holiday camp) because it's closed in, you know what I mean, it doesn't matter if she gets lost. So it gives me a break . . . and it gives her a break, because she can do her own thing'.

Even parents of typical young children find such things difficult, and when a child is mobile, excitable, likes to run off or can't stop touching things, life can be difficult. It can also be embarrassing. About half our parents experienced problems with this, and for a minority (around 16%), it prevented family outings almost entirely.

'Yes he prevents me going out. I can't leave him. You've got to be two weeks in front him to know what he's going to get up to next. He wears me out'.

'Who will baby sit? Will they cope in an emergency? What if she has a bad temper tantrum and they can't cope?'.

Half the parents did not experience such problems and enjoyed taking their children out. We found an increasing problem in the mid-childhood years, although still for a minority of parents. Behaviour that was easy to cope with, or not embarrassing in a young child, becomes much more challenging for parents of older and larger children.

> We did not find a relationship between the actual number of times parents managed to go out together and the level of behaviour problems. Some parents felt it prevented them going out and so felt their life was restricted, but others, whose child seemed just as difficult, did manage to get out. If parents are having problems leaving the child or going out, they may need to re-think whether this is due to their feelings, beliefs and personality. They do not have to be stoical and think that nothing can be done – it can help to actively seek out resources.

Feeling isolated

Many parents of children with a disability often say they feel isolated. There are two types of isolation: social and emotional. Social isolation is not being able to get out and do things because of the child. Emotional isolation is when parents feel they have no one to share their worries and concerns with, and no one who understands what it is like to have a child with a disability. The main source of emotional support comes from partners or close relatives, but support can come from many sources, such as contact with other parents.

> 'It took an effort but I rang up the local Down syndrome support group. M . . . came around the same day and it just lifted so many things off my mind. I then met other mums and we all help and support each. It has been my life-line'

Many parents are offered the chance of meeting with other parents of a child with Down syndrome in the first days or weeks after the birth. We found half did want to meet other parents fairly soon, but half wanted to wait for a few months or more, preferring to come to terms with things within their own familiar situation. Others never felt the need to meet other parents.

Support can come from friends and be a surprise. This is what a young single mother said:

> 'At first I just stayed in all the time. Then one of the lads from

the youth club came round. He's got no hand (Thalidomide) and said, "What's up with you!" I could have hit him, but I just cried. After I told him why I hadn't been out he said, "Don't be bloody stupid! . . . Look at me, I've got no hand and they've accepted me all right. 'Course they'll accept the baby, there's not much wrong with him!" That night they all came round. Now they spoil him rotten! I've no trouble getting baby-sitters, but I wouldn't leave him with them – they're all mad!'

An older mother described how she found it difficult:

'I kept finding excuses why I couldn't go out. One night my husband looked at me and said – "Are we going to sit at home like this with him for the rest of our lives? We have to make a move sometime". I could see he was right, so there and then we asked our neighbour if she would just come in for an hour or two. She was so pleased I had asked her, as she had wanted to suggest it but didn't like to. I worried for the whole two hours we were out. Now we get out just the same as we did for the other children, and most of our friends or relatives are quite happy to sit for us. They usually say he's easier than the other kids'.

Does having a child with Down syndrome affect the employment of parents?

Overall, there does not appear to be any effect on the employment of fathers. Some do not seek or take on work that would mean moving away from their area if they have special facilities. This happens with any child, but it is often a more difficult decision when children have a disability. Others find they want to move in order to be near such facilities, and this can mean a change in employment. It is important to balance the advantages and disadvantages of such a major decision for all members of the family.

The best place for a child with a disability is in a cohesive and caring family with resources. I believe, these things impact on the child's welfare and attainments more than special facilities and specific treatment programmes. Staying close to some facility assumes that the programme provided is effective, but this may not be the case (Chapter 11).

Some parents find they can't work or work full-time or do shift work. It may be that they can't find (or afford) special childcare, especially if the child has challenging behaviour or medical problems. I know of several parents who gave up their employment to focus on the child's disability and ensure he or she got all the help and treatments possible. But I am not sure that the benefits outweighed the losses. Others have become very involved in the world of disability and have changed jobs or re-qualified to work in the field.

Most of this research has been on mothers, and this differs to that for fathers. We found that at the preschool age, the mothers in our research group were less likely to have a job than mothers of typical children, and this is backed up by national studies of mothers of children with disabilities. When we looked at the employment of our mothers when the children were over five years of age and attending school, we found no difference compared to the national figures – around 40-45% were employed in some way.

These figures were obtain in the 1980's and early 1990's and may not reflect changes in female employment and variations between countries and cultures. A recent study in Australia found that around 54% of mothers of similarly aged children with Down syndrome were in the workforce. Like mothers of typical children, those of children with Down syndrome usually find part-time work initially, and as the children got older, more took full-time jobs. A difference was fewer mothers of children with Down syndrome went into full-time employment and many moved to full-time later in life when the children were older. Significantly more mothers in *our* group had jobs than in a similar group who had not received regular early support. Since there were no differences in the children or type of school attended, we felt that this difference in mothers' work was due to the support from the early home visiting and their changes in confidence and organising of resources.

We also found that the mothers who worked had lower stress and felt more content. This was particularly true of the 25% who had gone back into work quite soon after the birth and continued to work into the teenage years of the child. But of course these same mothers had the resources to cope with the child, and many of these resources act as a buffer to stress. Their additional earnings certainly help the financial resources of the family.

Only a few mothers say they took the job to *'get away from the baby'*. The majority worked for financial reasons, or because they were anxious not to lose touch with a profession. All the mothers in our studies felt that having a job was beneficial to themselves and the family. Most said it helped them not to get *'too engrossed in the child and problems'*, and that work gave them a wider range of interests. The lower levels of child related stress felt by fathers is possibly due to the same thing. Many mothers also felt that going out to work also helped to keep things in perspective:

'People react to children with disability very differently now. The first job I went to, they just wouldn't talk to me after I told them. I had to tell them 'cause I feel that I'm deceiving them in one way, making them believe that nothing was wrong and you feel as if you're not telling them the whole truth . . . But in my new job they're great! I don't feel like an outcast'

Overall, having a baby with Down syndrome does not by itself restrain mothers from employment, and that work helps with personal feelings and practical resources. Unfortunately some parents find restrictions on the type of employment they are able to take because of the child's behaviour problems and supervision demands. This again is a problem of resources.

Taking breaks from the child

As described in Chapter 1 many problems and the stress they cause the family can be reduced if we understand the issues and then provide the resources to meet the needs of individual families.

There are times in most families, however, when problems occur, and coping with the child's disability is just too much. For example, elderly parents or another family member can become ill or need special attention. There may be times when parents want to take their other children on an active holiday such as walking, fishing or boating, and the child with the disability may not be able to take part. In some families, the siblings lose out on parental attention as the child with Down syndrome has such complex needs and demands.

The choices are:

- You sacrifice your own needs or those of other members of the family.
- You carry on until you become too tired to cope and a crisis arises. By then you may be too tired to make any decisions.
- Or, you try to plan ahead, and get resources in place to help.

The importance of taking regular breaks

Some parents find the idea of being away from their child difficult. In Chapter 2, I described the strong feelings of protectiveness towards a child with a disability. Such feelings and the parent's personality will influence how ready they are to 'take risks'. These include giving the children more freedom and letting other people look after them. It is not easy, and parents of all children are frequently examining situations and making risk assessments. Unlike professionals, few parents get training in how to do such assessments, and the consequences of getting it wrong are greater. It is important to let the children be with others, and to think about setting up alternative places for them to stay at times.

Fortunately, the majority of children with Down syndrome do not need respite care in terms of breaks for families in crisis. But it is worth finding out about support services, getting the name of a contact person, and then making yourself known to them – just in case. The same applies for nursery and school places. Associations for Down syndrome and local parent groups usually have information about these facilities.

Many areas have small residential homes that can offer regular breaks for the child depending on assessed family need. Social services or voluntary associations run most of these facilities. Other alternatives in your area may include specially trained 'foster' parents who will get to know the family and the child, and look after him or her for weekends or holidays. Some places have 'buddy' schemes when volunteers get to know the young person and take them out for day trips. There are never enough for the demand, and often these services simply react to crises. You may have to emphasise your support needs and respite care may not be available unless your child has behaviour problems or you are ill or have some other difficult event.

It is a pity that such services are often called 'respite care', and seen as some kind of last resort for tired or desperate parents. They certainly can be, but this image means that many parents refuse to think about the possibility. Parents can feel guilt that they may be rejecting the child; or they may think others will see them as inadequate or rejecting. It doesn't help if relatives condemn parents for thinking about, or trying to arrange regular breaks using such services. Many of these ideas arise from outdated attitudes to disability and justifiable concerns about large institutions or homes for children. This is why I think it is important to look objectively at the benefits of breaks.

The benefits of breaks

For the family
- They give parents the opportunity to re-examine how things are going and recharge their sources of energy.
- They provide the opportunity for parents to give attention to other members of the family, and themselves.
- Parents can get to know their other children again. I found my children changed so quickly I had to make space to be with them individually, rather than just knowing them as a group.
- Parents can assess their home life best away from the everyday routine. It is nice after a break to look forward to having all the children together again. If parents don't feel this, it is a signal that there is a problem and help is needed. It is better than waiting until a crisis overwhelms the family.
- Regular breaks can help brothers and sisters for the same reasons as parents. In addition they can learn that their brother or sister with Down syndrome can live away from home and often likes it. This can help with any concerns they may have about looking after them in later life.

For the child with Down syndrome
- People often forget that there are great benefits for the child with Down syndrome when they have a break away from the family and everyday routine. We can all get stuck in routines, especially children with Down syndrome (Chapter 9). Living somewhere else for short periods, can stimulate their

development and improve their adaptability. I have often heard mothers marvel about how much the child 'came on' after staying with grandmother for a week. Changes challenge the child's behaviour by providing different routines and experiences. Some planning and preparation may be needed to make sure the challenge is not so great that the child becomes confused or cannot make sense of what is happening. Start when the child is quite young and build up to vacations, stays in residential settings and eventually independent living.

Taking breaks and using respite care is similar to what happens with many typical children. They may get looked after by someone other than their parent when they are very young, then stay over with a relative and have sleepovers with friends, short holidays with relatives and the school. Older children and young adults go off on their own holidays and may have exchanges with children from other countries. Many children with a disability are denied this type of normal life-style because of our fears about them getting upset or not being cared for properly, or the feeling that others would not cope with or want to cope with them. But I have found many very successful examples for all these. It takes planning and a belief that it is worthwhile and can work. It is not as easy as with typical children; there is a limited number of other families or places available, especially if some extra understanding is needed. Sometimes, a local group of parents of children with a disability are willing to set up sleepover arrangements. The Internet is providing a very useful way of searching for other families and places.

These ideas on breaks are all part of the plan needed to help the child toward independence. By this I do not mean just teaching him to dress and feed himself, but also encouraging emotional independence. The importance of this is seen most clearly in the question ask by all parents, '*What will happen when we die?*' It is no good ignoring this question, and no good worrying about it. All we can do for any child is to try to help them achieve independence. This means they have not only to learn how to look after themselves but how to live with other people. We start from birth (Chapter 8) and continue for as long as we are able. Most typical children and young adults have a strong inner drive for independence, but this may be less, or more easily suppressed in many children with Down syndrome. I am reminded of a conversation I had with a 28-year-old women with Down syndrome. When I asked her how she was getting on, and how her mother and father were, she replied:

> 'Just the same, thank you. They still won't let me get my own place. I look after them too well. I do all the shopping and tidying. They'd be lost without me – that's what they keep saying'.

Just as families have to learn to adapt to disability and care and love the new member with Down syndrome, they also have to think about the future and learn how to let-go when the time is right (Chapter 10). Planning this can be one of the most difficult but rewarding aspects for families.

Summary

1   The majority of parents and siblings feel that the child with Down syndrome in their family has been a positive experience. Rather than being passive recipients of family resources, they have been active participants in family life and added to family well-being.

2   There is no evidence that having a child with Down syndrome in the family automatically produces ill effects in the other children.

3   Parents are less likely to separate than couples in general. A very small number do separate when one parent cannot come to terms with the disability and the other can, and wants to raise the child.

4   There is no evidence to show that the social life of most parents of young children with Down syndrome is restricted and different from other families of young children. If the child has additional medical or behavioural problems this adds extra demands but many parents organise the resources needed to cope and reduce restrictions.

5   As the child grows, more families can experience restrictions, and parents experience higher than 'normal' levels

of fatigue and stress, although these are not within clinical levels unless there are additional pressures. Again the stress experienced is reduced if parents have the resources to meet the demands. It also decreased with older children and teenagers as they become more independent and self-controlled.

6 Stress is not inevitable because the child has Down syndrome; the level of the child's intellectual disability is not directly related to problems for the family. It relates to a much wider set of factors and resources.

7 A small group of families have major long-term difficulties with high levels of fatigue and stress. These families have inadequate resources to cope and the children usually have major health problems, very slow development and low independence, and are particularly difficult to manage (Chapter 9). These difficulties are more likely if parents have an anxious personality and low feelings of self–esteem. Some have not really come to terms with the child's disability and so live in a state of resentment and wishing things were different. Other families simply do not have many resources like finances, adequate housing and practical support to meet the demands of the child.

Causes, Risks and Prevalence of Down Syndrome

I want to stress here that Down syndrome is not caused by anything that happened during pregnancy. It began when either the egg or the sperm cells were being produced, or just after the egg was fertilised by the sperm. The new egg had extra genetic material from chromosome 21. This altered the plan and produced the differences between a child with Down syndrome and other children. Down syndrome is not an illness or disease. You don't catch it, and the children with Down syndrome do not suffer from it. It is far more common than many people think and people with Down syndrome now lead long and full lives.

4

What causes Down syndrome?

- **Are there different types of Down syndrome?**
- **How and why did it happen to me?**
- **How many babies have Down syndrome?**

Deciding on how much detail to put into this Chapter has been difficult. I have chosen what I feel is needed to make sense of Down syndrome. Some of it is detailed and complex. My hope is that you will get a feel for the complexity of producing new human beings and why the plan sometimes gets altered. The last half-century has seen rapid advances in genetics, which have brought us closer to some answers; but the issues are complicated and we cannot expect easy solutions. When describing how the extra chromosome occurs I have used the commonly used term 'chromosomal fault' or 'error'. I do not want to suggest any person is at fault or trigger feelings of guilt. As you read these chapters, I believe you will see that there is no factual reason why any parent should feel guilty that they have produced a child with Down syndrome.

This chapter is in three parts; the first is about chromosomes and genes; the second part is about how the extra chromosome got there, what factors may have caused it and the different types of trisomy 21. The third part is about incidence – the number of Down syndrome pregnancies and births and influential factors.

What produces the condition in the baby?

To answer this we need to know some basic facts about cells, chromosomes and genes and how we, like all living things, produce offspring similar to all human beings but uniquely different from each other.

Cells

Just like bricks make up a building, our bodies are made up of thousands of cells. Unlike bricks, cells are living things. They are not just small bags of chemicals, but are purposeful and 'know' what to do. With the exception of red blood cells, each cell has two parts – the nucleus, which is the control centre, and the cytoplasm, which is like a storage and energy producing area (Figure 1). There are many different types of cells – skin cells, blood cells, nerve cells, muscle cells – all with different structures and functions. Cells group together and form the major systems of the body – skeletal, digestive, circulatory, respiratory, hormonal and nervous system. All these cells fit and work together in harmony in a healthy body. How this complex set of systems develops from a single, tiny cell is a constant source of wonder. It starts as soon as a sperm and egg combine and form a fertilised cell. This divides and then the new cells divide and so on, forming specialised cell lines and body parts.

Chromosomes

How do the cells know when to divide and what sort of cells to become? How do the legs, arms, heart and eyes get into the right place? Why do babies usually sit up and walk and talk around the same age? Why do family members look the same? Why do different races have their own characteristics?

There has to be a master plan that controls and programmes this development. It is the **chromosomes** that carry this plan, as **genes,** from generation to generation and from cell to cell. They ensure that human beings produce human beings and equip the new being to survive in the environment on our planet. As we will see, if something does not go according to plan and we get more or less chromosomal material, the person is different. However, they are

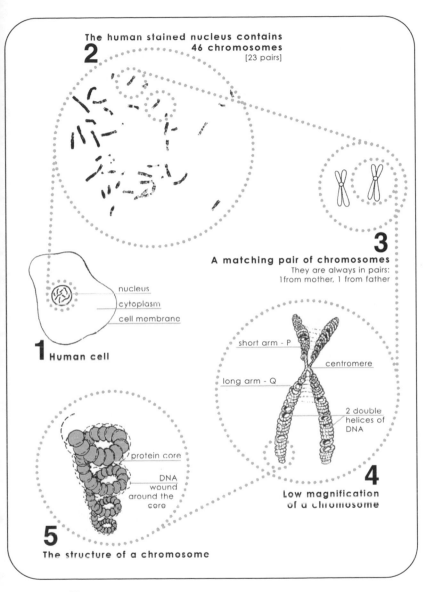

The human stained nucleus contains
2 **46 chromosomes**
[23 pairs]

3
A matching pair of chromosomes
They are always in pairs:
1 from mother, 1 from father

nucleus
cytoplasm
cell membrane

1 Human cell

short arm - P
centromere
long arm - Q
2 double
helices of
DNA

4
Low magnification
of a chromosome

protein core
DNA
wound
around the
core

5
The structure of a chromosome

Figure 1 Chromosomes

still human beings because they are produced from human chromosomes.

A sample of blood or skin cells is used to find the number and arrangement of chromosomes, or the **karyotype** of a person. Cells in the sample can be stimulated to divide and make new cells. The division is stopped, the cell is broken down, the chromosomes are released and stained. This is where the name came from; chromo meaning colour and soma meaning body part. They can then be examined under the microscope and photographed (Figure 1).

The chromosomes come in different sizes and have different patterns of segments or bands (Figures 1 and 4). Human beings have 46 chromosomes consisting of 22 matched pairs (one from each parent) and two sex chromosomes. The set of chromosomes is called the **genome** – in our case the human genome. Figure 2 shows a normal set of chromosomes for a female and Figure 3 shows those of a male. You can see the two female sex chromosomes, one from each parent, look similar and are called XX. The male sex chromosomes are called XY; the smaller Y chromosome is from the father and the X from the mother. For the purposes of identification, the chromosomes are put into groups, A to G, depending on size and numbered 1 to 22.

If you look at figure 1 you can see that each chromosomes is made of two long chains of chemical chunks (DNA molecules) – like a ladder that is twisted into a spiral. They are wound around a central core of protein and joined together at a specific junction point – the **centromere** – though it is not usually in the centre (Figure 1). They look like a cross with two short arms, known as p and two long arms – q. When magnified, segments of light and dark bands can be seen. These are important as they show specific pieces of the chromosome that do specific jobs. Each segment and even smaller regions has been given a number to help identification. Therefore 21q 11 means segment 11 on the long arm of chromosome 21. As new information about the segments was discovered, they were further labelled into sub segments e.g. 21q22.2, which is chromosome 21, long arm, segment 22, sub segment 2 (Figure 4).

Chromosome 21 and Down syndrome
Down syndrome is produced because there is either an extra chromosome 21 or extra material from chromosome 21. It is called

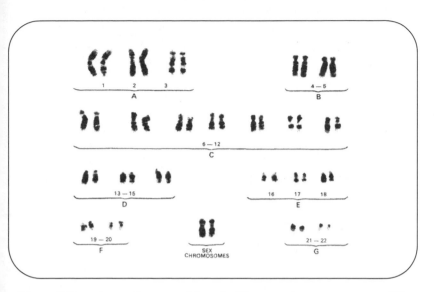

Figure 2 Karyotype of a normal female. The sex chromosomes are XX

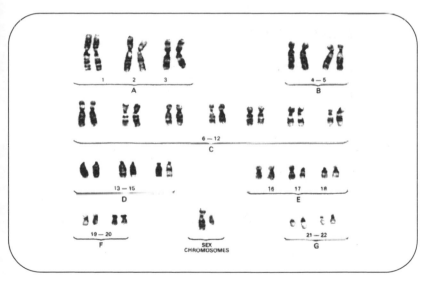

Figure 3 Karyotype of a normal male. The sex chromosomes are XY

trisomy 21 because there are three (tri) chromosome 21's instead of two. Figure 5 shows the chromosomes of a boy with Down syndrome; you can see three chromosome 21's in the G group.

Chromosome 21 is the smallest chromosome, but it contains about 40 million bits of code (see later, genes and codons). Recent estimates report that chromosome 21 contains 329 genes, around 1% of the total human genome.

Not all the genes on chromosome 21 are associated with Down syndrome. Most of the physical characteristics of Down syndrome result from extra copies of the end of the long arm of chromosome 21, around segment q22.2 and may involve between 50 and 100 genes. Given the millions of codes in the genome, this is a relatively small proportion. As shown in Figure 6, some of the extra genetic material has been shown to be associated with some frequent characteristics of Down syndrome such as heart defects, physical characteristics of face, hand, foot, 'looser' joints (hyperlaxity), lower muscle tone (hypotonia), slower development and learning difficulties (all discussed in later chapters). Genes just outside the region have been associated with some aspects of ageing and Alzheimer-like brain modifications that are also part of the syndrome (Chapter 7). Recent work has shown that there are 10 genes that influence the structure and function of the central nervous system, and 16 genes with a role in energy and reactive oxygen metabolism – see later.

One effect of the extra genetic material is that from conception the cells do not divide as rapidly as typical cells. This results in fewer cells and smaller babies. It also disrupts the migration of cells and the formation of different parts of the body. For example, some parts of the brain are smaller than usual, and overall there are fewer cells and connections (Chapter 7).

Types of Trisomy 21 (Down syndrome)

I talk about types of trisomy 21, because once you are born with trisomy and the features recognised as Down syndrome, what happens next to 'make' you a person with Down syndrome has a lot to do with environmental factors, like how you are treated by others and society as a whole (Sections 3 and 4).

There are three distinctive karyotypes of Down syndrome: **Free Trisomy 21**, **Translocation** and **Mosaicism**. Within these one can find different types of translocation and, very rarely, mosaic translocation and partial trisomies.

Free Trisomy 21
This is the most common type of Down syndrome where every cell in the person has an extra chromosome 21; between 90 to 95% of all people with Down syndrome have free trisomy 21. It is usually noted as 47XX + 21 for females and 47XY + 21 for males.

Translocation
In this type, the extra copy of chromosome 21 is not free, but has attached to one of the other chromosomes – it has **trans**ferred to a new **location**. The most recent studies suggest just over 3% of people with Down syndrome have the translocated type. As with free trisomy 21, each cell has 46 separate chromosomes but one of them is a translocation chromosome with the extra copy of chromosome 21 fused to another chromosome. To complete the picture and give some idea of how complicated this is, around 0.5% of babies born with Down syndrome have a mix of two trisomies. For example, some boys with Down syndrome have an extra female sex chromosome, known as Klinefelter syndrome after the doctor who discovered it. To complicate it further, some people have been found with translocated mosaicism.

Mosaicism
This type of Down syndrome is when there is a pattern of some trisomic cells and some normal cells. Most recent studies find that just over 1% of people with Down syndrome have the mosaic type, although some earlier studies report up to 5%.

All these different types of Down syndrome, and any additional chromosomal problems, can be detected by chromosome analysis.

Do the different types of Trisomy 21 have different characteristics?

This question has been investigated because of the wide range of differences in the physical and mental abilities, and personality of people with Down syndrome. As noted above, people with partial trisomy 21 can be different because they do not have all the extra genes or same set of genes as in full trisomy 21. However these are

The search to find out which parts of the chromosome cause the characteristics of Down syndrome has partly relied upon those rare people with an extra copy of only some of the chromosome – partial trisomy 21. By identifying the genotype of these people, or the extra genetic material they have, one can then try to match it to the features and characteristics of Down syndrome (their phenotype). If a match is found, it points to that particular gene (or genes) being involved in coding for that particular characteristic. At the present time, identification of genes and gene fragments is going on at a rapid pace.

Although most species cannot reproduce with another species (they have different numbers of chromosomes and arrangements of genes), the genetic material or biochemicals that make up the chromosome is similar. Some mice chromosomes, particularly chromosome 16, have segments or genes the same as those found on the human chromosome 21. By creating a trisomy of this chromosome in mice, many of the features seen in Down syndrome have been found; structure of the skull, learning difficulties and processes associated with Alzheimer's disease. This is also helping to unravel our understanding of how the extra chromosome material changes the plan.

very rare. Both free trisomy 21 and translocated trisomy 21 have the full extra set of genes; and studies have failed to find any conclusive evidence of difference between the two types.

The picture for mosaicism is different. As we will see in the later section, the extra chromosome can appear very early or quite late in the division of the cells. If late, people have very few trisomic cells and if early, they have nearly 100%. This may appear in skin cells, but not blood cells, or in neither, but in another system completely. It is possible that only the ovaries or testes are mosaic. To complicate matters even further, there is evidence that the percentage of trisomic cells can reduce or increase over time. This is because the cells in many of our systems are dying and need constant replacement, and the chromosome appears during cell division.

Because of this variability and the small numbers of people with mosaic Down syndrome, it is difficult to discover if they differ from others with Down syndrome. Most studies indicate that, as a group, people with mosaicism have fewer and less marked physical characteristics, possibly less health problems and slightly higher intellectual and linguistic abilities, than those with standard trisomy 21. But this difference is largely accounted for by people with less than 50% trisomic cells, most of whom are notably less disabled than the majority of people with Down syndrome. Some people with mosaicism are far more disabled than some of those with trisomy 21. This tells us that it is not just the amount of trisomic cells or the 'dose'. Complex interactions are involved and they act upon the inherited variability of the person.

Environmental factors will also play a part in promoting individual differences. I have often heard people who are surprised about the achievements of someone with Down syndrome say 'they must be mosaic.' This surprise shows a lack of understanding of the capabilities of many people with Down syndrome who are given support and opportunities; as well as a lack of knowledge about the genetic and biological basis of the syndrome.

Some people may have no obvious physical characteristics of Down syndrome, but they may have some trisomic cells – undiagnosed mosaic Down syndrome. They are more likely to have children with Down syndrome – there are reports of undiagnosed mosaicism in women who have had two children with Down syndrome.

A final historical note: Down syndrome is associated with distinctive finger, palm and footprints (called dermatoglyphics, see also Chapter 7). Before we understood the genetics, these were used to distinguish between what may have been different types of Down syndrome and to trace family lines. Studies up to the 1960's indicated that as many as 10% of births of Down syndrome infants may be related to undiagnosed mosaic Down syndrome. This dropped to around 2 to 3 % by the mid 1980's, but this approach has received little attention since then.

A Digression into Past explanations and labels for Down syndrome

Human beings constantly try to explain why things happen and how they work. We usually feel less uncertain, more in control and less anxious if we can name or explain something. But explanations may not be true – what looks like superstition today was yesterday's explanation.

Before genetic discoveries were made there were scientific beliefs that Down syndrome was a throwback to a more primitive type of human being, even monkeys! The nick-name 'mongol' for people with Down syndrome came from a belief that they were a sub-species, or a throwback to more primitive non-European races. In 1866 Dr. Langdon Down first identified a group of people with common characteristics including an apparently oriental look; and he called them 'Mongolian idiots'. The condition was soon called mongolism. At this time, 'Idiot' was a respected scientific term, and not a term abuse as used to-day. Langdon Down used other racial labels for different conditions such as 'Aztec idiots' and 'Malaysian idiots'; others' called Down syndrome 'Kalmuck Idiocy' after a race of small Asiatic-oriental people. At this time, the science of classification and Darwin's theories of evolution were foremost. Langdon Down was apparently related to Darwin by marriage. I do not know if they ever met, but I cannot resist the idea of the two of them chatting over a glass of wine on some family occasion. Langdon Down is searching for an explanation of a new group of people he has identified – could it be that different ethnic races represent different evolutionary stages of man? He called it 'racial retrogression'. Given what little was known at this time, and the confident superiority most Victorians felt, it is easy to see how the idea became popular. But it is less easy to understand how, as late as 1924, a book published in England called '*The Mongol in Our Midst*' argued that the condition was a reversion to the Orang-utan!

Fortunately, the discovery of the extra chromosome 21 in 1959 by Lejeune in France, and the growing understanding of genetics, have meant that such theories have been dispelled. This includes many that blame events during pregnancy. Past explanations include sin and immoral behaviour, alcoholism, inherited syphilis, problems with the reproductive system and hormonal imbalance. Even around the time of Lejeune's discovery, scientific papers were suggesting that the cause might be anoxia (lack of oxygen at birth) or maternal stress prior to conception. Although, with hindsight, these appear bizarre, they were serious efforts by serious people to find a cause. It is likely that future generations will look back on our current explanations in the same way. In fact the age of the mother is the only major factor that has been consistently found to be associated with a higher likelihood of having a child with Down syndrome (Chapter 5). *A fascinating historical perspective of Down syndrome can be found in Brian Stratford's book listed in the Bibliography.*

LABELS AND NAMES

Despite the evidence against the 'throw-back' theory, the term 'mongolism' and 'mongol' established itself in our language. It was still being used in scientific papers published in the UK well into the late 1970's, and it is still common in some parts of the world. I still hear it used by children as a term of abuse, although when questioned they have no idea of its origins or the offence it causes. For me, it is associated with an image of people in large institutions projecting no sense of self or initiative. This image is far removed from people with Down syndrome today who have benefited from positive expectations, inclusion in the community, good health care, a stimulating environment and efforts to educate the public. I am reminded, however, of a conversation with a mother of a baby with Down syndrome. I had, rather badly, tried to explain we no longer said 'mongol' but instead used the name Down syndrome. 'If I talk about Down's babies,' I said, 'that is what I mean.' She replied, ' I don't think that's very nice all babies have their ups and downs.' This forced me once more to realise that a label is a label whatever you try to do with it. These are not 'Down's' babies or children; they are first and foremost babies and children – children with Down syndrome. The People First movement has spread very quickly and today we always talk about people with . . . a disability or condition and not put the label first. It is about seeing the person not the syndrome.

How do chromosomes work?

Earlier, we have seen that the chromosome is a long chain of complex chemical chunks, called **molecules**, like a ladder that is twisted into a spiral called a **double helix** (Figure 4). If straightened out, it would be almost 10,000 times longer. It carries millions of bits of coded information, and is twisted to pack it all into a small space. The long chain of chemicals making the sides of the ladder is called **DNA (deoxyribonucleic acid)**. It was discovered in the mid-20th century and hailed as opening up the secrets of life. It triggered a rapid expansion in the study of human genetics and advanced our knowledge of Down syndrome.

The sides of the ladder are made up of two molecules. One is a sugar molecule (deoxyribose) and the other is a phosphate molecule. The rungs that join the sides of the ladder are made up of four base chemicals called Adenine, Thymine, Guanine and Cytosine – for convenience they are labelled as A, T, G and C.

One of these bases (A, T, G, or C) attaches itself to the sugar. The sugar is attached to the phosphate and these three parts make the basic unit in the ladder, called a **nucleotide.** These then link together to make very long strands – one side of the ladder. This produces a code or sequence of bases – A, A, G, C, T, T, A and so on.

To join the two sides of the ladder together the bases must join together. But base A will only join up to base T, and G always pairs up with a C. This mechanism results in two special properties:

- The sequence or code of instructions on either side of the ladder is matched.
- If the bases forming one side of the ladder separate and then find new nucleotides to join up with, they will make an exact copy of the first ladder.

So you get two ladders from one, the code is replicated and the plan (the human genome) can be passed on.

Codons and genes

This next bit is complicated but hopefully will give some insight into why and how things don't always go according to plan.

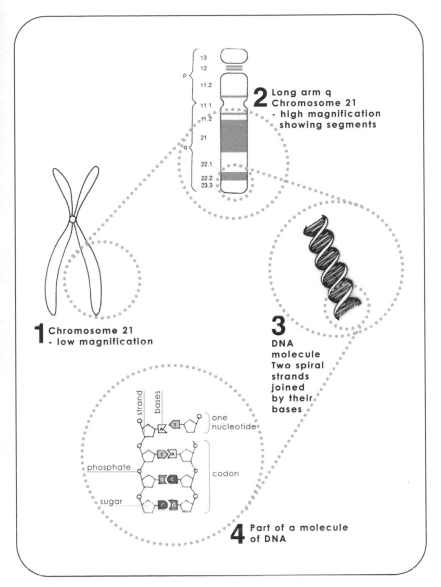

Figure 4 Structure of chromosomes and DNA

The bases work in threes, e.g. AAG, CTG, GCA, and are called **codons** (Figure 4). They are a special unit of DNA because a codon encodes one **amino acid**; amino acids are the basic building blocks that make **proteins**; and proteins are the building blocks of the body. There are 20 amino acids in the human body and they link together to form over 50,000 proteins. Some proteins form the structure of the body and others, called enzymes, control the chemical activity of the cell. The different codes therefore, carry the instructions for both the structure of the cell and its' function. For example, nerve cells have their own shape and structure, making up the brain and nerves; and their function is to transmit information and store information in specialised groups of cells (Chapter 7). Their structure includes 'gates' in the cell membrane that can open and close allowing chemical messages through at the right time and intensity. For example, a seizure or fit happens if the gates malfunction or too much of a specific chemical messenger gets through and 'floods' the system.

Just as the length of DNA that codes an amino acid is called a codon, the length that codes a protein is called a **gene**. So a gene is a long line of codons (often running into thousands) in a particular order, which carries the information to produce essential proteins (some genes encode RNA molecules, see later). According to the Human Genome Project that has been mapping the genes, there are between 30 and 40,000 genes making up the human **genetic code**.

Each chromosome is made up of a string of genes. Some chromosomes have less than a hundred and others have over 2000 genes. For example, the small Y chromosome that programmes the new baby to be a male, only has 78 genes. As was noted earlier, Chromosome 21 has 329 genes which carry over 40 million bits of code yet only 50 to 100 result in the many characteristics of Down syndrome. This is because of the millions of possible interactions between proteins as the new human being develops from the single cell and set of chromosomes. The same set of genes is always found on the same chromosome and, except very rarely, in the same sequence. This is the basic plan for the species. It can only happen because the DNA copies itself before a cell divides and makes new cells. Each new daughter cell should then receive an exact copy of the DNA sequence that was in the parent cell.

RNA is a key part of the process, and offers possible ways of

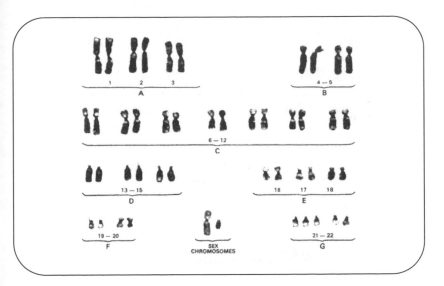

Figure 5 The chromosomes of a boy with Down syndrome. You can see the extra chromosome 21 in the G group.

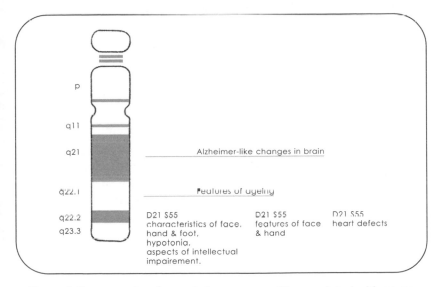

Figure 6 Genes and regions of chromosome 21 associated with some characteristics of Down syndrome

manipulating genes to prevent certain conditions. When a protein is needed the DNA ladder separates and exposes a gene. A copy of the gene is produced because of the way the bases link together. This copy is made of RNA. RNA is like DNA, except the sugar is ribose instead of deoxyribose, and the thiamine base (T) is replaced by Uracil (U). There are different types of RNA. One carries the information from the DNA and is called messenger RNA (mRNA). The mRNA molecules pass out of the nucleus into the cytoplasm where they travel to the protein-making factories, called ribosomes. Here the code is read through a series of intermediate molecules called transfer RNA. They transfer the information and assemble the amino acids that make up the protein. The amino acids are joined together in the same order and so a copy of the protein is made (Figure 7).

So far we have seen how these mechanisms try to make sure the code is kept the same. But as in all complex plans, things may not go as planned.

Genetic errors and possible treatments

When the DNA is replicating itself, hundreds of thousands of nucleotides are being added every second. Occasionally, the wrong base gets added into a sequence. The new DNA is therefore slightly different. This is called a mutation. Sometimes people think of Down syndrome as a mutation. But this is incorrect and misleading, as we will see in later sections. Mutations often arise by chance or through environmental factors such a radiation. Some chemicals (called mutagens) can cause faults in the cell's DNA. For example, cigarette smoke contains carcinogens (a mutagen) that cause the production of cancerous cells. Most mutations are harmless, like producing a few extra freckles. Some may be helpful and if they increase the chances of survival are more likely to survive and be passed on. If it seriously disrupts life, it will disappear when that person dies. Such mutations or upsets in the coding can start complex chain reactions by altering the amino acid, which changes the protein.

Some inherited genetic conditions may have started like this. Cystic fibrosis is an inherited condition that is well understood. It

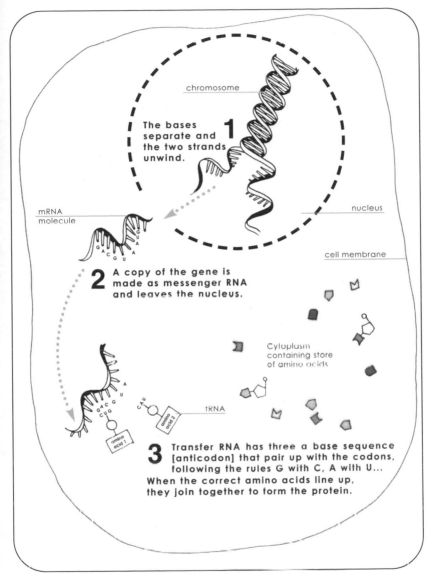

Figure 7 DNA replication

occurs because of a fault in one gene (discovered in 1989) that programs one protein and results in the production of a lot of thick
sticky mucus in the lungs. This illustrates that it is not just a matter
of how many extra genes are involved; it is how lack of a protein or
some extra protein interacts in the development and functioning of
the human being. Treatment for cystic fibrosis is a good example of
one type of gene therapy. The idea is to replace the faulty gene in
the hope of treating the condition. If a normal copy of the gene
could be inserted into the cells lining the air passages of the lungs,
it might direct the cells to make the normal protein that is missing.
Studies are being done where people with Cystic Fibrosis have been
asked to inhale either fat droplets or modified viruses containing
normal copies of the Cystic Fibrosis gene. These studies are at an
early stage – obvious problems are obtaining an adequate uptake of
the CF gene into the cells, and avoiding any side effects such as the
body's immune system reacting to a foreign virus. Even if these
problems are overcome, the question remains as to how often the
treatment would need to be repeated or whether there is any way
of permanently producing cells that contain the normal gene.

Similar ideas are being shared about potential gene replacement
with aspects of Down syndrome. But of course, in Down syndrome
we are dealing with more than one gene.

Genes that give rise to an over-expression of their protein have
been identified in people with Down sydnrome. Many others are
known, but not yet named and their function is unknown. One
example is a gene in bands q21.1–22.3 that encodes a protein (an
enzyme) called **superoxide dismutase**. This enzyme is about 50%
more active in people with Down syndrome. Its' job is to collect
toxic complex oxygen molecules that are a by-product of cell activity and turn them into hydrogen peroxide. This is also toxic but can
be acted upon by another enzyme, glutathione peroxidase to reduce
toxicity. Recent studies of people with Down syndrome have
found that the *extra* superoxide dismutase was not accompanied by
extra glutathione peroxidase. This in-balance means the extra hydrogen peroxide is not taken out, and being toxic, can cause damage.
Some of the studies found the in-balance in the brains of foetuses
with Down syndrome. So the damage may begin from the earliest
days of life. In later life extra hydrogen peroxide is associated with
premature ageing, another characteristic of Down syndrome.

In this case there is an over-expression of genetic material causing too much superoxide dismutase. One way to prevent this is to try to block the messenger RNA that tells the cell to make too much. As we saw in the earlier section this is a complex task working within the cell. **As yet it is all still more theoretical than practical.**

Another way is to try detoxification through diet and medication. This would not reduce the problem during pregnancy but might have an effect shortly after birth and reduce the damage caused to the growing brain, or later problems that are associated with some aspects of premature ageing (but see Chapter 11 on treatments)

How realistic is gene therapy in treating Down syndrome?

It was this question that prompted me to include a lot of the detail above. I hope it has shown that changing faulty genes through gene manipulation or genetic engineering is more common in fiction than in practice. Much of the current exploratory work in Down syndrome is on mice that have trisomic cells. But it is a long way from mice to people; and cancer research studies have found that what works in animals seldom transfers into humans. Also, it is a long process from the codons to the structure and function of cells and then body systems. Most of the characteristics of Down syndrome are not controlled by a single gene but by complex interactions between sets of genes. It will take a lot of time to understand these processes.

We also need far more detailed knowledge about the characteristics that are specific and unique to Down syndrome (phenotype) before the match can be made to the gene base (genotype). One way this is done is by comparing children and adults with different types of chromosomal errors or syndromes. There is a lot of current research in this area, but more is needed with the help of individuals with Down syndrome and their families. It is hoped that by discovering how and why people with Down syndrome are different from people with other conditions, a better understanding should emerge about how the genes work. This may lead to new ideas on how to prevent unwanted outcomes.

Variability – we are the same but we are all different

Before we leave this section on genes I think it worthwhile to talk about one more important function. Our individual genetic code allows for plenty of variation and is *unique* to each person – it is a particular combination of the chromosomes of the mother and the chromosomes of the father. That is why there are differences between races, families and individuals within a family. Identical replication would only come from a cloning procedure of one set of chromosomes. Some characteristics only appear in a limited number of forms e.g. blood group, eye colour, the ability to roll your tongue, or the shape of your earlobe (either fixed or free). This variation is called 'discontinuous' and only involves a few genes; a single gene is responsible for your ear lobes, or whether you have a straight or bent little finger, or hair on the second segment of your little finger. The other type of variation is called 'continuous' because there is a range of differences, such as in height, weight and intelligence. These characteristics involve many genes from different chromosomes; some are more dominant than others and have more influence. This allows for the range of variation in height – some races are taller than others and some families tend to be taller than other families. Within these races and families, you can get shorter and taller people depending on the genetic combinations. As we will see later, people with Down syndrome tend to be shorter than others in their family and race, but there is a wide range (Chapter 7).

I have often heard both parents and professionals note with surprise that the child with Down syndrome looks like his brothers or sisters or mother or father, yet take the resemblance for granted in other family members. This suggests that they have not fully understood the genetic basis of the condition, and are still thinking of the child as strange or even alien! Children with Down syndrome inherit their family's genetic code (but a bit extra of chromosome 21); they are of that family and so the likelihood of being like the family must be very high.

Well over 120 characteristics have been associated with Down syndrome (Chapter 7). Some involve discontinuous variations and others continuous variations and, as noted above, highlights the problems of finding solutions through genetic manipulations.

What we have with Down syndrome, are people who have some extra genetic material that makes them similar to each other and somewhat different to the typical 'model'. But they are still unique and **there is as much variation between people with Down syndrome as between people without Down syndrome.** To think of them as all being the same and, therefore, all needing the same treatment is to misunderstand the very basis of the make up of human beings.

What caused the extra chromosome? How and why did it happen to us?

So far we have seen how complex the mechanisms are to ensure that human beings turn out as human beings. We have also seen that small changes in the coding can have major effects, and that Down syndrome results from an extra chromosome 21, or more accurately, genetic material coded on 21.22q.1 to 22.3, with many modifications to the basic plan. One of the first questions parents ask is why it happened to them.

In order to answer the question of why it happened we need to understand how cells make new cells.

Cell division

Throughout life our cells are dying off and being replaced by new ones, by dividing into two – this is called **mitosis.** The long strands of DNA form into the 46 chromosomes, which then duplicate themselves as described above. The chromosomes line up along the centre of the cell where they are attached by their centromeres to a spindle consisting of a series of fibres. Each of the 46 duplicated chromosomes then divide into two and each of the two new sets of 46 chromosomes are drawn to opposite poles of the cell by the spindle fibres. The cell then divides making two identical copies of the original cell, each with 46 chromosomes (Figure 8).

This is fine for replacing cells in our bodies, but there is a logistical problem to start off a new human being. Human cells need 46 chromosomes, and to ensure uniqueness, half must come from the mother and half from the father. The first cell is made from the

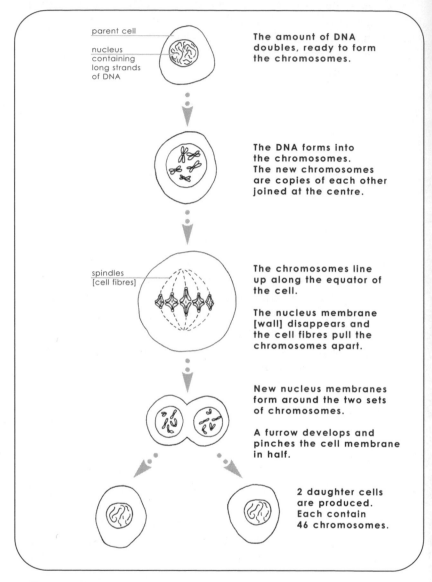

Figure 8 Ordinary cell devision – MITOSIS

fusion of an egg and a sperm which each contain 23 chromosomes (one each of chromosomes 1–22 plus an X or Y). Thus the 46 chromosomes represent 22 matched pairs – identical chromosomes both carrying the same genes (known as homologous pairs), plus the two sex chromosomes (an X chromosome from the mother and an X or Y chromosome from the father). The matching means they carry the same information such as a coded sequence for eye colour, but one of the pair comes from the father and the other from the mother.

To ensure that we all have 46 chromosomes, a special type of cell division is required in the testes and ovaries to produce sperm and egg cells that only contain 23 chromosomes. This reduction type of cell division is called **meiosis**. As we will see, it is problems in getting this reduction that leads to trisomy 21 and Down syndrome.

Meiosis actually involves two divisions, shown in Figure 9. In the first division known as meiosis I, the chromosomes first duplicate themselves, and then each member of the homologous pair goes to opposite poles of the cell. This means that when the cell divides each daughter cell contains 23 chromosomes (one of each pair). The second division, called meiosis II, is like mitosis with each of the duplicated chromosomes dividing and going to opposite poles. There are a number of differences between meiosis in the male and female. In the male, each cell entering meiosis results in four cells, each containing 23 chromosomes that go on to develop into mature sperm. In the female only one of the products becomes a mature egg, and the others (known as polar bodies) degenerate and are lost.

During meiosis I, another important event takes place known as **crossing-over or recombination.** Each chromosome pairs with its partner and they swap material, separating again before each one migrates to the opposite pole from its partner. This exchange of genetic material is very important as it creates the unique new person with genetic material from both mother and father. The joining points where the chromosome pairs are held together and then break in order to exchange material are called **chiasmata.** I shall return to these below as there is some evidence to suggest that the pattern of chiasmata at meiosis I, may have a role in the cause of Down syndrome.

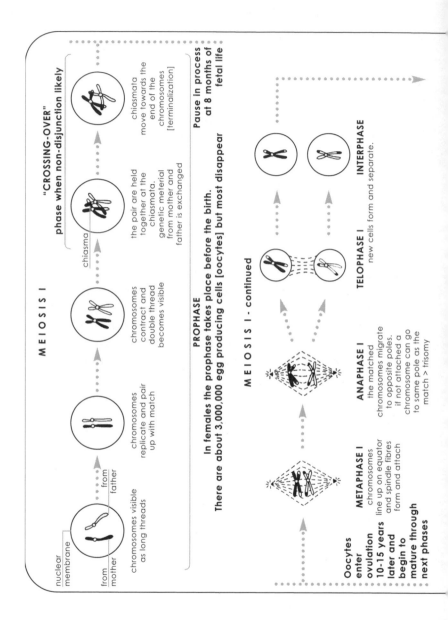

MEIOSIS I

nuclear membrane

from mother

chromosomes visible as long threads

from father

chromosomes replicate and pair up with match

chromosomes contract and double thread becomes visible

"CROSSING-OVER"
phase when non-disjunction likely

chiasma

the pair are held together at the chiasmata. genetic material from mother and father is exchanged

chiasmata move towards the end of the chromosomes [terminalization]

Pause in process at 8 months of fetal life

PROPHASE
In females the prophase takes place before the birth.
There are about 3,000,000 egg producing cells [oocytes] but most disappear

MEIOSIS I - continued

Oocytes enter ovulation 10-15 years later and begin to mature through next phases

METAPHASE I
chromosomes line up on equator and spindle fibres form and attach

ANAPHASE I
the matched chromosomes migrate to opposite poles. if not attached a chromosome can go to same pole as the match > trisomy

TELOPHASE I
new cells form and separate.

INTERPHASE

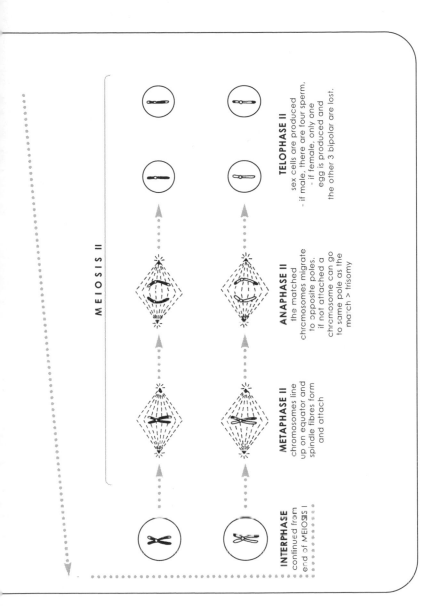

Figure 9 Reduction division – MEIOSIS (illustrated with 1 pair of chromosomes – 1 from mother, 1 from father)

How does the extra chromosome get into the cell?

Non-disjunction
The extra chromosome material gets into the cell because of the failure of chromosome 21 to separate during the division. This failure of separation is called **non-disjunction** (failure to disjoin). It varies somewhat between the different types of Down syndrome.

Free trisomy 21
In free trisomy 21 the extra chromosme 21 is lying free in the cell so that the cell has 47 chromosomes instead of 46 (Figure 10). In this case, the egg or the sperm must contain two copies of chromosome 21 instead of one. This error could arise at meiosis I. One possibility is that after forming chiasmata, the two copies of chromosome 21 fail to separate in time and so move together to the same pole, instead of going to opposite poles. Another possibility is that the two copies of chromosome 21 may not pair together at all, or they may separate too soon. They are not then controlled by the process that directs each of them to their respective opposite poles and may both make their way to the same pole.

There is some evidence for this latter process. All of the trisomies studied to date have shown a reduction in the numbers of chiasmata. Studies of trisomy 21 and 16 suggest that where the chiasmata only occur near to the tips of the chromosomes (distal-only exchanges), the likelihood of non-disjunction at meiosis I is increased. This could happen if the chiasmata near the tips of chromosomes are less stable. If released before the spindle attachment, the chromosome pair would just move about randomly.

So far, all these errors happen during meiosis 1 when the immature eggs are being formed in the foetus of the would-be mother. As we will see later, this is critical if we ask about any environmental factors that may have been the cause. We would have to find out what happened to the grandparent when she was expecting the mother. Some errors also occur at meiosis II; that is, after puberty when the eggs ripen and the menstrual cycle starts. Environmental factors could come into play.

Recent evidence indicates that some of these cases might originate during meiosis I. Studies have shown an increased number of exchanges (chiasmata) occurring near the centromere in people

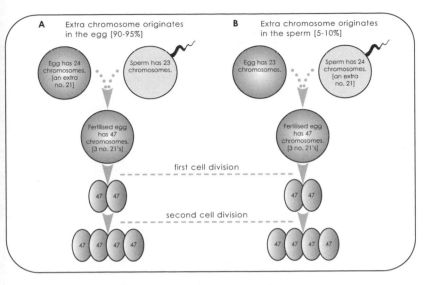

Figure 10 Faulty distribution of chromosome 21 leading to free trisomy 21

with Down syndrome where there has been meiosis II non-disjunction. These types of exchanges may somehow predispose the centromeric regions to separate prematurely at meiosis II. They would then move randomly, rather than being directed to opposite poles of the dividing cell. If, as this suggests, the non-disjunction causing free trisomy 21 is a two-stage process; it could explain why older mothers have more trisomic pregnancies (Chapter 5). What could be happening is that the chromosomes become susceptible to non-disjunction during the pairing process and chiasma formation in meiosis 1, but the actual disruption leading to non-disjunction occurs later. Advanced maternal age would not affect the frequency and distribution of chiasmata, but the ability of the compromised exchange to ensure a proper distribution of chromosomes to each pole.

The third occasion when non-disjunction might occur is after the fertilised egg has formed. In this case, the non-disjunction occurs during a mitotic division, either when the fertilised egg makes its first cell division, or later. The result would be a daughter cell with 47 chromosomes and one with 45 chromosomes. A

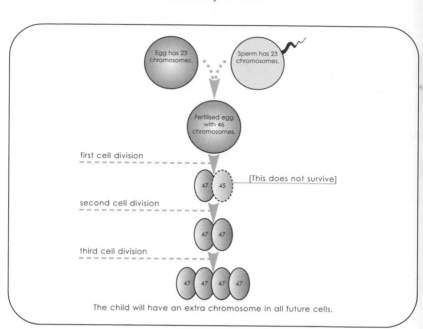

first cell division

second cell division

third cell division

[This does not survive]

The child will have an extra chromosome in all future cells.

Figure 11 Extra chromosome arises in the first division of the egg leading to free trisomy 21

cell with 45 chromosomes rarely survives for long because it does not have sufficient codes to plan a new being (Figure 11).

Mosaicism
If the non-disjunction comes after the fist division then a cell-line with 47 chromosome and one with 46 chromosomes will be produced. This develops into a mix of trisomic cells with 47 chromosomes, and cells with the typical 46 chromosomes. As noted earlier, a large variety of mixes can occur depending on when the non-disjunction occurs (Figure 12).

Translocation trisomy 21
The short or top arms of chromosomes 13, 14, 15, 21 and 22 (known as the acrocentric chromosomes) contain inactive genetic material or genes for which there are multiple copies. They can be lost without affecting the master plan. If the short arms of two

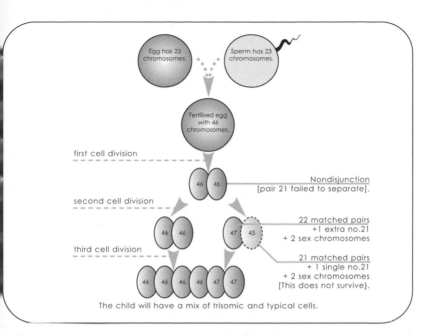

The child will have a mix of trisomic and typical cells.

Figure 12 Faulty chromosome distribution leading to mosaic trisomy 21. Found in 2–5% of all cases of Down syndrome.

acrocentric chromosomes break off during meiosis I, the remaining 'free' long arms can then attach themselves to each other. This is a translocation. If this happens to chromosome 21, the free long arm most commonly attaches to one of the D group chromosomes – 13, 14 or 15, most commonly 14. Less often it attaches to chromosome 22 or to the other chromosome 21.

Let us consider what might happen if a 14:21 translocation chromosome is formed during the first part of meiosis I in egg production. Normally as the chromosomes line up, the two number 14's will be opposite each other (paired) as will the two number 21's, ready to migrate to opposite poles when they separate. But if a 14:21 translocation has formed, the free copy of chromosome 14 will pair with the chromosome 14 section of the translocation chromosome. Similarly, the free chromosome 21 will pair with the chromosome 21 portion of the translocation. As the chromosomes separate, the free 14 and the free 21 might migrate to the same pole resulting in a daughter cell with one copy of each chromosome – a normal situation. In the same way, the translocation chromosome could migrate to the opposite pole. This would produce a cell with one copy of chromosome 14 and one copy of chromosome 21. Again, this would be functionally normal even though the two chromosomes are joined together. Under these circumstances, if this cell matures into an egg that is then fertilised, the resulting baby will have the equivalent of two copies of chromosome 14 (one free 14 from the sperm plus the copy of chromosome 14 as part of the translocation from the egg); and two copies of chromosome 21 (one free 21 from the sperm plus the copy of chromosome 21 as part of the translocation from the egg). The baby is said to carry a **balanced translocation**. He or she is healthy but is at risk of having a child with Down syndrome when they go on to reproduce (Chapter 5).

Alternatively, because of the unusual arrangement of the chromosomes produced by the translocation, it is possible that when they separate, the free copy of chromosome 21 and the translocation chromosome might migrate to the same pole. If this cell results in an egg, this egg will contain the equivalent of two copies of chromosome 21; if it is fertilised it will result in a baby with the equivalent of three copies of chromosome 21. This is termed an **unbalanced translocation** and the baby would have the translocation form of Down syndrome.

To sum up: the extra chromosome 21 material is the result of failure of separation (non-disjunction) during cell division. Mostly it occurs during meisosis 1 and this is important when asking what might have caused the non-disjunction. Some chromosomes are more likely to fail to separate and this may be because of the unstable chiasma (joining point). In a small number of cases the parent will be a carrier of a translocated trisomy 21, and so the child has inherited the condition. In Chapter 5 we look at what may have caused the non-disjunction and risks of conceiving a baby with trisomy.

How many babies with Down syndrome are there?

Many new parents of a baby with Down syndrome feel that they are the only ones it has happened to, as well as the 'why me or us?'

question. This is definitely not the case. I hope to show that the number of conceptions with too few or too many chromosomes (called aneuploidy) is so common, that we all have a high chance it could happen to us.

DIAGNOSING DOWN SYNDROME

Before chromosomal diagnosis, a diagnosis of Down syndrome was based on certain physical features, and called a clinical diagnosis – Chapter 7. There is little information on the accuracy of clinical diagnosis, but approximately 9 out of 10 babies with Down syndrome are recognised at birth or within hours of the birth. Clinical diagnosis may give a higher incidence figure. A recent study in England reported that as many as 30% of samples sent for chromosomal checking proved not to be trisomic. It is possible that as genetic testing has become routine and doctors are using it more frequently, even when they have a small suspicion about the baby. This may add to the delay that a number of parents experience between the birth of their baby and being told the diagnosis. Occasionally the diagnosis is not made for months or, exceptionally years, after the birth. These exceptions include all types of Down syndrome, not just people with mosaicism.

The Incidence of Down syndrome births

(Incidence is the total number of a particular condition per total number of births during a given period of time and in a given place).

For many years the incidence of babies born with Down syndrome was found to be between 1 in 600 to 1 in 700, although studies in different countries ranged from 1 in 500 to 1 in 1000. During the 1990's in most developed countries, the most quoted rate was around 1 in 1000. As we will see later, many factors can affect these incidence figures.

Births of babies with a trisomy

Down syndrome is a trisomy and around 1 in 300 babies born have a trisomy. Usually of chromosome 21 (Down syndrome), chromosome 18 (Edward syndrome) or chromosome 13 (Patau syndrome) – all named after the person who originally identified them; or a trisomy of the sex chromosomes (e.g. XXX, XXY, XYY). Each of these syndromes have their own set of distinctive characteristics because the extra genetic material comes from different chromosomes and so has different codes. For example, babies with Down syndrome are characteristically floppy whereas those with Patau syndrome are the opposite.

Pregnancies with a chromosome error

Down syndrome is an aneuploidy (too many or too few chromosomes). There are many types of aneuploidy following human conception, and the one resulting in Down syndrome may not be the most frequent. Current estimates indicate that over 5% or 1 in 20 of all clinically recognised human pregnancies involve a chromosomal error. Such estimates are difficult, and 5% is likely to be an underestimate because it is based on conceptions that do not survive (spontaneously abort), stillbirths and live births. Many conceptions are lost in the first 6–8 weeks of life, and before the pregnancy is clinically recognised. A more accurate estimate of how common such conceptions are is obtained from studies of chromosomes in samples of eggs and sperm. These indicate that as many as 20%, or 1 in 5 pregnancies may have a missing or an extra chromosome.

Between 6–8 and 20–28 weeks, an estimated 15 to 20% of pregnancies will spontaneously abort. Overall, spontaneous abortions are estimated at around 35% of pregnancies. Trisomic pregnancies are more likely to spontaneously abort, which may be why some reports suggest that couples with frequent miscarriages may have a slightly higher risk of having a child with Down syndrome. Around 1% to 4% of babies are stillborn.

As described in the earlier section some chromosomes are more susceptible to non-disjunction, and so result in a clinically recognised trisomic pregnancy. Half of these pregnancies are made up trisomies of Chromosomes 16, 21 and 22. The pregnancies with less extra chromosome material are more likely to survive.

Presumably there is less to disrupt the master plan. This is probably why Down syndrome, which originates from one of the smallest chromosomes, is the commonest trisomy to survive. For example, trisomy 16 appears to be the most common as it makes up around 7–8% of all spontaneous abortions, but it is never seen among live-born babies.

I find this information useful when I meet people who suggest that producing a child with a chromosomal error could not happen to them, or that 'nature' failed to eliminate the child before it was born. Most of us carry the potential for chromosomal errors, and the babies that make it through this system are viable and survivors.

Factors influencing the number of babies born with Down syndrome

Social, economic and health factors
The incidence of live births is influenced by social and health factors that support pregnant women, so different countries can report different numbers of birth. The numbers also depend on making and recording the diagnosis.

Family Planning
The greatest influence on the incidence of Down syndrome has been family planning. This is because trisomic conceptions and births are related to the age of the parents (Chapter 5). As the contraceptive pill became widely used, women had smaller families, and fewer babies were born to older women. In the 1960's, the average age of a mother of a baby with Down syndrome in England was about 36 years. By the mid –1970's the age had dropped to around 30 years and the number of births reduced. The incidence figures reported were between 1 in 800 to 1 in 1000. It remained around 1 in 550 in Ireland, where contraception was difficult to obtain. In the 1980's many women in developed countries began to delay starting a family. In Switzerland, the mean maternal age rose from

28 to 30 between 1980 and 1996, and the incidence of babies with Down syndrome increased. The same trend was reported in several large studies in other countries (e.g. North of England, New York, Norway, Hawaii). Recent studies found rates of Down syndrome pregnancies falling between 1.35 to 1.52 in 1000 births.

Prenatal Diagnosis

Prenatal tests can detect Down syndrome during pregnancy (Chapter 6). The first tests (Amniocentesis) started in the early 1970's. Little change in incidence rates occurred because it was only available to older mothers (initially over 38 years) and to those who had had a child or close relative with Down syndrome, and over half the births of babies with Down syndrome are to mothers younger than this. In the 1980's, blood screening tests and improved ultrasound scanning started to be used. The incidence figures stayed much the same because the reduction in births due to termination was partly balanced by the trend for mothers to start their family later. For example, a large North of England study found no reduction in the rates of live births of babies with Down syndrome between 1985 and 1999, although the rate of terminations of Down syndrome pregnancies rose from 15 to 38%, with the majority to women over 35 years of age.

The number of Down syndrome pregnancies and the number of births has been moving apart since the late 1980's. This is due to more accurate tests and a wider use of tests by mothers who are at low risk.

When such factors are taken into account, **very similar rates of incidence of trisomic pregnancies and births have been reported across all races, countries, cultures, and for the richest or poorest parents.**

Summary

1   Down syndrome is a *trisomy* caused by extra genetic material from the long arm of chromosome 21. With any human being, chromosomes come from the child's mother and father and so there will be many family characteristics. Down syndrome is not caused by an 'alien'

chromosome or a 'throwback' to a more primitive evolutionary stage; neither is it a disease that you can catch or give to other people.

2 Down syndrome is one of several trisomies and they are found in all races of people from all countries and social and economic conditions. About 1 in 300 babies are born with a trisomy, however as many as 1 in 5 conceptions are estimated to have a chromosomal 'fault'. Currently about 1 in 1000 babies are born with Down syndrome in developed countries. We all have a high chance of producing sperm or eggs with a chromosomal fault. Many do not survive the pregnancy, but those that do are viable human beings.

3 Trisomy 21, which results in Down syndrome, is caused by a non-disjunction during cell division. This happens most often during meisosis 1 cell division in the mother and so rules out many of the past explanations of causes from environmental factors. We do not actually know what causes chromosome non-disjunction (Chapter 5)

4 Research has started to trace the links between the characteristics of Down syndrome – such as distinctive facial and head features, ageing, heart problems and intelligence – and specific genes. Because genes program proteins, many current studies are investigating the patterns of protein in Down syndrome. With over 50,000 all interacting in a complex way, it is a long job.

5 Although the possibilities of genetic manipulations and treatments are becoming clearer, the actual possibilities in Down syndrome is more fiction than fact at the present time.

6 Pre-natcl testing and termination is beginning to reduce incidence in many countries.

Risks and prevalence of Down syndrome

- What factors increase the risk of having a baby with Down syndrome?
- What are the chances of having another baby with Down syndrome?
- How many people have Down syndrome?

What factors increase the risk of having a baby with Down syndrome?

When I first began working with people with Down syndrome it was generally believed that the extra chromosome came from the mother. This often put pressure on those mothers caught in a 'who to blame' situation. Advances in genetic research then showed that the nondisjunction, which produces the extra chromosome (Chapter 4), could also happen in the production of sperm. I have strong recollections of the difficulties that some very supportive fathers got into when they realised they may have contributed the extra chromosome. This is part of the 'shame and blame' mentality that arises in a society that does not value people with differences, and then extends this judgement to others who are associated with such difference. In turn, this promotes feelings of guilt. This is less likely when causes and risk factors are understood.

Uncertainty can be stressful, and parents often need to find a cause for their child's Down syndrome. When we give something a name, or understand the cause, feelings of uncertainty are reduced – as long as we believe the explanation. This is one reason why there are so many theories and beliefs about the causes of Down syndrome, often despite scientific evidence to the contrary.

Before describing the actual factors for which there is good evidence, I will briefly outline more recent speculations and theories that have failed to be supported. Hopefully this, together with the section in the last chapter, will help you to put any speculations of your own into some factual framework.

Environmental factors

There are many reports of possible associations between chromosomal errors and environmental exposure such as radiation and X-rays, pesticides, heavy metals, toxic waste, electromagnetic fields and anaesthetics. All have been investigated to varying degrees but none have been substantiated.

Contraceptives, hormones and fertility drugs

The contraceptive pill, spermicides and fertility drugs have all been suggested as risk factors for Down syndrome. For example, some studies showed a possible rise in the incidence of Down syndrome in younger mothers and suggested that the pill upset the hormonal balance and so the first eggs produced after the women came off the pill had a greater likelihood of chromosomal errors. Hormonal inbalance, in one form or another and particularly thyroid problems, has been suggested as a risk factor for over 100 years. But despite several studies no evidence has yet found a link.

Seasonality

Another observation is that more infants with Down syndrome are born in some seasons than in others and that the pattern of births is different to that found for all births. This has produced many speculations as to why, but again no solid evidence has shown hat conceiving a child at certain times of the year increases the risk of Down syndrome.

DOWN SYNDROME 'CLUSTERS'

Occasionally, 'clusters' of babies with Down syndrome are found. In the late 1970's I met a group of six mothers from Salisbury, Rhodesia (now Zimbabwe), whose babies, all under a year old, had Down syndrome. They speculated that the stress caused by the uncertainties at the time they were seeking Independence from the UK might have caused the births. A well-documented case occurred in Ireland. Six babies with Down syndrome were born between 1963 and 1972 to mothers who had been teenagers together when radioactive fallout from a fire at a nuclear power station might have reached them. Subsequent studies on radiation and Down syndrome failed to prove a connection. Similar ideas emerged in Europe following the release of toxic radiation from the Chernobyl nuclear accident in 1986. But no increase in Down syndrome births was found in affected areas. Nor have more Down syndrome births been found in survivors of the Japanese atomic bomb. Down syndrome is quite common in all parts of the world, and because people live in dense populations, small clusters of births will occur by chance.

Smoking, alcohol, drugs and fluoride

Recent speculations about smoking, alcohol, caffeine, and drugs reflect the moral explanations of the past (Chapter 4). While these activities certainly affect the healthy development of the foetus, they have nothing to do with causing the trisomy. Speculations often arise with new developments. For example, several reports have suggested increased rates of Down syndrome births in areas where fluoride is added to drinking water to prevent dental problems in children. Of the five studies that investigated this recently, only one found a possible increase, and all the studies had major design problems.

Related parents and health problems

If parents are related, cousins for example, then their children are at risk for many disorders. But Down syndrome is not one of them. Health problems are often thought to be a risk factor. The main ones have been the presence of thyroid antibodies in the mother's blood, illness such as hepatitis or even influenza. Again, studies have failed to find supportive evidence. Confusion can occur with some of the characteristics of Down syndrome. For example, a recent study from Egypt, suggested an increased risk of cardiac problems in the children with Down syndrome, if the parents were related, if the mothers had used oral contraception, had diabetes or used antibiotics during pregnancy. But this about the risk of cardiac problems in Down syndrome, not about what caused the nondisjunction and extra chromosomal material.

Folate metabolism

A more promising recent idea comes from observations in some studies, of an increased frequency of neural tube defect in Down syndrome pregnancies. These mothers may have genetic errors that cause problems with folate metabolism. The suggestion is that folate (folic acid) is required for adding methyl groups to DNA. If DNA is 'unmethylated', this might result in less stable chromosomes and the process of separation describe in the last chapter. Giving folic acid supplements has reduced the risks of neural tube defects, but as yet there is no strong evidence for the link in Down syndrome, or to my knowledge at this time, any clinical trials to test the idea.

Father's Age

Over the last twenty years, some studies have reported that older fathers were more likely to have a child with Down syndrome. Other studies have failed to find a link, and many people dispute the possibility. Recently, two quite large studies (one from Norway and another from the USA) suggest a possible association but it is very weak. Therefore, even if paternal age is a factor it is probably not very important.

A different approach is to investigate the sperm of older men, not just their age. Trisomy of the sex chromosomes has been reported as more frequent in older men, but as far as I can ascertain, no studies have revealed that older men are more likely to generate sperm with an extra chromosome 21. Sperm is produced in a continual 10-week cycle. Some studies with animals have shown that the longer the sperm is kept in the body before being ejaculated, the more trisomic sperms are found. This may also be the case in men, and there may be a decrease in ejaculation with age that could explain the father-age findings.

A recent study investigated the length of time that the sperm or egg was retained in the female reproductive tract before fertilisation. No effect was found. Of course the length of time before ejaculation and the length of time from ejaculation to conception are different factors. But this study failed to find any age effects.

There is little support for the age of father theory or the speculation about the frequency of intercourse and age of sperm. This should reassure couples who use natural family planning, or who have intercourse less frequently for any reason.

Mother's age

The one undisputed factor that has been linked to trisomic births is the mother's age. Approximately 2–3% of mothers in their early twenties will have a clinically recognised pregnancy with the foetus having too many or too few chromosomes (aneuploidy). Not all survive, and this figure is based on spontaneous abortions, stillbirths and live births. The number rises to 35% for mothers in their midforties. This age effect is found in all races, cultures, geographic locations and economic circumstances, indicating that it is part of the normal ageing process. It also partly explains why older women have more miscarriages, although social circumstances and medical care affect miscarriage rates at all ages.

Table 2 shows the increasing chance of having a live born baby with Down syndrome; there is a sharp rise in risk at around 35 to 40 years. It is important to note that over half the babies who are born with Down syndrome are born to mothers under 35. Recent reports indicate that between 65 to 80% of mothers of babies with Down syndrome are under 35, and at least a quarter are under 25.

This is mainly due to fewer births to older mothers as a result of family planning and screening. Such effects are seen less in countries or cultures that do not have screening and family planning.

There are slightly more first-born babies with Down syndrome for teenage mothers than young adult mothers. It may be that these mothers have a slightly higher risk, or are translocated carriers, or have undiagnosed mosaicism (Chapter 4).

Table 2 Number of babies born with Down syndrome as mothers get older

Under 20 years	less than 1 in 2000
20–25	less than 1 in 1200
26–30	between 1 in 1000 to 900
31–33	between 1 in 700 to 600
34	1 in 450
35–36	between 1 in 350 to 300
37–8	between 1 in 250 to 200
39	1 in 150
40	1 in 100
44	1 in 40
46–47	1 in 25
49+	1 in 12

Why should older mothers have more babies with Down syndrome?

At this moment in time we do not really know. The mystery has yet to be solved, but my guess is that we should have clear idea in the next decade. For those who are interested I will outline recent developments that have captured my attention.

Firstly, recent estimates show that around 95% of births of babies with Down syndrome originate from maternal nondisjunction (this excludes translocation and mosaicism). DNA analysis has also shown that the 'mother's age' effect is only found when the trisomy originates from the mother. This negates one early explanation; namely, that with increasing age, a woman's uterus does not recognise that the foetus has a chromosomal error, and so does not spontaneously abort. If this were true, one would expect equal rates of spontaneous abortion for trisomies originating from the father.

Secondly, all the eggs that a mother will produce are present in her ovaries in an immature form when she is born. The eggs remain 'suspended' in the meiosis 1 process until puberty, and then around 500 ripen at monthly intervals up to middle age (Chapter 4). This raises the question of whether environmental factors damage the egg while it waits to ripen, or around the time of fertilisation. However, as described above, none have been found that are associated with a higher incidence of Down syndrome pregnancies. This is not surprising, because around 75% of maternal non-disjunctions occur very early in the process during meiosis I, and as described in the last chapter there is reason to believe that the non-disjunctions occurring during meiosis II may actual originate in meiosis I. It may be that during meiosis I, chromosome 21 becomes susceptible and at-risk for non-disjunction, but there is no actual non-disjunction. Then, in the later phase of cell division, factors to do with the age of the mother cause the non-disjunction. The reduced number of egg producing cells (**oocytes**) that comes with advancing age may be the important factor. A recent study of women who have fewer oocytes for other reasons, such as the surgical removal of an ovary, has reported that they may have a higher risk of having a child with Down syndrome. One theory is that if there are fewer oocytes available, the oocyte selected may be less advanced in the cell division and more likely to undergo chromosomal changes. Again more studies are needed to unravel this possibility.

Environmental factors are unlikely to answer the question of why older mothers have more babies with Down syndrome. It is thought to be due to something in the egg and the ageing process of the mother.

It is also unclear what may cause the small number of trisomies that originate in the father. Different trisomies have different rates of maternal or paternal origin. For example, trisomy 16 always arises from maternal nondisjunction whereas 50% of the sex chromosome trisomies originate from the father. Studies looking at such differences are likely to help answer this question.

Can Down syndrome be inherited?

The quick answer is only in a few cases. Less than 1 in 10 Down syndrome pregnancies have a family history related to Down syndrome. Fewer than 1 in 100 people with Down syndrome have inherited the extra genetic material from a parent, and these have the translocated type and their parent is a carrier with a 'balanced translocation' (Chapter 4). If one of the parents is found to carry a balanced translocation, they should inform close relatives so that they can be tested or seek advice from a specialist geneticist, if they wish. If a chromosome analysis has shown that the baby has trisomy 21 or mosaic trisomy 21, there is no need to check the chromosomes of the parents. These parents have a small increased risk of having another child with Down syndrome in a future pregnancy, but the risk of relatives, including siblings, having offspring with Down syndrome is the same as for the population as a whole.

As described in Chapter 4, there are several variations of translocation and each carries a different level of risk (table 3). In the case of a D/G translocation or a G/G 21–22 translocation (D and G denote the chromosome group – see Figure 2), the couple could have:

- A baby with a normal set of 46 chromosomes.
- A baby who is a balanced carrier like the parent.
- A baby with Down syndrome.
- A fertilised egg with a missing chromosome that does not survive.

Their chance of conceiving a baby with Down syndrome is one in four. Because of the non-survival of some conceptions, the chances are one in 8 to 10 of having a live born child with Down syndrome if the mother is the carrier. If father is the carrier the odds are less, around one in 50 to 100. It is suggested that fathers with translocation are more likely to have lower levels of sperm production.

If the translocation is a G/G 21–21 the extra chromosome is always present and attached and all the offspring will have trisomy 21. This is very rare. More babies with translocation are born to parents under 30 years of age (up to 9%) than to older parents (1 to 2 %). This may partly explain the slightly higher risks in teenage parents.

Two out of three babies with translocation trisomy 21 are 'de novo' – the parent did not pass on the translocation. The risk here is less than 1%, but parents should be offered prenatal diagnosis in any future pregnancy, because of the small risk of gonadal mosaicism.

In free trisomy 21, the risk is calculated using mother's age and previous trisomic pregnancies or births. There are different ways of calculating the risk, but there is little difference between them. I have used the method used by the Down Syndrome Association:

- For woman under 30 years of age, the risk of having another live-born child with Down syndrome is approximately 0.7% (1 in 150). Some couples may have had a different trisomy in another pregnancy, and it is usual to quote an overall figure of 1% (1 in 100) for any trisomy. This risk is also quoted if a trisomy has been detected in a foetus that has been lost.
- For woman over 30, the increasing risk with age is added to this 1% risk. Using this method, the total risk would be about 1.5% at 37 years of age, 2% at 40, 3% at 43, 5% at 45.

If the baby has mosaicism, then the chances of another baby with Down syndrome are less than for free trisomy 21, but accurate figures are not available, due to the small numbers.

Why should the risk be more if the mother already has a child with Down syndrome?

There is no conclusive answer to this question and it is probably a combination of factors. As discussed earlier, we do not know what causes the trisomy. It might be something in the egg or the physiological status of the ovaries. It might be about the ability to carry the fertilised egg to full-term. It could be due to some mosaicism of the testes and ovaries, although this is speculative. Whatever the reason, unless the Down syndrome results from a translocation, the added risk of having a second child with the trisomy 21 is very small.

Table 3 Risk of having a second baby with Down syndrome
(Figures based on method used by the UK Down Syndrome Association)

Couple had a previous pregnancy involving a trisomy	usually an overall risk of 1 in 100 (1%)	
Present baby has:	**Risk:**	
1 Free trisomy 21 (add age risk to 1%)		
a) mother is under 30	1 in 150	(0.7%)
b) mother is around 35–37		
c) mother is around 40	1 in 75	(1.5%)
d) mother is around 43	1 in 36	(3%)
e) mother is around 45	1 in 20	(5%)
2 Mosaicism		
accurate figures not available	small, less than 1%	
3 'de novo' translocation	about 1 in 100	
(parent not a carrier)		
4. translocation		
of D/G or G/G (g 21/22)		
a) when mother is carrier	1 in 8 to 1 in 10	
b) when father is carrier	1 in 50 to 1 in 100	
of GG 21/21 for either parent	1 in 1	

Is there a tendency for some families to have babies with Down syndrome?

Several early studies of families with a child with Down syndrome found that between 5 and 10% of the parents' close relatives also had a baby with Down syndrome. When chromosome testing became widely available, some of these were found to be translocations. Because Down syndrome is quite frequent, one would expect more than one birth in close relatives to occur by chance. As noted above, the current view is that there is no discernable increased risk for other family members if the baby has free trisomy 21 or mosaicism; the risk is the same for the population without any family history.

GENETIC COUNSELLING

If you have a baby with Down syndrome you should be offered genetic counselling. This should include an explanation of why and how it happened, and your options for future pregnancies. The relevant information is contained in this book, but you should check it is up-to-date and accurate, by discussing it with an appropriate professional. If you are older potential parents, or you have a relative with Down syndrome, your obstetrician (pregnancy and birth specialist) will usually be able to give you the information you need. If you are the parent of a child with a trisomy, your paediatrician (child health specialist) can usually provide the information. If the child has a translocation, or there is a history of pregnancies with chromosomal problems in your family, it may be advisable to seek the more specialist advice of a clinical geneticist or genetic counsellor.

How many people have Down syndrome?

The number of living people with a condition at a given time in a given place is called the **prevalence**. It depends upon births and survival.

Using 1983 prevalence figures in two regions of England, of around 4.6 persons with Down syndrome for every 10,000 in the population, Brian Stratford (see Resources) projected (with some speculation) that there were at least 26,000 individuals in the UK with Down syndrome in 1985. He then estimated that the UK population in 2021 would be just over 59 million, of whom 27,000 would have Down syndrome. Other sources suggest that by 2010 in England, the number of people with Down syndrome over 40 years of age will increase by around 70 to 75%, and those over 50 by as much as 200%! With around 450 people with Down syndrome in a million it is quite easy to see that there are many distributed around our planet at this time and will be around well into the future.

How long do people with Down syndrome live?

This may be a painful subject for parents, but most of those I know say they prefer the facts. As seen above survival and life expectancy for people with Down syndrome has greatly improved in recent years.

Life expectancy or survival age is the average number of years that specified groups of people live. Overall survival figures and life expectancy includes babies and people with Down syndrome who are very ill from birth, and who have medical complications as well as Down syndrome. If you have a thriving, energetic baby with Down syndrome, the chances of survival into their later years will be higher than these figures indicate.

Figures for survival age in Down syndrome began to appear in the early 1900's. In England in the 1920–30's, the average age was 9 years, rising to 12 years in the late 1940's. During the 1950's, the survival age in Australia rose from 10 to 18 years and to 36 years in England. This four-fold increase was due to medical advances and improvement in living conditions. Immunisation for childhood illness such as diphtheria, measles, whooping cough and tuberculosis reduced the risk of death to almost zero. Deaths of all babies in England and Wales less than one year of age dropped from 30 per 1000 to 16 per 1000 by 1974. Other developed countries had similar reductions. These reductions were also seen in the survival of young children with Down syndrome.

Recent Australian figures for children with Down syndrome born between 1980 and 1996, found that over 90% lived beyond their first year and 85% over ten years. The biggest cause of death was severe heart problems. Similar figures from the North of England found that 45% of babies had an additional health or medical problem at birth· 78% of these babies survived to one year of age compared to 96% who had no additional problems. Advances in cardiac surgery for babies have significantly increased the chances of survival for those with heart problems.

We do not know why, but girls with Down syndrome tend to have a slightly higher mortality rate than boys and, consequently a slightly shorter life expectancy, which is the opposite of typical children.

Despite this increased survival, there was a popular belief well

into the late 1960's and 70's that most babies with Down syndrome
would not live beyond their teenage years. This was often used to
argue that even if they could learn skills there was not much point.
The situation has changed dramatically, but it is still common to
hear reasonably educated people say 'they don't live long'. I read in
a Science Foundations textbook for school examinations which,
although published in 1988 is still in some libraries, that people
with Down syndrome do not normally live beyond their 30's. This
hardly prepares the citizens of tomorrow for the fact that there will
be many adults with Down syndrome in their communities who
will live well beyond middle age.

LIFE EXPECTANCY FIGURES

By the 1980's, reports in England concluded that the
expected average survival age for existing 20 year olds with
Down syndrome, would be 56 years; and for those who were
already 50 at that time, 61 years. Similar figures were reported
in Holland; 20 year olds had a 57% chance of reaching 54
years of age, a 34% chance of reaching 59 and a 7 % chance
of being alive at 64. In Denmark, an overall life expectancy of
55 years was reported, with those people living at home
surviving longer than those in large institutions. In the USA,
reports concluded that 44% of people with Down syndrome
born between 1952 and 1981 would survive to 60 years of
age and 14% to 68 years. A large study in California
estimated that most people with Down syndrome would live
to over 50 years of age if they did not have congenital heart
disease or significant health problems.

In the 1990's a further report from California examined
survival age between 1986 and 1991 for people with Down
syndrome and other forms of intellectual disability aged
between 1 and 80 years. They projected that life expectancy
for most 1 year olds with Down syndrome would be 55 years.
For the small number with profound intellectual disability
(Chapter 10), it was 42 years. Often those with high levels of
disability also have other medical and health problems and
poor mobility. Most studies reported the major cause of death

in later life was due to a lack of mobility and eating problems, resulting in respiratory infection. In children and young adults the most common cause of death is congenital heart problems followed, as in all children, by accidents.

In the 1990's cases were documented of people with Down syndrome aged 74, 75 and 86 years. Another was surviving at 78 with no significant health problems. An 83 year old woman had mosaicism in which 75% of her cells were trisomy 21. Her health had been good with no severe heart problems and only one noted serious infection. She had never lived in a large institution, where there is increased risk of infection. These are just a few examples; more and more cases are being recognised and noted in many countries.

Life expectancy in the future

What can we predict for the 21st century? The figures will differ between different geographic areas because of climate, health facilities and overall quality of life. The rise in life expectancy was slow up to the 1940 and 50's, but from then on, improvement has been rapid in most developed countries, and more so for people with Down syndrome than for the general population. This is because of the impact of immunisation, antibiotics to control respiratory problems, more children with Down syndrome being raised at home, and young adults living in community housing. My current estimation is that the life expectancy of people with Down syndrome is around 20 to 30 years less than that for the general population. The extra genetic material affects the growth 'time-table' of people with Down syndrome who have slow early growth and development, and after the age of 40, a more rapid onset of ageing and death (Chapters 7 and 10). Chromosome studies have shown a region of chromosome 21 to be associated with Alzheimer's disease (Chapter 4), which reduces life expectancy. Current advances in understanding the processes of Alzheimer's disease and ageing in all people will be of particular benefit to many people with Down syndrome. Hence, the current survival age difference between typical people and those with Down syndrome may continue to shorten.

I estimate that the average survival age of babies with Down syndrome born around 1990 to 2000, will be about 57 – 60 years. 80% to 90% can be expected to survive until 10 years, and possibly more, as treatment of congenital heart problems in infancy improves. About three quarters will live to at least 30 years of age and 25% to the late sixties and hopefully early 70's.

Summary

1   Nothing that happened at the time of conception or during pregnancy was the cause of Down syndrome. It is caused by extra genetic material that arises during cell division. At present I am only aware of one idea about preventing this non-disjunction and this concerns exploratory work on folate metabolism.

2   The only factors that have consistently been found to be related to the incidence of Down syndrome are:
    • The age of the mother – older mothers, especially after the age of 35, are more likely to have a baby with Down syndrome,
    • Problems with crossing-over of genetic material during the meiosis phase in cell division – but as yet we do not know why this happens.

3   Fewer than 1 in 10 parents who have a pregnancy diagnosed as Down syndrome, have a family history related to Down syndrome. Less than 1 in every 100 people with Down syndrome have inherited the extra genetic material from a parent.

4   More people with Down syndrome are surviving for longer. The average current life expectancy is around 55 to 60 years. 95% of new babies with no serious medical complications can be expected to survive their first year, as can 75% of those with complications. At least 25% will reach their late 60's and there are people with Down syndrome alive now who are well over 70 years of age.

5   Current estimates are that in the next ten years the number of people in England with Down syndrome who are over 50 will have increased by 200%.

Children with Down syndrome must be prepared for a long and fulfilled life. To do this we must ensure we develop and maintain the provision of high quality health care, education and leisure facilities across their life span. In the coming years there will be many adults with Down syndrome and many more living to old age. Like the rest of us they need all opportunities to lead a fulfilled life of quality.

'It is not enough for a great nation to have added new years to life, our objective must be to add life to those years'. John F Kennedy – President USA

6

Prenatal diagnosis: tests for Down syndrome during pregnancy

- Why have prenatal tests?
- What prenatal tests are available?
- Prenatal tests and terminating a pregnancy

There has been a rapid development in tests in early pregnancy for chromosomal errors; and these tests bring with them increasing issues for many parents or parents to be. Deciding whether or not to have the tests, and what to do following the results, is a very individual and often difficult decision. We all need accurate information and space to consider our choices without pressure. People who have a relative with Down syndrome, and are at high risk of having a baby with Down syndrome themselves, may benefit from seeing a genetic counsellor (Chapter 4).

There are two types of prenatal tests. 'Screening' tests give a risk figure for the likelihood of having a baby with a chromosomal condition, and 'Diagnostic' tests show if the foetus has Down syndrome. The screening tests use mother's blood and ultrasound scanning, and the diagnostic tests are chorionic villus sampling or amniocentesis. Screening tests are not intrusive and carry no risk to the foetus. Diagnostic tests are intrusive, have a risk of miscarriage and have a small chance of failing. They cannot guarantee your child will not have other conditions that were not tested for, but they can tell you if the baby has Down syndrome.

Why have prenatal tests?

Most parents of children with Down syndrome, and many without, want prenatal tests in order to know as soon as possible if they have conceived a child with Down syndrome. They want to know this:

- to put their mind at rest
- to prepare themselves and learn about Down syndrome,
- or to terminate the pregnancy

I have listened to parents describe a lack of counselling about Down syndrome when they are offered these tests. Others say how they felt pressured to have the tests on the assumption they would terminate if the results were positive. I have talked with women who were given a high-risk result from the screening test, and who then faced the decision of whether to have the more intrusive diagnostic test. It is not easy for those mothers who have had a history of miscarriages, or those who are older or do not conceive quickly.

Other mothers have told me how they decided to terminate their pregnancy and only later became aware of children with Down syndrome. Some described regrets and mixed feelings, because they had no idea how 'delightful' these children could be. Equally, some parents who were not offered the tests were extremely distressed when they had a child with Down syndrome. Some never seem to resolve the bitter feelings they felt about this.

I think it is important for people who are thinking of having a baby to demand accurate information about prenatal tests and Down syndrome, and to carefully work through the process and consequences. Partners should try to discuss it openly and accurately.

Making decisions about prenatal tests and termination

Current estimates indicate that over 90% of UK women who have tests and discover that the foetus has Down syndrome decide to terminate their pregnancy. These figures do not include women who refused, or for other reasons failed, to have the tests. Figures for other countries are difficult to find, but they will differ depending upon culture and beliefs and the efficiency of the screening programmes. There is little research about the feelings and needs of parents who decide to end the pregnancy.

Most of the parents in these estimates will have very little experience of children with Down syndrome. The 'model' of Down syndrome in their culture will largely influence their decision, as will the information provided by professionals and family at the time. There is very little research with people who have experience of children with Down syndrome and how they make decisions. I interviewed the parents in our studies and have some small studies from others.

About three quarters of mothers in our group who had recently had a baby with Down syndrome said they would not terminate. This included a number who would never terminate any pregnancy because of their beliefs. Things changed when the mothers began to think of another pregnancy; more said they would consider having tests with a view to terminating. By the time they became pregnant, very few did not have prenatal tests. Most had decided on termination on the grounds that having more than one child with Down syndrome – or a severe disability – would shift the balance within the family from having one member with a disability to being more of a 'handicapped family.' Parents with other children felt it would be unfair on them to have two siblings with Down syndrome, as well as a strain on family resources. I think for many families this is probably true, but I do know very happy families with more than one child with Down syndrome – twins or families who have fostered or adopted.

Another source of information comes from a recent study of sisters of people with Down syndrome. Over half said they would have prenatal tests, a third that they would not, and the rest were unsure. Asked if they would consider termination, just over half would not, a third would, and the rest were unsure. This was a theoretical situation, and based on what I found with the mothers, I think the closer the person gets to having the child, the more likely they are consider to termination. Factors influencing the decision include religious and moral beliefs, practical circumstances for caring for the baby, whereabouts in the family life-cycle the pregnancy occurs, views of partners and experience and understanding of Down syndrome. My impression from talking with many people over the years, is that siblings whose brother or sister with Down syndrome caused major problems for the family, were more likely to decide on tests with a view to termination.

The shift in the decision about termination as people move from a theoretical to a real situation, suggests it might be sensible not to take too strong a view of what you would do until you find yourself in the actual situation of being at high risk or having conceived a baby with Down syndrome. As described in Chapter 2, we often do not know how we will react until faced with the reality.

What prenatal tests are available?

Diagnostic tests

The only way to find out for sure if a foetus has Down syndrome – or another chromosomal condition – is to take a sample of cells and analyze the chromosomes. This is done by chorionic villus sampling or amniocentesis tests, carried out by a specialist obstetrician at an outpatients' clinic. These tests are normally offered to 'higher risk' mothers, those who have had a child with Down syndrome, those over 35–38 years of age and those who appear at high risk from a screening test.

Chorionic villus sampling (CVS)

This is also called a chorionic villus biopsy, and it is done in the first three months of pregnancy – the first trimester – ideally between eight and ten weeks. The miscarriage risk is 3 to 4% for chorionic villus sampling; but this includes a 2% risk of spontaneous abortion, which occurs anyway, this early in pregnancy.

Using an ultrasound scan as a guide, a thin, flexible tube is inserted through the cervix into the uterus, and a small sample of villi is extracted (Figure 13). The villi are small finger-like projections that attach the placenta to the wall of the womb. The cells in the sample are examined, and the chromosomes analysed. Because these cells are dividing rapidly, the sample quickly grows more cells, which are then stained and the chromosomes are counted (Chapter 4). Results can be available in a few days, although it takes longer for the most thorough investigation. Occasionally the cells do not grow, and the test has to be repeated. Because this test is done early in pregnancy, repeating the test does not usually cause problems.

Early testing and early results may mean that a termination is easier medically and psychologically, not least because women have not yet experienced many of the physical sensations of being pregnant. But losing a wanted baby is always an enormous psychological trauma, how ever and whenever it happens.

Amniocentesis

This can only be done in the second trimester, usually between 14 and 16 weeks. The miscarriage risk is less than 1%. Before the test, the woman is asked to drink plenty of water, and not to pass urine. This enables the preliminary ultrasound scan to clearly map out the position of the foetus and placenta. The woman is then asked to empty her bladder, and the lower abdomen just below the navel is numbed using a local anaesthetic. A thin needle attached to a syringe is inserted into the amniotic sac and a small amount of amniotic fluid is withdrawn, containing cells from the foetus (Figure 13). As with CVS, the cells are grown, stained and checked. However, in this case the growth is slower and the results are available about two to three weeks later. Occasionally, the fluid contains no cells or the culture fails. It may be two to three weeks before this is known. At such a late date there may be problems repeating the test and, if positive, deciding on termination. Fortunately the chances of an amniocentesis test failing are small.

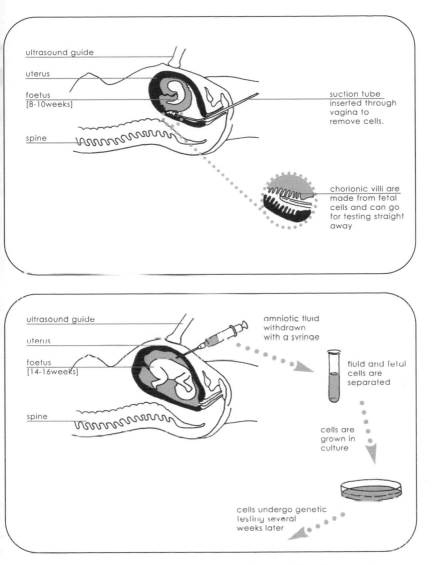

Figure 13 *(top)* Chorionic villus sampling *(bottom)* Amniocentesis

Screening Tests

Screening tests such as blood tests and ultrasound scanning, have developed rapidly in recent years. They are less intrusive than diagnostic tests, and carry no risk to the foetus. They are also cheaper and are being made available to all mothers in many countries. About 90% of mothers in developed countries such as Europe, USA, Canada and Australia choose to have an early screening test, even if they are at low risk. However, these tests only indicate the possibility of risk, and cannot detect whether or not a baby has Down syndrome.

Biochemical or blood tests – maternal serum screening
Certain bio-chemicals are more likely to be found in the blood of mothers whose foetus has Down syndrome. The risk of the foetus having Down syndrome is calculated by using the levels of chemical found in the blood, and the mother's age. This individual risk figure can then be used to decide whether or not to go for further testing. Initially, the measurement of these bio-chemicals was not reliable until after the 16th week of pregnancy, but recent advances have pushed this down to the first trimester. Other potentially useful bio-chemicals are now being identified that might be equally accurate earlier on. Current figures suggest these tests have a 69% detection rate; they miss 1 in 3 pregnancies that result in a Down syndrome birth. In 5% of cases they will say the foetus has Down syndrome when it has not. This is called a false-positive result.

Rapid improvements in screening are being made and parents should seek the most up-to-date information for their area. Attempts are being made to trace and isolate cells from the foetus in the mother's blood. It might then be possible to test the chromosomes of these cells, eliminating the need for the intrusive diagnostic tests. For parents using in-vitro fertilisation, it is possible to screen before implantation.

Ultrasound scanning
Ultrasound scanning is rapidly become more sophisticated and widely used in pregnancy screening. In most developed countries all pregnant women are screened. An ultrasound examination involves an experienced operator looking for characteristics of Down

syndrome in the foetus – specifically the shape of the head, a thickened skin fold at the back of the neck (nuchal fold), length of the thighbone and possible heart defects. It can detect about 80% of Down syndrome pregnancies. Ultrasound scanning is very time-consuming and costly, and at present, it is usually available after 12 to 14 weeks. Again, this is an area of rapid changes and parents should find out the current situation in their area. Early scans of the nuchal fold (called nuchal translucency scans) are available in some areas.

By combining maternal serum screening and ultrasound scanning, the detection rates for Down syndrome are 80 to 85% and rising. Each year more 'markers' – bio-chemicals that indicate the possibility of Down syndrome – are being detected at earlier ages. Some are found n the first 3 months of pregnancy. When combined with improved ultrasound scanning, in the hands of well-trained people, these early screening tests will soon detect around 90% of Down syndrome pregnancies.

MULTIPLE PREGNANCIES

Some multiple pregnancies, mostly twins, involve Down syndrome. Maternal serum screening tests cannot detect which foetus is affected, and ultrasound scanning is made more complicated. Amniocentesis or chorionic villus sampling can be performed but will be more complicated as every foetus has to be tested. It is possible to terminate individual foetuses leaving the other(s) to develop.

Summary

Screening tests using mother's blood and ultrasound scanning are improving rapidly and becoming available to all women in many countries. There is no risk of miscarriage.

1   In combination, they detect around 8 out 10 Down syndrome pregnancies, but sometimes show the foetus has Down syndrome when it does not.

2 Down syndrome is confirmed with diagnostic tests –
   amniocentesis or chorionic villus sampling, done by a
   specialist obstetrician in an outpatient clinic. There is a
   small risk of miscarriage.

3 The majority of women tested who find the expected
   baby has Down syndrome choose to terminate their
   pregnancy, but a sizeable minority do not, for a wide
   range of personal reasons.

4 These tests have brought difficult choices and parents
   need accurate information and time and space, without
   pressure, to come to their own decisions.

As prenatal screening and diagnosis becomes more accessible
and accurate many future parents will face the difficulties of
choosing whether to continue with a pregnancy. It is predicted
that the number of babies born with Down syndrome will
reduce, possibly quite dramatically. But having these tests
should not be conditional upon deciding to terminate the
pregnancy. Parents should be given information, counselling,
choice and support to make their own decision.

Characteristics of Down syndrome

CHAPTER 7
Physical characteristics and health

CHAPTER 8
Personality and socialisation

CHAPTER 9
Behaviour and psychological problems

CHAPTER 10
Intelligence, development and attainments

Much of this Section is about what is different in people with Down syndrome compared to 'the norm'. Remember that people with Down syndrome have far more characteristics that are typical of human beings, than of the syndrome. Most children with Down syndrome will not have every characteristic, nor will they necessarily have any of the health, medical or behaviour problems described in this section. Characteristics can change as the child grows.

Many parents have told me that they want to know all the possible physical and behavioural characteristics so they can then stop asking themselves if a particular aspect is due to the Down syndrome. They can forget about the syndrome and get on with the job of caring for and helping their baby.

7

Physical characteristics and health

- What are the main physical characteristics of Down syndrome?
- What are the main health and medical problems?
- How can they affect the child's development?
- How can we help our child with Down syndrome?

In 1866, when Dr Langdon Down first recognised Down syndrome, he identified fewer than a dozen characteristics. Since then, the number of clinical signs associated with it has multiplied at a great rate. Most textbooks suggest over 50 signs; many studies list over 80; one Polish study identified 120 clinical characteristics, another study up to 300; many concern the fine structure and biochemistry of the body.

The number of signs identified has increased with developments in medicine. For example, when X-rays became available, many differences were found in the skeletons of people with Down syndrome. As late as 1966, one study reported that about 18% of adults with the syndrome, mainly women, did not have a twelfth rib. As medical techniques advance we can certainly expect more discoveries about Down syndrome. Many of the signs are not common and are of minor importance – they do not really affect the child's growth, health or functioning. For example, fewer than one in 100 children with Down syndrome will have a webbed toe.

While this is more common than in typical children, it is still rare and has little or no effect on the child. It is neither possible nor useful to discuss all these signs here.

WHAT IS NORMAL?

I use the word normal in the statistical sense of measuring things about a population of people and plotting norms. If the population is made up of people with Down syndrome I would say, for example, the average height is 62 inches and this is normal for men with Down syndrome. There are many things that are 'abnormal' in people with Down syndrome when compared to 'normal' findings, but they may be 'normal' for people who have Down syndrome.

Physical characteristics and the newborn baby

Parents often ask how the doctor could tell their baby had Down syndrome. They have a strong need to see what the doctor sees and accept the diagnosis. Down syndrome is only present when an individual has a collection of the more common signs – that is what 'syndrome' means – plus the extra chromosome 21 material.

Common signs of Down syndrome in a baby

Many studies have identified the most common observable signs of Down syndrome; these were used to make the diagnosis before the discovery of the extra chromosome. Listed below are the major signs seen at birth, in at least 50% of young babies with Down syndrome, and usually in 60–80%.

If the baby has six to ten of these common signs, Down syndrome is almost certainly present. There are very few cases when the signs are present but the trisomy is not found in the chromosome test (Chapter 4).

- The eyes slant upward and outward – often exaggerated by a fold of skin on the inner side of the eye (the epicanthal fold). This fold is seen in 60–70% of adults with Down syndrome, and 80–90% have the upward slant of the eyes
- The eye slit is narrow and short – 30 to 70% of the babies have small white patches (called Brushfield spots) on the edge of their iris
- The face has a flat appearance – the bridge of the nose tends to be low and the cheekbones high. This makes the nose look small and stubby
- The head is usually smaller than average and the back of the head, called the occiput, tends to be flattened – giving it a round appearance
- The soft spots on the head – the fontanels – are larger than usual –occasionally there is an extra soft spot in the middle. Because the baby is growing more slowly than ordinary babies, the bones of the skull take longer to grow together
- The ears tend to be small and are usually low-set – the top of the ear may be folded over or, in just under half of the babies, the earlobe is very small or absent, which can also be a family trait
- The mouth looks smaller and the lips are thinner than usual – there is less room inside the baby's mouth, the roof of the mouth is flatter, with a high arch in the middle – called a 'cathedral' or 'steeple' palate. Because of this smaller mouth space, the tongue has less room and so tends to stick out. The mouth is often open because the jaw and tongue muscles tend to be floppy
- The baby's neck appears slightly short with loose folds of skin at the sides and back. These disappear as the child grows
- The legs and arms are often short in comparison to the length of the torso
- The baby's hands are often broad and flat and the fingers short – the little finger is often short, with a single crease; it may curve in towards the other fingers (called clinodactyly)
- About half of the children have a single crease across the palm – the simian line – on one or both hands. They may also have a crease on the sole of the foot running from the gap between the big toe and the other toes

- The feet tend to be broad and the toes rather short. Often there is a larger space than normal between the big toe and the other toes, and between the thumb and the fingers
- The baby may have poor muscle tone (*hypotonia*) and floppiness at birth – a tendency for loose-jointedness (*hyperflexibility*) adds to this feeling of floppiness
- The baby's reflexes tend to be weaker
- Two-thirds of babies have a shorter or weaker cry – many cry very little and may not cry for food or when they are uncomfortable. Parents need to check on them, rather than wait until they cry

Babies with Down syndrome tend to be born a week or two earlier than expected; their birth weight, while in the normal range, tends to be lower than average – about 6.6 pounds (3.0kg).

Parents can become worried when they 'see' physical signs of Down syndrome in their other children or themselves. But many typical children and adults will have some of the signs. For example, many newborn babies and 20% of typical Caucasian people will have a fold of skin on the inner side of the eye, and about 14% will have the slant of the eye that is characteristic of Down syndrome.

Muscle tone and floppiness

About half the babies with Down syndrome have very poor muscle tone in the first months of life, and less than five percent have good muscle tone. At 18 months to two years old, less than five percent have extremely poor muscle tone and over half have mild to normal muscle tone.

Because of poor muscle tone, the young children often have a rounded belly that sticks out for longer than normal. Many babies with Down syndrome also have a protruding navel called an umbilical hernia. Estimates of frequency range from 12 to 90 % depending on the criteria used. Only a few cases require surgery; most close by themselves as the child grows and muscle tone improves.

It is not how floppy the baby is that matters, but how quickly they improve. Very poor muscle tone at or after one year of age is associated with slow development.

WHAT YOU CAN DO TO IMPROVE YOUR BABY'S MUSCLE TONE?

Muscle tone can be improved by physical activities such as handling and playing with the baby. We found that when parents carried out physical activities to stimulate the babies' muscles and motor skills, the babies had sharper reflexes and sat up and stood up a few weeks earlier than babies with less stimulation (Chapter 11). Babies with severe heart problems usually have poorer muscle tone, as do babies who fail to thrive and who have other medical complications. Some studies have found slower development in these babies; possibly because their parents are less likely to physically stimulate the baby. It is difficult to be certain whether it is poor muscle tone or the heart problems plus less stimulation, that influences later physical development. We found plenty of handling and physical play was beneficial, and those with severe heart problems only had slower physical development.

Some characteristics change as the child grows. For example, the floppiness reduces, the inner folds of skin on the eyes becomes less obvious; the mouth changes shape as teeth appear; and many of the children are more able to keep their tongue in their mouth as the muscle tone of the jaws and tongue improve. They can also be helped to learn to control their tongue (see later).

Do more features of Down syndrome mean the baby will be more disabled?

Parents often feel that the more obvious the physical features, the worse the condition, and the greater the degree of disability. Doctors and researchers have been studying and arguing about this since the turn of the century. The answer, in terms of a baby with Down syndrome, is a definite no.

In the late 1950s and 1960s, several studies of adults with Down syndrome (mainly those living in large institutions) investigated the relationship between physical features and mental functioning. Some found a small association; some found the opposite, but most found no relationship.

Overall, no significant relationship has been found between the physical characteristics and the person's mental functioning or behaviour and personality.

When the children in our study were between 7 and 14 years, we used our own and teachers' ratings of facial features, posture and appearance. We did not find any link with measures of intellectual ability, academic attainments like reading and writing, self-help and social skills, attachment to the child by family members, or stress on parents.

Some studies of children with severe intellectual disability, including some with Down syndrome, have found the child's appearance was associated with higher stress in some mothers. Studies of adults with disabilities, find that appearance becomes more important with age and that 'unattractiveness' does affect social life and employment. But this is not a problem for the majority of children and possibly many adults with Down syndrome. My view is that the facial features of children with Down syndrome, are not unattractive to people. The widespread eyes maintain a younger look for longer; it is an open faced and non-threatening look. 'Baby' features are thought to be attractive and important to ensure that all infants are cared for. Few of the children with Down syndrome develop what might be thought of as 'ugly' features. I will return to this later when we discuss plastic surgery (Chapter 11).

Physical and medical characteristics of Down syndrome in children and adults

This section is structured around the main systems of the body but of course they interact all the time and it is necessary to discuss some issues across systems.

The Skull and Face

Many of the features of Down syndrome are due to differences in the skeleton, and show how the extra genes can have a wide affect on the structure and growth of the body.

The different growth of the skull results in egg shaped orbit holes for the eyes, giving them a slanting appearance. The nasal bone remains underdeveloped, giving the face a flat look. The bones of the jaw tend to be small, producing a small mouth and the cathedral shaped palate; although fewer than one in 200 will have a cleft palate. Often, the upper jaw is smaller than the lower jaw, which affects the bite and encourages mouth breathing. The canals in the ear, sinuses, and around the eyes can be narrow and become blocked, causing hearing, visual and breathing problems.

In a few cases the physical abnormalities result in a protruding tongue, excess dribbling and problems with breathing, speech and chewing. As the child grows and the teeth appear, there can be improvements.

The combination of larger lower jaw, small sinuses, relatively large tongue and low muscle tone causes many children to breathe through their mouths. Mouth breathing encourages the 'open-mouth, protruding-tongue' look, often associated with Down syndrome, and also causes chapped lips, inflamed corners of the lips, dry tongue and possible infection.

Speech and language therapists can advise on increasing the tone and movement of the mouth area. These techniques are worth trying as long as they are fun for parent and child. They do not work with all children with Down syndrome. The use of dental plates is being investigated (see below).

Low muscle tone also causes less sharp facial expressions. Studies, and parent's comments, have highlighted that this lack of expression can make it difficult to 'read' the emotions of these babies or

---

WHAT YOU CAN DO ABOUT MOUTH BREATHING

Try to keep the nose and sinuses clean and free. Get advice on nasal drops and nose cleaning for a baby from your doctor, health visitor or nurse; babies can build up resistance to nasal drops from continual use. As the child grows older, encourage them to use a handkerchief frequently and remind them to' keep your mouth closed', 'breathe through your nose'. Play 'push the tongue in' games with an infant, or gently push their jaw up – many times a day and for many months.

These early efforts will reduce the mouth breathing and 'tongue out' problem for quite a lot of children. This can prevent later social problems, because most people do not feel attracted to a gaping mouth or a protruding tongue.

---

children. It is important not to just rely on facial cues as we do with most people, but to learn other ways of 'reading' the child (Chapter 8). Stimulating facial muscles (e.g. tickling, face pulling games etc.) can reduce this to some extent.

Like other children, those with Down syndrome can have an extra large tongue – called **macroglossia**. Medical treatment, including surgery is used to treat this, but this is not to be confused with cosmetic surgery (Chapter 11. Some children, with and without Down syndrome, produce excess saliva and dribbling. Sometimes one salivary gland is removed, the nerves to it are cut, or the ducts are re-routed so the saliva runs down the back of the throat. Such procedures are usually successful.

The Lungs and Respiratory System

There are usually no lung abnormalities associated with Down syndrome. But the limited information we have, indicates that, up to the age of 5, the rate of severe infection is about twice as high as among typical children. **This leaves half the children with Down syndrome with no more serious infections than typical children.**

PALATAL PLATE THERAPY

A recent development is Palatal Plate Therapy. A dental plate is made for the child, which they use for several hours a day. 9 children who had the plates, and 11 similar ones who did not have them, have been followed for four years. Those who used the plates are reported as having less tongue protrusion, less open mouths, and better lip-rounding during speech. Parents said they snored less, and overall their facial expression was considered to be better. There were no differences in articulation. This is probably because problems with articulation and speech are due more to differences in the brain than in the physical aspects of the mouth. This early work needs further examination. Some children with Down syndrome may not cooperate with using dental plates and we need to ask which children need it and how early should it start, rather than make all children with Down syndrome use plates.

Some children with Down syndrome are more likely to inhale mucus or food than typical children: partly because the floppiness in their muscles makes swallowing less efficient and partly because the mechanisms which respond to inhalation, and stimulate coughing and expectoration of inhaled materials, are less responsive. Lots of handling and physical activity will help expectoration and muscle strength.

As the children get older the frequency of infection reduces; about 1 in 5 pre-school children with Down syndrome are likely to have a short stay in hospital for respiratory problems, compared to 1 in 10 teenagers. Respiratory infections can lead to pneumonia, which was a major cause of death in the past. Antibiotics have considerably reduced this risk, but those with severe heart conditions are still at higher risk.

In the middle of the last century, many infants in large institutions succumbed to Sompe syndrome – infections in the ear, sinus and lungs – probably caused by foods and fluids getting into the ears via the Eustachian tube (see 'Ears and Hearing' below), because the

---

IMMUNO-DEFICIENCY

A number of reasons have been put forward to explain this proneness to infection. The main one is immune-deficiency related to an intrinsic T-cell immune defect. T-cells are produced in the thymus gland in the upper part of the chest. Their job is to recognise foreign substances in the body and then start a response. B-cells produce antibodies and have a memory of the foreign protein causing the infection. If the foreign protein returns the B cells multiply very quickly to form clones of the cells that neutralise the invader. Why it fails to work well in Down syndrome is not fully understood, but it seems that the extra genetic material from chromosome 21 results in excess production of T-cells. In turn this reduces their efficiency in dealing with infections.

---

babies had long periods lying on their back and being inactive, especially during feeding. Immobility and respiratory infection is still a major problem for adults with severe physical and intellectual disability who are or become immobile.

PREVENTING PROBLEMS

Apart from plenty of exercise and handling and keeping the nose clean, some medical professionals encourage tipping an infant head down, and then tapping gently on the back. Excess mucus is likely to run out. When feeding, it can help some babies if you hold them half-upright or almost upright with the head well supported and not tilted too far backwards. If there are problems swallowing, gently stroking the throat can help. Maternity nurses or the health clinic will advise on help.

We compared the children with Down syndrome in our group at 5 to 10 years of age, with a similar group whose parents did not have the type of early support and guidance we offered. We found that those in our group had less serious health problems – mainly respiratory ones – and higher attendance for hearing, visual and health checks. It is difficult to be certain, but we think that this was because parents were more knowledgeable about health problems, and were more likely to seek help and advice quickly. We also think that the early physical activities and good diet might have helped to produce a healthier life-style.

A number of claims have been made that 'jackets' which inflate and deflate to control breathing, can enhance development in Down syndrome. One theory is that they increase the amount of oxygen in the blood, which in turn helps the brain. Unless the child has cyanotic heart disease, however, there will already be a normal amount of oxygen in the blood, and it would be impossible to increase it by this means. The children in our research who had heart problems did not have slower mental development than the rest. The original claim for benefits of this treatment was based on trivial interpretations and a lack of knowledge about the development children with Down syndrome.

Upper airway obstruction and sleeping problems

Around 60% of children with Down syndrome breathe through their mouths and are restless when asleep. Between 30 to 50% may have an obstruction of the upper airway. Sucking air into the lungs becomes difficult because large tonsils, adenoids or a floppy tongue, obstruct the narrow passages behind the nose and tongue. If the child's muscle tone is poor it adds to the problem.

When the airway becomes blocked you can see the pressure as the breastbone is pulled in at each breath. When the child is asleep, and their breathing is more relaxed, difficulties can arise if they are unable to suck in as much oxygen as is needed. As the oxygen in the blood becomes low, the child will wake, often with a start. Sometimes the throat is sucked closed; if this happens for more than

10 seconds it is called **sleep apnoea.** About 12% of children with Down syndrome have apnoeic episodes. If the child has severe heart problems, there is more urgency to check that the airway is clear.

The signs of apnoea
- mouth breathing and sleeping with neck extended
- very noisy breathing, especially at night with heavy snoring
- the caving in of the lower end of the breastbone on each inhalation
- frequent waking up at night with a start
- excessive daytime sleepiness, lack of energy, and failure to thrive
- unusual sleeping positions, such as sitting up, or bent forward with head on knees

Some of these signs are also likely when the child has a cold and blocked nasal passages; it is best to monitor the situation for a few months before getting too concerned. Obstructive sleep apnoea is constant; it is associated with larger tonsils and adenoids and possibly mal-development of the upper airway structure. If you think there is a problem, talk to your medical advisor who may refer you to an Ear, Nose and Throat (ENT) specialist. Studies of adults with Down syndrome have found that sleep disturbance and apnoea is quite common and that it increases with age. It is also more likely in obese people, another reason to invest in good nutritional habits from early on and a life-style that includes regular physical exercise.

How does sleep disturbance affect children?
Studies have found that children with major sleep disturbance, including apnoea, are more likely to have behaviour problems, which can be detrimental to their learning. A recent study suggested a direct relationship with the number of apnoeic episodes and non-verbal measures of intelligence, but this needs confirmation. Sleep disturbance can put pressure on families and make it difficult to establish bedtime routines. It is worth keeping an eye on your child's breathing and sleeping from the early weeks. Treating sleep apnoea can prevent quite serious problems later on. But the condition is complex, there is no guaranteed cure and not all restlessness and sleep problems are due to airway obstruction.

What can be done about it?

To find out if the child has an obstruction, their sleep is monitored with small sensors. This is not an intrusive or uncomfortable procedure, although some children object if they become fearful. In exceptional cases it is recommended that the tonsils and adenoids be removed. Removal of tonsils and adenoids used to be more common for all children, and was often thought to help breathing, ear infections and hearing problems in those with Down syndrome. The evidence to support this is weak, and given the potential complications of an operation, it is very much a last resort.

If the tongue is the main problem, surgery is possible. Current limited information suggests that surgical treatments (e.g. adeno-tonsillectomy) are not effective. The best approach for most sleeping problems, and that preferred by parents, is behaviour management (Chapter 9). Sometimes this is used with drugs, but side effects need to be considered.

Ears and hearing

Nearly all children with Down syndrome have problems with language development and speech (Chapter 10). Much of this is due to differences in the brain, but my rather crude estimate is that about 10 to 20% is due to hearing problems – far more for those with severe hearing impairment. Even mild hearing problems can affect speech and communication, learning to read, and children's social behaviour. Mild and moderate losses can go undetected. All too often communication or behaviour problems are assumed to result from brain impairment without the person's hearing having been checked.

Between 50 and 90% of young children with Down syndrome have some type of ear problem, or hearing loss in one or both ears, especially when they have a cold. A recent Australian study found that 64% of children with Down syndrome had a hearing problem, and that 75% of these had 'glue' ear (conductive hearing loss, see later). A German study found that 56% had a hearing problem, and 88% of these had a conductive hearing loss. About a third of these involve relatively mild hearing loss, and do not appear to hinder the child's development.

Around 50 to 60% of adults with Down syndrome have hearing

problems that increase with age, as they do in many people. If adults, and older children start to fail to respond to sound, become withdrawn and quiet, or develop emotional and behavioural difficulties, their hearing must be checked.

A young boy in our study was born with severe deafness that became apparent by four or five months of age; but it took longer to convince medical practitioners to investigate it. Many parents used to complain about this before more refined methods of testing young babies' hearing were developed. Because this boy's intellectual impairment was quite mild, and his main disability was being hearing impaired, he attended a school for the deaf. He has just got a job as an assistant caretaker.

If the child has hearing problems then anyone working with them should be informed so that they can speak clearly. If they are in a group or a class the child should sit close to the speaker and be able to see them face on.

HOW WE HEAR

The ear has three parts: outer, middle and inner. The outer ear catches the sounds, which then travel down the ear canal to the eardrum. The drum separates the outer and middle ear. The middle ear is a chamber with three bones forming a bridge to the inner ear or cochlea. Sound waves pass down the ear canal and vibrate the eardrum. This vibrates the bridge and the sound wave passes into the cochlea. Here they are processed and sent to the hearing centres in the brain along the auditory nerve. The middle ear is joined to the throat by a tube called the Eustachian tube?

Types of hearing problems

There are two main types of hearing loss. People can have a mixture of the two. Both types of loss can range from mild to severe. The types of problems relate to the structure of the ear (see box above).

- **Conductive loss** is when there are difficulties conducting the sounds waves through the outer and middle ear to the inner ear.
- **Sensorineural** loss is when there are problems in the cochlea or nerves; it is usually permanent and difficult to treat.

Sensorineural hearing loss is rare in people with Down syndrome affecting about 5 in 100 young children and 15 to 20 % of adults. This later loss may be more likely if there has been continued conductive loss in childhood. A frequent explanation is that this loss reflects the earlier ageing process found in many people with Down syndrome (see later). But it has to be more complicated because the deterioration in hearing found in teenagers and young adults, especially at high frequencies, does not continue at the same rate into middle adulthood. This suggests different causes for hearing deterioration at different ages.

Conductive hearing loss is common, but it is often mild and can be treated.

It is often caused by a blockage of the smaller than normal ear canals. Studies have indicated that the bones of the middle ear are different, there is less flexibility of the eardrum, and the cochlea may be different. We can add possible differences in the nerve cells to this list and problems with the Eustachian tube, whose job it is to let air into the middle chamber and drain secretions. Dilation of the drum appears to be different in Down syndrome and affects the pressure in the middle ear needed to allow the vibrations to pass through. These differences in the tube also increase the likelihood of infections and blockage, which are more frequent with heavy colds. Large adenoids can also partially block the tube.

As many as a third of children with Down syndrome produce excessive wax which can block the outer ear canal. In extreme cases this can cause a significant loss in hearing. Wax-removing eardrops for five days in each month is often recommended but do check with your medical advisor.

Many people with Down syndrome produce thicker than the typical mucus that lines the middle ear found in most people. This mucus, plus the increased infections and blocked Eustachian tube, all result in conductive hearing loss and particularly 'glue' ear (see below). People who have a cleft palate also seem to have thicker mucus, problems with 'glue' and later sensorineural hearing loss, which suggests there may be some common genetic problem associated with Down syndrome and with cleft palate.

GLUE EAR

Glue ear or Otitis Media with effusion can be found at any age – even in the first two weeks of life. It is often a temporary problem, brought on by colds and is common in all young children who average a cold about 5 to 7 times a year. In typical children, glue ear improves with age and usually disappears by around 8 to 9 years of age, partly because the Eustachian tube grows. In Down syndrome it takes longer, possibly due to slower physical growth, or lingers on for the reasons noted above. Children who live in polluted atmospheres, for example with parents who are heavy smokers, are reported as having more hearing problems.

What can we do to prevent problems and improve hearing?

Decongestants to control chronic catarrh are often used; they are not universally successful and seem less so for children with Down syndrome. They may be worth trying, but on a 'let's see if it helps' basis. The consensus of Ear Nose and Throat specialists is not to use decongestants on a long-term basis. If hay fever or allergic symptoms are observed, treatments can usually be tried for short periods, and again need to be closely monitored for changes in the child's behaviour.

Some people think that nasal congestion can be reduced with a milk free diet, but research has failed to support this idea. Despite a lack of conclusive evidence and ongoing debate many parents testify to the benefits of extra vitamin C or vitamin supplements to reduce the frequency and level of respiratory infections. Perhaps, like most things, some people will respond to a treatment and others will not. There is no reason why children with Down syndrome should react badly to vitamins, providing they are not excessive (Chapter 11).

Antibiotics can help discover if the problem is due to an infection. Most medical practitioners are cautious about overuse of antibiotics; if the hearing problem does not improve after say a month, then the child needs to be referred to an ENT specialist.

An operation can be used to drain the middle ear; it does not normally require an overnight stay. A small hole is made in the eardrum and the fluid drains out. A tiny silicon tube, called a grommet, is put in to keep the hole open and ventilate the middle ear. There can be problems because the ear canal can be quite small. The biggest problem is that the grommets can get blocked quite easily, and they usually fall out after six to twelve months. Replacement is limited to two or three times because of the damage to the eardrum.

After the operation, some parents observe quite marked changes and improvements in the child, indicating that blockage was the main problem. Often, speech, language and behaviour improve very quickly, showing that the problem involved hearing, rather than 'something else in the brain'. Unfortunately, the improvement may only last for a few weeks, or very rarely, up to a year. Other children may not show any changes, but their hearing should be tested in case there are some small improvements. This line of treatment is being advised less often because of the poor long-term results.

Hearing aids are increasingly being used, especially for children with moderate to severe hearing loss. Some years ago these aids were so big and the ears of the children with Down syndrome so small, that it was very difficult to fit them. Fortunately, modern aids are small, light and comfortable, and most parents find that the child accepts them well.

A teacher of the hearing impaired, or similar person, should be involved, as levels have to be set and often changed as the hearing changes. Parents and teachers need to know how to observe and check the child is hearing. This is why six monthly check-ups are advised for children with hearing aids.

An advantage of aids is that they can be fitted to young children whose language and communication skills are developing. My impression, from talking with parents, is that many young children with Down syndrome benefit from hearing aids, but I have not found any studies of their use at present. The benefits for older children and adults are the same as for any of us. Methods of augmenting hearing are improving, as is our understanding of the biochemical nature of 'glue' ear. We can expect further improvements.

Signing is another way of coping with hearing problems, and signing systems have been developed for children with intellectual disability. Infants with Down syndrome can start using them from around six to 9 months onwards. Signing can compensate for hearing problems and slow language development, and they can help parents and young children to communicate (Chapter 8 – Socialisation). Good communication helps to build good social skills, reduces frustration and prevents some behaviour problems. It was thought that signing would delay speech, but this has not been found. Children are far too sensible to use signs when they can talk, because speech is so much more efficient.

LISTENING AND PREFERENCES FOR SOUND

Babies are very attracted to rhythms, which then help them pay attention to words. This is probably why nursery rhymes are found in most cultures and have a long history. We did a study in which the baby could touch either of two touch detector switches that switched on a tape recorder. If the baby touched one a lot more than the other, we gained some idea as to what he or she liked to listen to. At the developmental level of six to nine months, typical babies and babies with Down syndrome preferred to listen to speech or song, rather than musical noises, and to familiar nursery rhymes rather than the same rhymes sung backwards. This showed that by this level of development, babies were recognizing many familiar words and so beginning to comprehend language and the using the rhymes gave lots of repetition and practice.

Hearing Assessments

Early detection of hearing problems is very important to avoid developmental and behaviour problems. The child should have an objective test before the age of six months using auditory brainstem responses. Behavioural tests, where the child responds to various sounds while being distracted, should start between 7 and 14 months of age (6–8 months developmental level). Further assessments should be done yearly up to three years of age and every two years after that. As the child develops, and especially as they start to listen to words, tests become more specific. It is not just a case of observing if the child responds to noises; some hearing losses only cause problems with high or low frequency noises. For example, 'G' as in go, is low frequency and 'SS' as in snake is high frequency.

Objective tests that measure pressure in the middle ear can be done at 4 to 5 years for most children with Down syndrome.

Should the child have a specialist hearing assessment?

A child with Down syndrome may need to be seen by an ENT specialist because of their small ear canals. Some can be difficult to test because of their slower reaction times and attention problems. Ideally, a skilled paediatric audiologist should carry out the hearing assessments.

Some years ago we found that the usual hearing checks conducted in child health clinics by skilled, but not specialist nurses, often failed to detect problems in children with Down syndrome. This is not to say there are not very skilled people in these clinics, but parents should not be afraid to ask for a second opinion or a referral to a specialist. It helps if parents have monitored the child's behaviour and reactions to sound and made notes and questions before the assessment.

Eyes and vision

Appearance of the eyes

Some of the characteristics of Down syndrome affect the appearance of the eyes, but not the person's vision. These include the distinctive shape of the eye, 'Brushfield' spots (see below), the folds of skin in the corners of the eye (epicanthal folds), and the broad, flat nasal bridge mentioned at the beginning of this chapter.

A common problem in babies is the canal draining the tears to the back of the nose becoming blocked resulting in watery eyes. This usually improves as the bones of the face develop. In most cases it is not advisable to try to unblock these tear channels until the baby is 9 to 12 months old. If the channels are blocked the tears run down the face and cause chapping and dry eyelids. The dry skin flakes, bits get into the eye and the child rubs the eye.

This problem is associated with a condition called **blepharitis,** which is an irritation of the eyelashes and lid margins that gives rise to specks of skin and debris on the lashes. It happens in around 60% of people with Down syndrome, but is easily treated by keeping the eyelids clean. They can be wiped with a weak solution of salt or sodium bicarbonate, or baby shampoo. If these do not work, antibiotic ointment usually will. If the problem is persistent ask you local optometrist for advice. It is important to control blepharitis because constant rubbing of the eyes, or turned in eyelashes, can cause infections and permanent damage.

Some typical children have a slight asymmetry in the structure around the eyes, which looks like a squint – the eyes not looking in the same direction – but in fact is not a squint and does not effect their vision. This **'pseudosquint'** is more common in babies with Down syndrome, and usually disappears as the face changes. Sometimes it is due the floppiness of the eye-muscles and because it takes babies with Down syndrome longer to get their eye coordination under control. As this improves with age and experience, so the crossing disappears. Giving the baby practice in focusing on and tracking slow moving objects, from around two to three months, is thought to speed up this coordination.

Problems with vision

Around 60 to 80% of children with Down syndrome have some sort of visual problem. They don't all need glasses: about 50 to 60% of the girls and 35 to 45% of the boys have glasses. As with hearing, it is important to observe the child closely and have regular eye-checks, starting in the first year of life. Visual problems do not

correct themselves, and the consequences for later development can
be serious.

Should my child have a specialist vision assessment?

As we found for hearing, other studies report that the staff of child
development clinics, including paediatricians, miss more visual disorders in children with Down syndrome than specialist
ophthalmologists, optometrists and orthoptists (see box). These specialists have a much wider range of methods and equipment for
assessing visual problems than most child clinics.

Bring your own observations to the assessment. You may have
noticed that the baby seems to have a squint or poor eye coordination. It is helpful with older children to observe how they look at
picture books and road signs. Sitting close to the television may be
a sign of a visual problem, but many children with Down syndrome
without visual problems seem to do this. I think it helps them shut
out distractions and get closer to the action – or they may have a
hearing problem.

WHO ARE THE SPECIALISTS?

An ophthalmologist is a medically qualified eye specialist
based in a hospital eye department. You will need a referral
from your doctor or paediatrician.

An orthoptist usually works alongside an ophthalmologist
and specialises in assessing vision, especially children with
squints.

An optometrist used to be called an optician and works in
a hospital or local practice. They test vision, prescribe and fit
glasses. As more individuals with disabilities live in the
community and use community services, optometrists and
dentists are becoming more skilled in working with them.

Types of vision problem

Squints (strabismus) or lazy eye

Around 20 to 27% of children with Down syndrome have a gen-
uine squint (as opposed to a pseudosquint). A squint does not mean

the child inevitably has problems with vision. Where there is no visual problem, surgical correction can be done for cosmetic reasons when the child is older. If there is a visual problem there are several ways to treat it.

Sometimes the brain selects either eye to process information from, alternating between them; this is more common in children with Down syndrome. Sometimes, one eye is used and the other is ignored, causing 'lazy eye'. About 12 % of children with Down syndrome have a lazy eye. If it is left untreated, the eye can lose vision for detail; this is irreversible after the age of 8 years.

Treatment using glasses, will usually straighten up the eyes. In more serious cases, the good eye is covered up (or occluded) for short periods each day to get the other eye working, and to develop the pathways needed by the brain to use it. Getting children with Down syndrome to cooperate is not always easy − they will not be happy with suddenly losing their visual ability − and when they are very young or developmentally young, it is difficult to explain it. If these treatments fail, surgical correction, where the muscles that control the eye are shortened and the eye is straightened, may be necessary for a small number of children with Down syndrome. These operations do not normally require an overnight stay. Often the child needs glasses and sometimes the squint can return, and a second operation may be needed.

Nystagmus
Nystagmus is rapid eye movements from side to side, caused by a lack of control of the eye muscles. 3 to 15% of children with Down syndrome have this condition; it sometimes disappears as the baby matures. Sometimes children will adopt a slightly different way of holding their head to compensate for the movement, and this is best left alone.

Long-sightedness (hypermetropia) and short-sightedness (myopia)
These conditions are more frequent in children with Down syndrome. Around half of the children in our research were prescribed glasses for these conditions by the time they went to secondary school. Short sightedness is the most common problem; recent research indicates that 80% of young children with Down syndrome

may have reduced ability to change focus between distant and close objects (called 'accommodation'). Reduced accommodation causes difficulties focusing on close objects and sorting figures from a background, but it can be corrected with bifocal glasses. It used to be thought of as a problem with the elasticity of the lens, but recent research has disproved this theory.

Cataracts

A protein associated with cataract formation, is coded at segment 21q22 (Chapter 5), which is probably why cataracts are more common in people with Down syndrome and can appear at any age, though more often in later life.

Between 1 to 3 % of babies with Down syndrome are born with congenital cataracts − a clouding of the lens. Surgical treatment is needed within the first months, or if the vision is severely impaired. A recent study found that just over 3 % of children had had cataracts; but estimates range from 12 to 83% for all people with Down syndrome. This difference in estimates reflects the problems of collecting data and the fact that some cataracts have little effect on vision and are ignored. Implanted lenses are fitted for older children and adults, and it is becoming more common for babies to have this treatment. We can expect to see more people with Down syndrome who need such treatment because more are living longer. All adults should have regular eye-checks from their mid-20's onwards.

Keratoconus

This is found when the cornea − the transparent cover of the front of the eye − becomes conical in shape. It is more common in Down syndrome and more likely to appear around puberty. It is thought that increased eye rubbing may increase the chances of this disease occurring. Keratoconus always impairs vision, unless it can be treated with contact lenses. Lenses may be feasible for some children, but can be problematic with dry eyes. Keratoconus affects a minority of people with Down syndrome.

PERSUADING CHILDREN TO WEAR GLASSES

It can be difficult getting young children to tolerate glasses, but even babies can get used to them. Light-weight frames and well formed wire clips around the ear have made it easier. The small ears and flatter nose bridge of many children with Down syndrome means that special attention is needed in selecting and fitting glasses. It helps not to over-emphasise or draw too much attention to the glasses – silly remarks about how they look can take a long time to correct. Suggesting the child looks like a favourite character or a relative who wears glasses can help. At first, encourage the child to wear their glasses to watch a favourite TV programme, then gradually increase the length of time they are worn. Don't turn it into a battle. It is very important that the school is aware that the child needs glasses. Some children associate glasses with school and wear them happily there – often it will do no harm if the child removes them at home. Ask your ophthalmologist or optometrist for advice. Make sure your child has his or her glasses with them when they need them.

Many parents find that the professional has not given them appropriate advice when a child is reluctant to wear glasses, or has not taken sufficient care in fitting them. No child wants to wear glasses that are uncomfortable or that slip down the nose or fall off when they run. Insist that the glasses fit well and have them adjusted regularly. Getting this right from the start is vital – it can take a long time to re-learn things that have gone wrong.

Growth

A baby's length and weight is a good indicator of their general health and medical condition – growth is controlled by our genes, our nutrition and, to some extent, how active we are. If there are problems they need to found and treated as quickly as possible.

It is easy to become anxious and a bit obsessive about growth and feeding in any baby, and more so when there are complications. Later there are concerns about being underweight or overweight. Some parents get confused and concerned, sometimes as a result of professionals who do not understand about growth when it comes to babies and children with Down syndrome. This can continue throughout childhood and can make mealtimes very tense, when they should be happy and relaxed. (See 'Feeding and weight gain' below).

For this reason, I have gone into a lot of detail, starting with typical growth and then looking at Down syndrome. But I don't want to overemphasise the issue. For most babies and children with Down syndrome, once the early checks of growth have been made, and they are feeding, that is enough. Train yourself to be alert but relaxed about their eating and growth.

HOW IS GROWTH MEASURED?

Height (or length in babies) and weight are the two standard measures of growth. Head circumference is also important in the early months. The growth of typical children falls into a 'normal' range and increases at a normal rate with periods of faster growth or growth spurts, around adolescence for example, and then slows down until it peaks in early adulthood. Weight increases in proportion to height, but is far more controlled by our diet and activity level and it continues into later years. Measurements of large numbers of children at different ages are used to make standard growth charts. They show the percent of children who have that weight or height at the same age. This is a percentile: if a boy of 5 years is 109 centimetres (43 inches) tall he would be at the 50th percentile: 50 out of 100 five year old boys would be shorter and 50 would be taller. If his height is 101 centimetres (40 inches) he would be at the 5th percentile: 95 in 100 boys would be taller and 5 would be smaller. Males and females grow at different rates and separate charts are used.

Growth and inheritance

When a child's height is compared to the normal growth charts, the parent's height is taken into account because we inherit the genes from our parents that control height, weight and body shape. For a boy, the father's height is looked at and for a girl, the mother's. This inherited factor explains why height and growth varies between races, different nationalities and geographic regions. Economic circumstances, diet and life-style also affect these measures. People are taller now because of improved diet and health care. In some countries, more people are overweight because they eat high calorie foods and are less active.

Only when the child's height or weight falls below the 3rd percentile is there cause for serious concern, unless of course the parents and most other family members are at the other end of the range.

Body Mass Index and Ideal Body Weight

By comparing weight to height we can find out the body mass of a person and compare this to the normal ranges to decide if the person is over or underweight. You divide the weight in kilograms by the height in metres, and then again by the height in metres. This gives the Body Mass Index (BMI= weight/ height squared). If the result is under 21 the person is underweight and their health may be at risk (although some feel that below 19 is a health risk); between 21 and 24 is considered a desirable weight, and between 25 and 30 is considered overweight. Above this there is a health risk. There are problems with simply using the formula; if someone is short but very muscular you would not think they were overweight, and this formula does not work well with children.

For children with or without Down syndrome it is better to work out the Ideal Body Weight (IBW) also called Desirable Body Weight (DBW). To do this you:

- Take the height/length of the child and find where this height falls at the 50th percentile on the standard male or female growth chart for typical children. Note down the age that corresponds to this.

- On the weight chart, find what the 50th percentile weight is for that age. Note this down.
- Then divide the child's actual weight by this weight and multiply by 100. This gives the percent IBW.

Ideally it will fall between 90 and100. Between 111 and 120 is considered overweight and if it is over 120, the person is considered to be obese.

NORMAL DISTRIBUTIONS

When you look at a person their height, weight, lengths of arms and legs and size of head are normally related – there is a normal range for this balance of parts. For each part there is a set of measurements that make up the 'norms' for that group of people. For example, if you measure the height of a typical large group of 10-year old English children you will have a range and an average height. If you draw these on graph paper you get a bell-shaped curve which shows the how the different heights of the children were distributed. This is called a normal distribution curve. But it is only for the children measured. If the group that was used are typical of all 10 year old English children at that time – the population of such children – then you can compare other 10 year old English children to the graph and work out were they fit in. If they were at the extremes, or outside of the range you would say they are not fitting in the 'normal' range. This will happen for most children with Down syndrome.

However the range of differences in height among children with Down syndrome is just as great as in typical children and if you draw them you also get a normal distribution curve, but for the population of 10 year old children with Down syndrome. So, you can use 'norms' to see where someone fits into that specific population. The important thing is to make sure that you are comparing them with the correct population. As we will see later this holds true for lots of measures including, mental development, energy levels and speed of response.

Growth patterns in Down syndrome

Children with Down syndrome have different growth patterns and balance of parts. This is because the extra genes affect their metabolism, growth and possibly activity levels. (Metabolism is the chemical process that breaks down and builds up organic bio–chemicals after they have been digested.)

Ultrasound studies have shown a smaller thighbone compared to 'normal' lengths of foetuses of the same age. Newborns with Down syndrome are slightly smaller in height, weight and head circumference; many are born two to three weeks before their due date. Clothes marked for younger babies still fit or have space in the arms and legs; their arms and legs are often proportionally shorter than their trunk. The same is found in older children and adults; they appear to be normal height when sitting, but look short when they stand.

The growth of children with Down syndrome does not follow the typical curve. They grow more slowly in the first two to three years, and many will be light and slim for their length or height. Height then speeds up and most start to put on weight. Some studies suggest the slowest growth rate is around 5 years, with relatively fast growth after this age, and a spurt in adolescence (not quite as strong or obvious as typical children). Like all children, the growth is not continuous but full of small stops and starts. As we will see in Chapter 10 the same pattern is found in their general development. Some studies have suggested that the peak in height is achieved earlier than typical people but others suggest it might be later. A recent study in England of over two hundred young adults with Down syndrome, suggests that after the rapid growth in the adolescent years, height still increases between 28–35 years, some 5 to 10 years later than in the general population. My own impressions agree with study. Again, this slower but longer growth is reflected in their intellectual development (Chapter 10).

This atypical growth can be seen in the relationship between height and weight. Infants with Down syndrome tend to fall in the 80 to 100% IBW level in the first two or so years. The ratio then increases and more become overweight, some showing signs by 3 years but most during the adolescent years. Some figures suggest that less than one in five young adults with Down syndrome are at the desirable weight. Figures for obesity (BMI greater than 30) vary between a quarter and nearly a half; many adults fall into the 'medically significant' category. We should note, that if you have shorter legs, and therefore, shorter height, the BMI and the IBW methods may be inaccurate; other indicators, such as levels of body fat should be considered.

Girls are more likely to be overweight than boys. Current USA charts show that at 18 years of age the average women with Down syndrome is about 18 centimetres (7 inches) shorter than typical women of that age, but that she weighs about 3 kilograms more. The average height for young men with Down syndrome at this age is about 21 centimetres (10 inches) shorter than the typical male who also weigh around 6 kilograms less. Using the IBW method, and taking the 50th percentile as the actual weight, the men have a 130% IBW and the women 156% IBW. These clearly exceed the 120% figure that indicates obesity in typical people, but as noted we may need to make some adjustment for shorter limbs.

Some Dutch studies of children with Down syndrome born around ten years later and active in sports, found that the men were on average 10 centimetres taller than the USA figures, and the women 7 centimetres taller; the IBW for the men was 110 and the women 126. Dutch people are amongst the tallest in the world and so, naturally, Dutch people with Down syndrome are taller than other nationalities. This comparison may also indicate that active children with Down syndrome may be taller or have a more balanced height-weight ratio. Recent figures from Northern France show children with Down syndrome to be taller than the early USA figures, and a study from Sicily found the children were shorter than the Dutch and French groups. It may be that the sample in the USA in the 1980's had more children from shorter races and nationalities. A recent study has provided data on children in Saudi Arabia that falls between these ranges. Neither the Dutch nor the French studies included people with severe heart problems, but it is unlikely that this alone explains the difference. Looking at the height of the Dutch and French studies, the 50th percentile is falling around the 70 –75th percentile for the USA charts.

This all suggests, that when using growth charts adjustment must be made for nationality and carefully take into account if the family is generally well built and muscular rather than tall and slim. Also look at the balance between torso length and limbs.

OBESITY

Even taking into account short stature, there is a risk of obesity for many people with Down syndrome, and it begins early in life. Obesity is associated with social problems – less friends, less activity and joining in – and health problems such as hypertension, lung disease, arthritis and strain on joints, strokes, diabetes, thyroid dysfunction and digestive problems. It makes sense to try to prevent obesity in children with Down syndrome. Ideally, this is done through an active lifestyle, understanding nutrition and diet, and emotional support. In a perfect world, this begins early in childhood, but it can be difficult to put it into practice.

Keeping an eye on growth

The baby should have regular health checks at the baby clinic. Their length (height) and weight are compared to growth charts and plotted over time to track changes in the child's growth curve. This includes rapid changes in height or weight and the relationship between the two (IBW). It is important to use growth charts for children with Down syndrome, and not charts for typical children, because of the differences in growth. These can be obtained from your health advisor or directly from various websites (Resource section). As we have seen above, even these special charts are not as accurate as we would want. If parents or carers have concerns it is useful to plot the height and weight on a growth chart (Down syndrome or typical) and do the IBW calculations. Before concluding the child is over or under weight, think through the issues outlined above.

Why do children with Down syndrome have different growth patterns?

As yet we do not know the full answer to this question. I will describe the ones that have quite good support from research. They involve differences in the endocrine system. The Endocrine System is made up of several glands that make hormones. Hormones are the chemical messengers used by the body to stimulate changes in other systems. Several hormones are closely related to growth; and people with Down syndrome have been found to have too much or too little of the specific hormones.

Human growth hormone

Children with Down syndrome generally have a deficiency in insulin-like growth factor 1 (IGF-1) which may partially account for them being shorter in height. In other children with short stature, growth hormone injections has been used to some effect.

Growth hormone injections have been tried in a few controlled studies for children with Down syndrome, but with little benefit. Like typical children of short stature, those with Down syndrome respond but the improvements in growth have been short-term; the children appear to mature and enter puberty earlier but do not show much difference in final height. No positive advances were found in social and intellectual development. The treatment is intrusive and demands daily injections over several years. There appears to be a heightened risk of leukaemia with human growth hormone, so until further research is done, it is not recommended as a treatment for children with Down syndrome. If the child is exceptional short for children with Down syndrome it may be worth considering.

Thyroid disorders

The thyroid gland is found in the front part of the neck, beneath the Adam's apple. It produces two main hormones thyroxine (T4) and tri-iodothyronine (T3) both of which partially control the rate at which the body burns-up its energy stores (metabolism). It can be overactive (**hyperthyroidism**) and so more energy is consumed and weight is lost, despite eating normally. Or, more common in Down syndrome, it can be under-active (**hypothyroidism**); less energy is used, weight is gained and the person slows down. Deficient thyroid hormones will also result in shorter height and intellectual impairment because the brain cells need the hormones to stimulate energy release and growth. This partially explains why levels of mental impairment in past samples of children and adults with Down syndrome, a proportion of whom had untreated thyroid problems, are lower than current estimates.

Signs of hypothyroidism

In younger children – poor growth, weight gain, very poor feeding, constipation, hoarse cry, prolonged hypotonia. In teenagers and adults – dry skin, increased weight, reduced appetite, hair falling out, lethargic movements, weakness, slow pulse, mental slowness, hearing problems, constipation, hoarseness, puffiness around the eyes.

A blood test will show the levels of the hormones T4 and T3 which can signal the need for treatment. When the body detects falling levels of T4 and T3, the pituitary gland compensates by sending out Thyroid Stimulating Hormones (TSH). So the tests can also detect higher levels of TSH if the thyroid is failing, often accompanied antibodies.

Screening for thyroid problems

All newborns are screened for thyroid and treated where appropriate. Between 1 and 4 % of babies with Down syndrome are born with a thyroid disorder; it is a short-term problem in about a third. The numbers increase relatively quickly in the teenage years – between 10 to 25% of adults, and as many as 35% of older people have problems.

Because thyroid problems can impair intellectual development and functioning and are linked to many other health problems, it is important to monitor the signs. Regular blood tests are needed because thyroid problems can be difficult to detect and can be confused with other behaviours of people with Down syndrome.

There is some dispute about how often to do blood tests. Current advice is to test every year or two from birth. But the necessity of such frequent testing has been questioned, especially as the majority of children and adults with Down syndrome will not develop thyroid problems, and many become distressed about giving blood samples. The issue is about finding those children with Down syndrome who are at risk and require frequent tests, and those who do not. Many people with Down syndrome have different levels of thyroid hormones compared to typical people, but do not appear to suffer from problems. This problem of assuming that what is 'normal' for typical people can be applied to those with Down syndrome is noted elsewhere in this chapter.

A recent study with our cohort attempted to investigate these issues. Thyroid function was tested in the children at 6 to 14 years of age and again ten years later. The results showed that many had lower levels of thyroid hormones but no physical symptoms. About a quarter appeared at risk because of raised levels of TSH, but ten years later 70% of these had normal levels of all the thyroid hormones and had not shown any physical signs of symptoms.

These results suggest that if the child has not shown any signs in the initial screening test, nor has any physical symptoms, they only need testing again between 5 to 10 years of age. Those with raised TSH levels and antibodies at this time, should be considered at risk and tested every year or two, until their results indicate no problem or otherwise. Around adulthood all young adults with Down syndrome should be tested again and the same risk factors applied. It would seem prudent to do the same with older people given the increase with age, but more research is needed. New research about the issue of 'who to test and how often' may change this advice.

My advice at this time is that, in the absence of physical signs, parents should question their medical advisor if they recommend very frequent blood tests and treatment.

The Digestive System and Metabolism

Most children with Down syndrome have a structurally normal gut. About 2 to 8% have problems. These include blockages in the tube leading to the stomach, or more often, in the duodenum (called congenital duodenal atresia). The blockages usually cause the baby to vomit a lot at most feeds.

Another condition is Hirschsprung's disease, an abnormality of the large bowel. These serious conditions are discovered in the first days of life, and generally require surgery if the baby is to survive. The outcome is good, the same as for typical babies.

Metabolic rate

Your metabolic rate affects how quickly your body breaks down and builds up organic bio-chemicals after they have been digested. Studies have shown that most children with Down syndrome have a lower basal metabolic rate (BMR) than typical children of the same age. This means they use fewer calories (between 10 and 15%) when asleep. Despite lower metabolism the research showed that the children were just as active as typical children of the same age.

If it is felt necessary to control the weight gain of a child with Down syndrome, calculate the daily calories needed as for anyone of the same age, sex and activity level and subtract 10 to 15 percent. But remember some children are leaner and may eat less. You should always look for ways of promoting the child's activity levels.

Vitamins and mineral supplements

Dietary supplements are becoming popular with the general public; but giving a supplement just because a child has Down syndrome is not helpful or necessary (Chapter 11). A supplement may be helpful if the child is ill or having a reduced diet.

Research has shown that, like many typical children, those with Down syndrome will choose foods that meet their calorific needs and are nutritionally balanced, without adult direction. But because they need fewer calories the total amount of food they eat is less.

This suggests that some may not be getting enough vitamins and minerals and may need a supplement. Some children with Down syndrome can be 'picky' eaters, have problems chewing and prefer softer foods and again not getting a balanced intake. If they appear to be more than usually tired, fatigued or frequently 'run out of steam' it may be helpful to consider a multivitamin supplement. In these cases it is worth talking this over with your health advisor.

Coeliac disease

About 4 to 5 % of people with Down syndrome have coeliac disease. It is a genetic condition causing intolerance to gluten – a protein found in wheat, barley, oats and rye. Gluten prevents the person from absorbing nutrients; the bowel wall becomes inflamed and its' lining becomes flat, reducing the area for absorbing food. The effects can be sudden, or they can appear gradually over months or years. The most common symptoms are diarrhoea, foul-smelling stools, vomiting, abdominal discomfort, excessive gas and unexplained weight loss in adults, or slow growth in children despite eating a good diet. It is also associated with fatigue and anaemia.

Coeliac disease is becoming increasingly recognised and a one-off test at two to three years of age is becoming common. This can be a blood test or a tissue test for children who don't like needles. If there is a possibility of Coeliac disease, a gluten free diet can be tried for six months, or a biopsy of the small bowel is needed. Since it is a genetic condition it is worth testing other members of the family. Because symptoms can appear slowly, it is worth testing any child with Down syndrome who has not been tested before, if they are showing many of the signs. This can be done as part of the regular checks for thyroid problems as both need a blood sample.

Diabetes

Diabetes is about seven times more common in children with Down syndrome than typical children – it develops in about 1 child with Down syndrome in 250. It is suggested that this may be due to an enzyme (phosfructokinase), which is coded at 21q21 (Chapter 4), and is involved in the process of glucose production and metabolism. Regular testing for diabetes is not done, so it is worth being vigilant. The symptoms are excessive urination, increased consumption of fluid and foods, and tiredness. Other symptoms include dry itchy skin, visual blurring, and headaches.

Type 1 Diabetes requires injections of insulin and often develops in childhood. Type 2 Diabetes appears later, and is associated with obesity, poor diet and a non-active life-style. Type 2 is on the increase in the general population. The relatively few children with Down syndrome and Type 1 diabetes usually need close supervision in managing the administration of insulin and controlling their medication.

Hepatitis

There is a misconception that people with Down syndrome are more likely to get Hepatitis. This arose when many lived in large institutions and the Hepatitis A infection was passed around because of poor hygiene. There is a suggestion that people with Down syndrome become persistent carriers of Hepatitis B, because of their poorer immune system. In countries or situations were there is a high risk of Hepatitis infection, immunisation is beginning to be recommended. Current carrier rate figures for North Europe and USA are 0.1%, South Europe and the Mediterranean countries 10% and Africa 20%.

Feeding and diet

Babies with Down syndrome grow more slowly and use fewer calories; they will not need the same amount of food as a baby of the same age. In fact, their chronological age is not very helpful in looking at their development over the coming years. It is the child's growth, developmental level and functioning that matter. They may take longer to learn to suck and then to chew. Their progression from bottle, to strained food, to mashed and chopped food takes longer. Low muscle tone and the shape of the mouth will cause difficulties in some children; they get tired quicker, the food can get stuck in the palate and the tongue does not shift it out as easily as in typical children. Despite this, most flourish and progress with minor problems. Feeding problems are more likely if the child has a severe heart problem, although most thrive after surgery. Hopefully parents are well supported by health staff; in many areas there are specialist staff to help with feeding and oral-motor development.

Most people with Down syndrome need the same diet as anyone else, unless they have medical complications. We all learn about food from birth and to some extent this forms the basis for what we like and what we don't like and how much we eat in later years. Although recent studies suggest children with Down syndrome are quite good at selecting a reasonable diet, there is much debate about the issue. Many certainly enjoy their food and appear to be very interested in it – possibly because they have a more limited range of interests than other children. Older people, who become less active and have fewer interests, appear to focus more attention around meals.

It has been suggested that people with Down syndrome have a marked preference for sweet foods, but again it is difficult to tell if this is more or less than typical people and whether it is a biologically driven preference or caused by habit. Perhaps it is another instance of focussing on the Down syndrome to explain typical individual differences. Some parents do appear to indulge their children – possibly to compensate for their disability or, in the early years, as an easy way to cope with frustration and demands for attention.

Breastfeeding

Several studies have found that many babies with Down syndrome will breastfeed. In our study about half of the families experienced some difficulties in feeding in the first days. This is more than with typical babies, and is usually due to immaturity and weakness of the sucking and swallowing reflexes and muscles. These problems can usually be overcome; in the past there was a tendency to assume that the baby could not do it, and to give up too soon. In one or two percent of cases, severe feeding difficulties are prolonged, and parents need special advice from medical staff.

Sometimes it is quite obvious the baby can't breastfeed well enough because their sucking reflex is weak. After giving it time, if breastfeeding is not working out and parents are getting distraught, it makes sense to use bottle-feeding. The most important thing is a relaxed relationship with your baby; as a father I liked being involved and feeding my children. Pumped breast milk or processed baby milk can be used for babies with Down syndrome, like other babies.

With the current emphasis on breast-feeding parents can feel guilty if it does not work out. Sometimes claims are made for benefits that are not justified. For example, it is claimed that breastfeeding will help speech by developing the baby's oral muscles. I have not seen any conclusive evidence for this. There are many factors associated with poor speech, and improved oral-muscle tone in the early months is likely to make a relatively small contribution – sucking on artificial teats should be just as useful. Some studies have indicated cognitive benefits of breastfeeding for low birth weight babies. Again the current evidence is weak and doesn't refer to babies with Down syndrome; it may be the breast-milk that is the key factor. Breast-milk has been shown to reduce the risk of allergic responses in typical children and may help in children with Down syndrome. However, while it may help immunity, it probably has little effect on the problem causing the impairment to the immune system discussed earlier.

Unfortunately, some babies with Down syndrome have to be tube fed for the first weeks of life. This used to prevent them going home but now parents are likely to be trained to do this themselves. Although this is a bit daunting at first, most parents are happier having the baby at home.

> There are lots of things to try to help breastfeeding – the 'football' hold, removing most of the child's clothes to keep them cool, and supporting the lower jaw while soothing the throat to help swallowing. Advice from a nurse specialist or another parent can help. If the child tends to go to sleep, get them aroused before you start feeding – massage, play, even a bath.

Bottle-feeding

If a baby is not growing at the expected rate, he or she will need less than average feeding. The average number of ounces given for bottle-feeding typical babies – their norms – will not be relevant for the slower growing baby with Down syndrome. As long as the baby is reasonably active and is not showing any signs of dehydration, there is no need for great concern if he or she does not take all the ounces stipulated for his or her age and weight at each feed. Keeping records is helpful. The main signs of dehydration are: the soft spot on the head (fontanel) begins to dip inwards, and the skin becomes loose – it does not return to its original position if it is pinched. If you are concerned, ask your health advisor to explain this more fully.

Solid foods

Most babies with Down syndrome will have no difficulty moving onto solids, but it may take longer for them to learn to use the tongue to push the food to the back of the mouth and swallow instead of thrusting the tongue back and forth as when sucking a teat. Don't be too quick to assume that the baby 'is not ready' or does not like the food. Use smaller steps in increasing the texture or solidness of the food, and allow longer periods at each step before moving on to more solid food. Unfortunately some children have a very low tolerance for more solid foods and parents will need professional help.

Try pressing the spoon gently down on the child's tongue and gently pressing the chin upwards. This usually causes the tongue to move backwards, taking the food with it and it encourages the child to close the mouth. If you still have difficulties after several days, try altering the size of the spoon, placing the food towards the edges of the tongue, or altering the texture and taste of the food.

Vomiting

Do not think there are problems because your baby vomits a little after a feed and has a round belly. Many babies with Down syndrome seem to vomit after feeds, and more so than typical children. This diminishes as they grow, and usually disappears by six months. It is probably due to floppy stomach muscles; and the vomiting reduces as these strengthen. Sometimes, the baby is allergic to milk, and needs a change of diet. Vomiting reduces as solids are gradually introduced at around six months. If the child is vomiting heavily and at every feed, you should consult your doctor or health clinic.

Constipation

Parents can get worried if the baby does not 'go' once a day, but babies and young children can be healthy and regular with bowel movements less often than this. Over three-quarters of our parents reported that their babies with Down syndrome seemed to strain a good deal when passing a bowel movement. Mothers were often worried although the babies were not in distress. For many, the difficulty was simply due to the low muscle tone (hypotonia) of gut muscles, and lack of activity. Usually it diminishes as the child gets older and moves around more, and it seldom becomes a serious problem. Several of our mothers found improvement when they increased the roughage in the child's diet. Other parents gave the babies mashed-up raw fruit, or gave older children some bran sprinkled on their cereal. For a young baby, a spoon of fruit juice or a prune soaked in a little water is sufficient. Some parents have found that increasing the fluid intake helps.

About 20% of children with Down syndrome have persistent constipation after these attempts. Mild laxatives may be needed; but they can become habit-forming and require increasingly larger doses. Get medical advice before using them, as the constipation may indicate a mild form of Hirschsprung disease or thyroid disorder. On the positive side, many mothers find their baby is so regular they can 'catch' the stools at certain times and avoid soiled nappies from nine to ten months onwards. Make sure that when older children sit on the toilet their feet are on the floor or supported.

Teeth and Dental Care

Children with Down syndrome cut their teeth later than typical children. Their teeth are often rather small, of irregular shape and can be in unusual positions. The first milk teeth usually appear between 12 and 20 months and may not be complete until the child is four or five years old. Often, the back teeth arrive before the front teeth. Some children are still cutting teeth in late childhood and like babies, can become irritable and moody. It is worth keeping a count of teeth and checking if they have arrived or started.

The permanent teeth tend to be shorter with smaller roots. 25 to 40 % of people with Down syndrome are reported to have one or more congenitally missing teeth. Some early studies suggested dental decay was less likely due to chemical differences in the saliva and more space between the teeth. But these studies were of people with Down syndrome living in large institutions, who probably had fewer sweets in their diet, regular checks and routines for teeth cleaning. Like all children, those with Down syndrome will get dental caries if they have a poor diet and poor dental hygiene.

Older children and adults with Down syndrome are more likely than most people to suffer from gum disorders. This could be due to their lower defences against infection (see immuno-deficiency above), and mouth breathing is thought to increase the chances of infection; the evidence for this theory is sparse. More likely, is that the shorter than normal root reduces the attachment into the jaw. Diet, and food which improves chewing and circulation in the gums, along with good oral health habits should be developed from the early months of life.

Some children with Down syndrome grind their teeth. This can be difficult to stop, especially if it is done during sleep. Sometimes

---

WHAT YOU CAN DO TO HELP YOUR CHILD DEVELOP GOOD ORAL HEALTH

Because of a small mouth and large tongue, some children with Down syndrome can find brushing the teeth more difficult. Using a smaller brush head or an electric brush can help. It might help to brush the tongue to remove bacteria and remnants for food from the deep furrows. Mouthwashes that control plaque are advised, and from around 5 to 6 years, flossing may help. The child should visit the dentist at around 18 to 24 months and then regularly – some say 3 to 4 times a year and others once a year. Your own dentist will advise you; but they may not have experience or knowledge of Down syndrome. Care should be taken when visiting the dentist to help the child understand what is happening and to prevent anxiety. Letting the child visit with parents or siblings so they can see what happens before actually being put in the chair and examined can help.

a bite plate can prevent the teeth becoming worn. Seek specialist advice.

Because of the shape of the jaw and mouth, older people with Down syndrome have more difficulties with dentures.

Bones, Muscles and Joints

People with Down syndrome have several differences in their skeleton and muscle system. I mentioned the absent twelfth rib and the shorter limbs earlier. 'Funnel chests,' where the chest bone is depressed, and 'pigeon chests,' where the chest bone sticks out, are more common, but do not cause any difficulties. The pelvis is rather small and the bones less developed; the iliac wings of the pelvis tend to be flatter and wider than in the general population. This smaller pelvis may result in more complications if a woman with Down syndrome gives birth.

Poor muscle tone and strength

The main problem is lower muscle tone (hypotonia) and 'looser' joints, due to the laxity of the ligaments. The ligaments attach muscles to bones, and if they are more easily stretched, the joint will be less tight.

Muscle strength is associated with muscle tone; this is reduced in adults with Down syndrome compared to typical adults and others with similar levels of intellectual disability. In typical children there is a steady increase in strength with a spurt in adolescence (around 13 to 15 years) related to hormonal changes and growth spurts in height. Teenagers with Down syndrome have less of a height growth spurt, and a recent study failed to find a spurt in muscle strength at this time. This corresponds to the relative increase in weight to height discussed earlier; becoming overweight and not stronger will put more tension on joints and may reduce mobility.

It is important to explore why the spurt in muscle strength is less. There is no difference in the levels of sex hormones and the onset of puberty (see later). Rather than a lack of hormones failing to 'switch' on the spurt, this suggests something may be preventing it.

It may be associated with the ageing process, and the interface between the nervous and muscular systems. There is a possible connection with excess of superoxide dismutase (see Chapter 4). Current research into the biochemistry of ageing may eventually find some treatment. For the present, the main treatment is the use of physical exercise to strengthen muscles, and improve coordination and good posture.

Types of problems

- Clicky hip – more babies with Down syndrome have a 'clicky' hip than typical babies because of the poor muscle tone and flexible joints. This is easily corrected early on.
- Strange postures – children and babies may lie on their front with their feet turned inwards, sit with very splayed legs, or with the legs in a W shape with the feet behind and the shins, thighs and bottom all touching the floor. There is a danger of abnormal growth if they stay like this for long periods. Floppy and inactive children are more at risk of such problems.
- Flat feet – due to poor muscle tone and flexibility in the tendons. It is used to be common for children with Down syndrome to be fitted with special shoes, supports and given special exercise. For most it is not needed, so ask why it is being advised and don't accept the answer –"because he or she has Down syndrome". The problem usually improves with age and physical activity.
- Clubfoot or a foot turned in or out – affects about one in 100 children with Down syndrome. It is diagnosed early and can be corrected with orthopoedic devices
- Spasticity – this is not associated with the genetics of Down syndrome, but like any baby, damage can occur at birth. This adds to the child's disability, and parents need to learn, not only about Down syndrome, but also about physical disabilities.
- Orthopaedic problems including degenerative arthritis are more common because of joint laxity and hypermobility in the feet, knees, hips and neck.

What can we do to help?

Over the years, many programmes of physical exercise have emerged for very young children with and without Down syndrome. There is some dispute as to how effective they are (Chapter 11). It is sufficient for many children if parents handle their baby and young child like any other, frequently changing their position until they can do it for themselves. They do not need physical therapy simply because they have Down syndrome. However their physical development can be helped with exercises. Once the child is mobile, it is important to give them lots of opportunities for regular physical exercise and attending gym clubs etc. is fun and a good social outing. A small number of children have severe problems and should be seen by a paediatric physiotherapist who will design an exercise programme.

Neck problems and atlanto-axial dislocation

Our spinal column (backbone) is a pile of small bones stacked on top of one another. They are held in place by muscles and ligaments. A hole in the middle of each one allows the nerves of the spinal cord to pass through. The top two bones in the neck are very specialized and allow the movement of the head. The top one is the atlas; it has a saucer-shaped surface that supports the skull. The other is the axis; it has a peg-like protrusion that sticks through the hole in the middle of the atlas along with the spinal cord.

The lower muscle tone and the lax ligaments of children with Down syndrome, allows one bone to move more freely than normal on the surface of the next. Usually this is unimportant, but occasionally the axis is able to move about too much on the atlas; this is called atlanto–axial instability and can result in dislocation. The peg-like protrusion of the bone can cause the spinal cord to become squashed as it passes through the atlas; this is known as spinal cord compression. Symptoms of trouble include difficulty with neck movements, a painful neck, stiff-legs, deterioration in walking, and gradual loss of bladder or bowel control.

These problems can come on suddenly as a result of a violent neck movement, or more often, they come on gradually over months or years. Laxity in other joints does not mean there will be laxity in the neck.

Neck X-rays were thought to be a reliable test, and were recommended for all people with Down syndrome. These suggested between 9 and 30% of children with Down syndrome were at risk for atlanto-axial dislocation. As a result many people were prevented from engaging in sports. Later studies, including a major one using the children from our Manchester sample, showed that X-rays are not as reliable as first thought. For example, three X-rays on a child over a few weeks resulted in three very different results. So the leisure activities of many children had been restricted unnecessarily, and for others a false sense of security was created. Routine neck x-rays are no longer recommended, but they are still required for some activities, including the Special Olympics.

The number of reported cases of spinal cord damage is quite small. If problems are suspected, an MRI scan of the lower brain stem and upper cervical spine needs to be obtained. Current estimates suggest that 1 to 2 people with Down syndrome in a 100 may have problems, and very rarely, surgery may be needed to stabilize the bones. In a recent survey of 27 people who underwent this surgery, 24 enjoyed good or excellent outcomes.

WHAT CAN YOU DO ABOUT ATLANTO-AXIAL DISLOCATION?

Be alert to the potential dangers, signs and symptoms. Support the neck if the child has to be anaesthetised for any operation or dental treatment; at this time they are even more relaxed and at risk for damage if the head swings around too much. It may give you peace of mind to have your child examined before activities that may put pressure on the neck, such as trampolining, diving and gymnastics. Get a medical examination immediately you notice any signs or symptoms, or any injury around the neck area. Always balance your concerns about the potential risk against the loss of the benefit to your child of the sporting activity. Finally, since many children with Down syndrome do have lax necks, it is even more important to ensure that he or she uses the correct car seat, a headrest and a seat belt when travelling.

Clicking knees and patella instability

There is far less research and information about this problem than neck problems. About 20% of people with Down syndrome have hypermobility of the kneecap (patella). This means the kneecap can slip out of place and dislocate, usually sideways. It can be detected in the first months of life, but more often when the child becomes mobile and in later years. It is due to:

- Laxity in the ligaments
- Minor differences in the bone structure, for example an underdeveloped groove into which the kneecap fits
- The kneecap being abnormally high on the joint
- A misalignment in the lower and upper leg that pulls the thigh muscles over to one side.

The problem can be mild, with clicking sounds and occasional dislocations that are easily pushed back in and do not seem to cause pain or problems with mobility. Moderate dislocations cause some pain and soreness, and then nothing happens for several weeks. Severe and frequent dislocations are called habitual dislocations. It can occur in one knee or both knees; the knee can just give way and the person falls. This has major implications for the child's lifestyle, can cause soreness and pain and can lead to arthritis. In the mild form, this problem can be overlooked in routine physical examinations. Even in more severe cases, the person can compensate for the problem by adjusting their gait, with no pain or obvious disability.

For most cases, the first line of treatment is physiotherapy with the aim of building up the thigh muscles to add strength and stability to the joint. For more serious problems elastic bandages and splints are used. In severe cases of habitual dislocations or abnormality, surgery is needed. The idea is to tighten up the tissues to stabilise the joint. Unfortunately there is a tendency for the tissues to stretch with use; for some children there is no major benefit and others need further operations. From the limited information available it is difficult to determine a consensus related to surgery; the surgeon's knowledge and experience of children with Down syndrome appears to affect practice.

WHAT CAN YOU DO ABOUT KNEE PROBLEMS?

Parents should be aware of potential knee problems; if you suspect your child has a weakness, seek medical advice and not just from one source. In some cases surgery is delayed, sometimes until the child has stopped growing. In other cases parents are told that damage has been done to the joint and that surgery should have been carried out sooner. Some say it took them time to convince their medical advisor to refer them to a specialist and others say there was disagreement between the physiotherapist and occupational therapist about treatment. Given the nature of the problem, this confusion is not surprising. Most Down Syndrome Associations have access to medical advisors if parents feel they need additional help. The advice from parents is to persist until you feel satisfied you have up-to -date accurate information and treatment from experienced professionals.

Much of the above is based on a collection of parent experiences in the UK obtained by Lynne Davies whose son has major problems with his knees and when she was the chair of the North Wales Branch of the Down Syndrome Association.

Posture and physical activities

The way we stand, hold ourselves and move sends out messages about how we think of ourselves. Certain postures are unattractive and do not send out the message that the person wants to engage socially. As one parent described her vision of people with Down syndrome before she had her child:

'I had a picture in my head of sack-like people with dropped heads, eyes on the floor, drooping shoulders and shuffling about.'

It is certainly an image I recall – usually the product of a poor exercise program or an inactive lifestyle – together with clothes that were too young, too sensible and unfashionable. It also resulted from living in an un-stimulating and non-challenging environment, where children and adults with Down syndrome received little respect, encouragement or opportunities to express themselves and make choices. Thankfully, we rarely see this in to-days young people with Down syndrome.

PHYSICAL ACTIVITIES AND THE CHILD
WITH DOWN SYNDROME

In recent years there has been considerable effort by parents, teachers and sports people to provide a range of activities for people with Down syndrome. These include swimming, athletics, gymnastics, dancing, horse riding, drama, ten-pin bowling, cycling, skiing, karate, weightlifting, canoeing, rock-climbing, and rambling and so on. Most recreational activities are available, and without looking too far, you can usually find someone with Down syndrome who has excelled in the activity. Many children with Down syndrome thoroughly enjoy swimming from the earliest years, and, depending on their health, some start when a few months old. Bear in mind that the child with Down syndrome is more likely to get cold quicker than his or her brothers and sisters, and may catch more colds. Many children start at gymnastic clubs for toddlers. Several of the girls in our research began dancing classes at three or four years, just like their friends, and went on to pass examinations and win grades. Horse riding is not only great fun, but it really helps to overcome the poor sense of balance that is common in people with Down syndrome. Most of these activities encourage a sense of confidence, competence and pride, and this is seen in the people who stand up straight and face the world. Providing these activities can make demands on family resources: not just financially, but time transporting children from place to place and waiting for them, which adds to the levels of fatigue for some parents.

Sometimes, the posture of children and adults with Down syndrome can be due to the differences in the skeleton and muscles, and their weight and height distribution. Recent work has shown that the posture and movement of children with Down syndrome can be improved with plenty of physical exercise and good training. A heart condition or respiratory problems do not preclude the child from physical activities, but a medical check-up is advisable if in doubt. One of the boys in our research took up gymnastics and was selected for the Special Olympics, even though he had a small hole in the heart.

Everyday activities not therapy

Many of the activities noted above are available for all children in the community. Years ago, I would have been more likely to talk about physical therapy, play therapy, hydrotherapy and other therapies. This is because we saw the child as a medical or developmental problem that needed fixing and so invented special ways to justify our efforts. We now know that most children with Down syndrome do not need 'therapy'; they need opportunity and encouragement to take part in these activities so they can benefit, like any child, within the limits of their abilities. Some will find they are good at something and continue with it, and others will move on to try different activities.

The Skin

Children with Down syndrome have distinctive creases on their hands and feet. Nearly all of them also have different lines and fingerprints (dermal ridges). The patterns made by these lines are called dermatoglyphs; they tend to be fewer than usual, and, looking at the palm of the hand, the loops open more often to the left side. These differences do not affect the child in any way; they are mainly of interest in diagnosis and study of the condition.

Dry skin and poor circulation

The skin of people with Down syndrome often has less elasticity than in typical people, and in places can be quite firm, dry and rough. This is not very noticeable in the young baby, but increases with age. The circulation of the blood in the skin also tends to be poor, even in children who do not have a severe heart condition. This can give the skin a "marbled" look (called marmoration), but does not have any serious consequences. The nature of the skin causes it to dry out and chap easily – particularly the lips, cheeks, hands and feet, and as noted earlier, the eyelids (see blepharitis). This is exacerbated by poor circulation, which also reduces sensitivity to temperature changes. Babies with Down syndrome are less likely to be in control of their 'cooling' and 'heating' system and so rely more on parents to regulate the temperature externally. Concern and anxiety can make parents go overboard. I often see babies so swamped with clothes that they cannot move and kick, they are unable to get themselves warm, even if they want to.

WHAT CAN YOU DO ABOUT SKIN AND CIRCULATION PROBLEMS?

Physical handling, such as rolling, rocking, bouncing and tickling, stroking and bathing, can stimulate the circulation of blood – it is a form of baby aerobics. Baby massage is becoming popular; this will certainly help the condition of the skin and circulation, and is very relaxing for fretful babies. It is worth trying to establish regular habits in diet, hygiene and skin care early on; these can compensate for some of the inherent problems of the condition. Dry skin and chapping can be treated with creams; good cosmetic care of hands, elbows and face should help combat the drying of the skin that occurs with age. About half the people with Down syndrome have tiny pinkish pimply eruptions, mainly on the trunk, upper thighs and buttocks – as do many typical people. These can get inflamed and infected, eventually causing boils. Good hygiene will prevent this.

Sensitivity to pain

Many people with Down syndrome have a higher pain threshold and less sensitivity to surface pain. They may be more able to tolerate things that would cause us to react, like chaffing, tight belts or shoes, and heat. This can be a particular problem for a few, but usually, once parents and carers are aware of it, it is not a serious issue.

Sometimes, poor verbal communication and a high pain threshold combine. Parents should be vigilant, but without becoming too concerned and fussy. We all have varying degrees of tolerance to pain; be concerned only if there are clear signs of very high pain thresholds and health problems.

Hair

The hair of children with Down syndrome can be rather fine and sparse. Since the scalp can also be dry, it is worthwhile consulting a good hairdresser for advice on the use of shampoos and hair conditioners. For some older children, try to find a hairdresser who can cut the hair well; this may not be as easy as for typical children. When girls begin to use makeup, get advice from a reputable beautician who understands skin. Appearance is important, and good skin and hair can help with this.

Facial cosmetic surgery

In the last 20 years, cosmetic surgery to alter the Down syndrome 'look' has been developed by some medical practitioners and supported by other professionals and parents. These operations remove the epicanthal fold on the inside of the eye, correct the slant of the eye, raise the flattened cheek bones, reduce the lower lip, make a small chin larger, shorten a very large tongue and reduce fatty tissue in the neck. The idea is to make the child's appearance more 'normal', with the assumption that this will improve their functioning long-term, because people will treat them more normally. While the evidence shows that the physical appearance of a child with Down syndrome can be altered, there is no real support for improved functioning. (See 'Cosmetic surgery' – Chapter 11).

Cosmetic surgery is becoming more widely used, even by young people. Some young people with Down syndrome may decide they would like to change their appearance. Providing they understand the risks and implications, and have discussed it with a competent professional, they have the same rights to do this as other young people.

The Heart

Between 30 to 60% of babies with Down syndrome have some form of heart defect; 10 to 15% of these have a severe heart defect.

No specific type of heart defect is characteristic – the whole range of possible problems has been reported. Some problems are mild, disappear with time, and do not seriously affect the child's growth and development. Others may be severe, or require major surgery, and some are inoperable. Some babies are unlikely to survive beyond the first months of life without surgery. Accurate figures are not available, as recent advances in surgical techniques have meant that many babies are now surviving who, just a few years ago, would have died. The chances of success of such operations are no lower for children with Down syndrome than for any other child.

Detecting a heart problem

Doctors can detect a heart problem in most babies soon after birth – especially a severe problem – but sometimes the defect is not found for several months. A heart murmur often alerts the doctor to the possibility, alongside other characteristics. These include: the colour of the skin (pale, grey or blue), swollen eyes and the effort required to breathe. About 5% of the babies with a severe heart problem appear to be doing well in the first 6 to 8 months of life, but serious damage is taking place in the heart-lung system. These babies often need surgery before six months of age and so specialist assessment soon after birth is important (see below).

Types of heart problem

- **Atrial Ventricular Canal Defect** – this is a hole in the centre of the heart, and is the most common problem in children with Down syndrome, accounting for about half of all severe heart defects. It can be corrected by surgery in infancy.

- **Ventricular Septal Defect** – this is a hole in the wall of the two ventricles (the two large, lower chambers of the heart). It is the second most common problem affecting just under a third of children with heart defects. Small holes do not cause any strain and often close by themselves. Larger ones may need surgery.

- **Patent Ductus** (2% of cases) and **Tetralogy of Fallot** (7% of cases), are the most severe types of heart defect. Tetralogy of Fallot is a combination of four defects, including a large hole between the ventricles and a narrowing in the pulmonary valve. The child's skin, lips and fingernails appear blue. Total correction is difficult in babies, but an operation is sometimes carried out to provide temporary relief. When the child is older there is a better chance of correcting the defect.

DOES MY BABY NEED AN ASSESSMENT BY A HEART SPECIALIST?

All babies with Down syndrome should be assessed by a paediatric cardiologist (child heart specialist) before the age of three months. This assessment should include an echocardiogram, which is like an ultra-sound scan used during pregnancy. If this shows problems, a small catheter is inserted into the system to give precise details of the extent and location of the problem. These examinations are becoming routine in many places when the baby is very young, but they do require attendance at a hospital. If your baby has these checks, there is little chance of a serious defect being found in the second year of life or later.

What effect will a heart defect have on my child with Down syndrome?

Children with Down syndrome who have major heart defects often have delayed growth and weight gain. They are also likely to have less muscle tone and be more floppy. Together, this causes an additional delay in their development of gross motor skills compared to children with Down syndrome without a severe heart problem. But there is no evidence that their mental development is any slower, or that they are less sociable.

Children with severe heart defects are more likely to get infections and so need antibiotics before operations or dental procedures such as drilling or extractions. The risks can be reduced with good dental care. We did find a slightly increased frequency of behaviour problems in the children with heart problems and frequent infections. We think this was due to parents managing the child differently when unwell (Chapter 9).

Should a child with a serious heart defect take part in physical activity?

Severe heart defects do not necessarily mean the child should not take part in physical activities. Of course, parents should always check this with their doctor, but we have found that many of the children in our sample, even those with inoperable defects, happily take part in physical activities with ordinary children in regular schools. As with any child who has a major health problem, parents can expect temporary setbacks, especially when the children are ill or receiving treatment.

Circulation and Blood

Studies have suggested that some children with Down syndrome have differences in their circulatory system, such as slightly narrower and thinner arteries with fewer branches and capillaries. But most people with Down syndrome have quite a normal circulatory system.

Through the blood, energy and food is transported around the body. If the body does not get these supplies in sufficient quantity, one might expect less activity, even a tendency towards lethargy, and possibly some effect on growth and development. This is another good reason to give babies and young children with Down syndrome plenty of handling and stimulation from the first weeks of life; it encourages circulation.

Leukaemia

About 1 in 100 to 150 children with Down syndrome develop leukaemia. This is about 10 to 15% more than in the general population. Leukaemia is a condition where there is an abnormal growth of white blood cells, and it usually occurs in early childhood. A first symptom is that the child bruises easily, and shows signs of excessive bruising. They are also pale, easily fatigued and get lots of infections.

Some types of leukaemia respond to treatment better than others. A very rare type, almost unique to Down syndrome, is Mega-Karyo-blastic leukaemia; it is sensitive to chemotherapy with a high chance of cure. The most common type is acute lymphoblastic leukaemia, occurring mostly between 2 and 9 years. Nowadays leukaemia can be brought under control, and affected children can remain well for long periods. In well over half, the disease can be permanently cured. During periods of illness and treatment, the child's development may slow down, but they catch up when they are well. Early detection and getting expert help from specialist centres for children with cancer is essential.

A recent study in Denmark found no cases of leukaemia over the age of 29 years in people with Down syndrome. Interestingly, it also found a decreased risk of other cancers in people with Down syndrome compared to the general population.

The brain and nervous system

The brain and skull of people with Down syndrome tends to be smaller in relation to the size of their body than found in typical people. By itself, this does not account for their intellectual disability. But specialised parts of the brain, particularly the brain stem and the cerebellum, are smaller relative to the size of the whole brain. Some of the nerve pathways, or bands of nerves that join different parts of the brain, are also smaller and less developed. There are fewer nerve cells and fewer connections (dendrites) between the nerve cells. There are also some differences in the chemicals in the nerve cells, and in the junctions (synapses) between nerve cells that form the complex pathways that make up the brain. These are general findings and, as discussed before, people with Down syndrome vary widely despite having the same extra genetic material.

Nerves and learning

Put simply, learning means something becomes established in our memory. Information from our senses is passed along the nerves as an electrochemical impulse. The impulse travels along the nerve fibre of a cell to a junction called a synapse. The impulse causes a chemical change that triggers a fresh impulse in the cell on the other side. The chemicals in the synapses are called neurotransmitters and can excite or inhibit the electrochemical activity in the adjoining cells.

With new information, the first electrochemical signal is unstable and stored in the short-term memory. If it is reinforced by other signals, it becomes stable and stored in the long-term memory, and the person has learned something new. The more we use and reinforce it the stronger it will become. If it has high emotion attached to it, it is likely to be stored immediately, often almost intact in every detail. The new information is tested to see if it is important and matches in with something else.

The stimulation of electromagnetic signals results in permanent changes to the brain and the nervous system. So, if the system or part of the system is not used, then links are not made. This means that we might learn something, but we lose it if we don't use it and consolidate it. The higher the volume of signals the more the pathways need to grow – like roadways with increased volume of traffic. It is the dendrites that link the nerve cells together and form complicated sets of pathways. As we grow and learn, we develop many pathways and junction points. As noted earlier, fewer dendrites and nerves cells are found in the brains of individuals with Down syndrome. But they can still benefit from experience.

It helps that different parts of the brain specialise in different functions and types of learning and memory. This means that brains can become different with different types of experience. For example, brain scans of London taxi drivers who spend hours learning the maps of London (called 'the Knowledge') have shown they have a larger specialised area of the brain to do with 'maps' than the rest of us.

Another clever device is that as a pattern of repeated signals build up in the brain, they form into a 'sub-programme' and begin to work automatically. This means we merely need to send a signal, without even thinking consciously about it, to a sub-programme and a whole action plan emerges. For example, a baby learning to reach for something has to concentrate on the object, watch their hand and constantly make adjustments by seeing if the hand has gone too far. It is quite a laborious process at first. After a period of practice, which involves repeated signals and a growth and reorganisation of nerve cells, it becomes automated; the baby reaches out and picks things up 'without thinking'. Another good example is a young child carrying a cup or glass filled with a liquid. If you speak to them they are likely to tell you to be quiet or they will spill it. The action of carrying and monitoring the level of the drink is not automatic, they need a lot of conscious control. Months later they are carrying things while chatting, singing, dancing or possibly riding a bicycle if that is what they want to practice. The action plan of carrying objects has been consolidated into an automatic sub-routine.

Learning a new word is another useful example. The child hears the word 'ambulance' and says it quite clearly. We are all delighted. The next day they can't quite get it right; we are disappointed and wonder why they have lost it. We may even think there is something wrong with them. Gradually they learn the correct pronunciation – by using and practicing the word and similar words and sounds. This is called generalisation or transfer of learning. You learn one thing, which helps you to learn something similar. You may have had similar experiences with learning a skill such as driving a car. You slowly learn the parts and gradually put them together. Then you find you can drive quite well. But the next day it all goes wrong. In the time between the driving lessons, your brain has been consolidating the nerve network for driving, making it more automated and more efficient and getting the links to other centres formed. But because some links were not that stable, they have been lost or interfered with. After your next lesson or two, driving suddenly 'clicks' for you. After using the skills for some time, they are so consolidated, it will take something quite traumatic to damage them. Equally, if you have learnt and consolidated a bad habit, it takes a great effort to change it. We need to ensure that we don't let children with Down syndrome learn 'bad habits' because it will take them even longer to correct them.

Learning is more difficult for children with Down syndrome because they have fewer nerves cells, differences in neuro-transmitters, and take longer to form new pathways and systems.

Development and sensory co-ordination

Children with Down syndrome may have specific problems with some areas, such as sensory coordination and muscle tone. This may be because they have a relatively smaller cerebellum compared to the rest of brain, or if the cerebellum fails to grow because of other problems in this area of the brain, leading to less growth of the nerve cells.

Babies and young children go through organised sequences of development. For example in motor development: holding their head steady, rolling over, sitting, pulling to a stand, standing, walking, running, standing on one leg, jumping, doing a head over heels. These sequences are found in all aspects of development – motor, social, emotional, language and cognition (Chapters 8 and 10). Some children develop more quickly than others. Some go through one area quickly, for example, walking at 9 months, but they may be slower to say their first word.

We do not really understand these differences in development, nor why some children are more gifted at some things than others. But we do know that you can't learn some things until the body, or the part of the system, is ready. So you can't learn to sit before you have the strength, and have learned to hold your head and upper part of your body steady. Children with Down syndrome have a mix of slower growth and development, and slower learning. Both might involve similar parts of the nervous system, but they are separate.

Growth and maturation can be delayed by depriving a child of nutrients and stimulation, but there is little evidence that their inner timetable can be speeded up by increasing the amount of nutrients or stimulation, or practice. The practice effect works mainly when the system is ready.

See Chapter 10 for more on Intelligence, development and attainment, and Chapter 11 for the effects of early stimulation.

We found that babies with Down syndrome started looking at and reaching for an object just a few weeks later than typical babies – which showed they had the strength and the intention – but it took them several weeks to co-ordinate the visual feedback, consolidate it and reach automatically. This suggested a particular problem with coordinating the visual information with the motor information. It also showed problems feeding information forward to anticipate the reach and adjust the reach. Problems with coordination and 'feed-forward' control are frequently described for people of all ages with Down syndrome. Watch how the children move about the playground or garden compared to typical children. Don't just see them as slower or clumsy, but look how they approach objects and navigate around barriers.

Another study involved looking at babies with Down syndrome learning to sit and walk. We found that the stage between sitting with some support and sitting and balancing on their own was more delayed than in typical children. The same happened for the stage between standing with support and standing alone, and walking with support and taking several independent steps. These stages involved the coordination of the automated plan for physical control with balance and other sensory inputs. This showed that children with Down syndrome had a problem when bringing these two aspects together to produce coordinated and skilled functioning. They are like little plateaus when no progress is seen (Chapter 10), but of course progress is taking place internally as the cells in the appropriate part of the brain set up connections. These plateaus are often seen at times when two or more senses need to become coordinated into a skilled action.

Since people with Down syndrome have slower growth of nerves, fewer nerve cells and dendrites, and differences in the electro-chemicals needed to operate the system, it is not surprising there are differences in their development and ability to learn. Some neurotransmitters (electro-chemicals) control muscle tone, coordination and responsiveness. Low levels and differences in the neurotransmitters cause mild physical problems. Hence many people with Down syndrome are both intellectually and physically disabled. Attempts to remedy these problems have resulted in many 'special' treatments and therapies for Down syndrome (Chapter 11).

Ageing and Deterioration

People with Down syndrome generally age earlier than typical people. They are more likely to suffer from dementia and a type of Alzheimer's Disease (see below). Other features of ageing, such as an increase in sensorineural hearing problems, or epilepsy, begin earlier, and suggest neurological deterioration. If an older person with Down syndrome starts to show signs of forgetfulness, withdrawal, slowing down and loss of skills, have their hearing and thyroid functioning checked before assuming it is old age.

A lack of skin elasticity can make some people with Down syndrome appear older than their years. There is a whole range of products to maintain healthy skin, and as far as I can discover, there is no reason why people with Down syndrome should not use them. They may not be as effective, because the factors causing the problem are different, but don't rule them out just because the person has Down syndrome. Decline is less in people with good health and those who remain active; about half of the 60 year olds with Down syndrome are active, alert and enjoying life.

Seizures and epilepsy

Seizures are also called convulsions, fits or infantile spasms. There are different types and different causes; children and adults can have a single seizure triggered by illness, fever, infection or drugs. Recurring seizures are called epilepsy. Parents should always seek medical advice if the child has a seizure; there may be a risk of disorders such as autism (Chapter 9). Always get advice from a paediatric neurologist who specialises in epilepsy before deciding that a child has epilepsy and starting treatment.

ALZHEIMER'S DISEASE

The first signs of dementia are forgetfulness, disorientation with time and routines, mood changes and withdrawal. Later, there is loss of self-care skills, slower walking and shuffling, sometimes delusions, psychomotor seizures (a sudden jerking of muscles called myoclonus), and eventually loss of mobility and cognitive functioning. There is debate about whether the cause of the dementia in Down syndrome is the same as that for Alzheimer's disease – and whether it should be called Alzheimer's disease in people with Down syndrome – but recent work has traced both to the same gene areas on chromosome 21 (see Chapter 4). There are some issues about the quality of research in this area, but recent studies are providing a consensus. Firstly, significant deterioration in function and cognitive ability only occurs in less than a quarter of people with Down syndrome before the age of 50 years. Between the ages of 50 and 60 years, significant decline in functional skills is reported in 20 to 40% of these people, and mild decline in up to 60%.

The incidence of epilepsy in people with Down syndrome is between 5 and 10%. This is a little higher than the general population, but lower than other categories of intellectual disability. There appear to be three peaks – infancy, teenage to young adults and people over 50 years old. The latter is related to ageing. Infantile spasms in babies – a sudden jerking of the muscles – are quite common, but respond well to treatment. Anticonvulsant therapy produces a marked improvement for most people with Down syndrome, particularly young children. A recent study found the prognosis to be better than in the general population, and most of the children continue to develop well. Unfortunately, where the seizures are severe, persistent or require major control, the children tend to have much slower intellectual development than other children with Down syndrome. Of course there are always exceptions.

The Reproductive system, Sexuality and Sex education

In the first edition of this book I said that the sexual development of people with Down syndrome was often delayed or never occurred. This observation was based on people who were institutionalised, and was incorrect. A different picture is emerging from more recent studies of people with Down syndrome living in the community. Many do have sexual needs and want intimate relationships with a partner. They have the same rights to this as any other person, and recognising this has led to a lot of work looking at how these needs are best met.

Males with Down syndrome

Recent studies comparing the sexual development of boys with Down syndrome living in the community with typical boys, found no major differences in the sequential emergence of primary and secondary sex characteristics. Puberty begins at around the same time; some boys enter puberty by 10 years, and they are physically quite mature before starting secondary school. The penis and testes may be smaller than average, especially in infants, but the range appears to be as great as for typical males. There is a higher likelihood that one, or occasionally both testes have not descended into the scrotum – this happens by around 7 months in typical babies – but it is easily corrected, normally during infancy. Increasing levels of sex hormones with age are also similar to the norm. The growth of facial hair however, is generally delayed, but some men with Down syndrome grow full beards. Minor urogenital abnormalities have been reported such as a double urinary opening on the underside of the penis. Again, surgical correction is usually done in the first year of life.

The consensus of studies indicates that the hormones controlling sexual maturation are normal, but that most males are sterile. Information on sperm production is limited because of problems in collecting sperm for analysis. This might become easier as more parents accept their sons may be sexually active and sex education becomes more available. At present studies report the sperm of males with Down syndrome are often less mobile, and more abnormal forms were found than in samples from typical males. Some men with Down syndrome are fertile. In 1989, the first confirmed pregnancy was reported of a father with Down syndrome.

Females with Down syndrome

Girls with Down syndrome usually develop secondary sex characteristics, although breast development is often moderate compared to the norm. Most studies report that girls begin to menstruate regularly at the normal age of 10 to 14 years. Obese girls often start menstruating earlier, and some studies have indicated that more girls with Down syndrome start earlier. If menstruation starts before 10 years or after 18 years, it may be related to a thyroid or cardiac problem and needs to be investigated. Periods are normally regular, occurring approximately every 28 days, but some studies suggest that females with Down syndrome experience less regularity, a shorter cycle and more prolonged flow, than typical women. The onset of menopause is reported to be about 5 to 6 years earlier than typical women. Unfortunately the research on many of these aspects is sparse, but the general picture is of normality.

There is some evidence for ovarian dysfunction and possibly higher levels of some hormones after puberty. However, ovulation occurs in around 90% of females with Down syndrome, and current estimates indicate that 70% can be assumed to be fertile. Over 30 births to females with Down syndrome are documented. About two thirds of the offspring were classified as physically and intellectually normal, just under one third had Down syndrome, and a small number had some other intellectual and physical disability.

The majority of girls and women with Down syndrome can learn to care for themselves reasonably well during menstruation, especially those who cope independently with the toilet (Chapter 10 – attainments). With patient and careful explanations about half the older girls with Down syndrome have some understanding that periods are part of the process of changing from a girl to a woman. Far fewer understand the relationship between periods, pregnancy and reproduction. Such understanding is highly related to their level of mental ability.

Many mothers find the best way is to let the girl become aware that older females in the family menstruate and, by openness, show that it is neither frightening nor mysterious. Any questions should be answered specifically and simply and not treated as a prompt for an in-depth lecture. Around the time that her periods are due to start, it helps to make occasional comments at appropriate times about the fact that she will soon be changing in readiness for womanhood. The secret of consolidating her learning is to provide gradual and natural preparation over a long time. A sudden crash course to cope with a crisis is unlikely to succeed.

PRE-MENSTRUAL SYNDROME (PMS)

PMS has received very little attention in women with Down syndrome. The limited research available suggests it may be a little more common than in typical women. It may go unrecognised by parents and professionals, as affected girls and women do not have the communication skills to explain it, or the symptoms are confused with other behaviour problems or conditions. The symptoms of PMS include headaches, irritability, mood changes, weight gain, fatigue, lethargy and pain. If parents or carers suspect PMS, then monitor the menstrual cycle over two to three months, and keep records of changes and symptoms. In our group of young women some mothers noted quite major emotional and behavioural changes in the week or so before their period. The usual PMS treatments, including oil of primrose, can work. One woman, who is amongst the most intellectually disabled of our group with very few communication skills, started her periods late, at around 18 years old, and they were irregular for some time. Her mother noticed that her usually very happy and sociable daughter was moody and showing problem behaviour, which she finally thought were due to PMS. When she used oil of primrose she found 'quite dramatic' changes.

'I no longer had to dread that time in the month with her.'

She also told us that on two occasions she failed to use the oil of primrose and the behaviours returned.

Sexual activity and people with Down syndrome

The main information on sexual functioning and activity in people with Down syndrome comes from parents. Most parents do not experience major problems. Regular masturbation was noted in about half of young people with Down syndrome in earlier reports. Our recent estimates, based on the young adults in our group, suggest it might be a lot higher. This may be because young people with Down syndrome have more access to sexual information through TV, sex education and inclusion; typical children often learn about masturbation and aspects of sex from their peers.

At first, children with Down syndrome can be quite uninhibited, playing with their genitalia, or boys may proudly show their erect penises to anybody present. But by the time they become sexually active, most are ready to understand the ideas of modesty and privacy – if that is the custom of the family. This occurs at the same developmental level as with typical children – around four to five years of age. They can also understand that they are growing up and changing into men and women, and 'big boys', 'men' or 'big girls' don't do that in company.

Such ideas and behaviour need to be taught. If the child is encouraged to develop independent skills with bathing and hygiene – as opposed to passive acceptance that others do it for you – then notions of body parts and touching will be developing. It helps if the young person has developed a sense of self. At first this is about toys, objects and clothes that are 'theirs'; it helps if they feel they had a part in choosing these things. With this, comes the responsibility to look after their things. It also helps if they choose what to wear and have a room of their own, or a designated space within the house, in which they are encouraged to express themselves in selecting decorations and organisation. This is part of self-identity and with it come ideas of how to behave and privacy. Most parents find that once the child starts to masturbate, it is relatively easy to ensure they understand they do it in private.

Parents need to move beyond the idea of the 'perpetual child', to acknowledge the 'potential adult' with sexual needs, and prepare the child for adulthood.

LEARNING APPROPRIATE BEHAVIOUR

The older literature tended to over-emphasise inappropriate sexual behaviour such as public masturbation, genital exposure and touching others genitalia or breasts; but these behaviours are not as common as was thought. Children with Down syndrome, like many typical children, need to learn about touching, hugging or kissing people, and about personal space – not getting too close physically when engaging in everyday interactions. Parents can reduce problems with relatively simple training; stop the child hugging and kissing everyone; teach them to judge the personal distance as an arms-length away; discuss differences between family members, close friends and others. There are programmes to teach appropriate sexual and social behaviours, both as part of protecting children from others and taking care when touching others (Resources).

Young people and sexual relationships

Several studies have reported that over half of the adolescents and young adults with Down syndrome are interested in the opposite sex, and that many have special friends. We found a major problem for this age group was difficulty finding someone who would be a close friend. Most people select special friends who share similar interests and abilities. Typical teenagers will have a great pool and range of other teenagers to get to know. If you have intellectual disability your potential choice of friends is vastly reduced, and they are spread over larger distances. This problem can be greater for those in mainstream settings who have little contact with similar children, and those who live in rural areas. In my experience, many parents try to ensure that their older sons and daughters have opportunities to mix socially with others who have an intellectual disability. But this is an added task that comes at a time when the parent's peer group are beginning to find, and possibly enjoy, more freedom from their children.

Wanting a boyfriend or girlfriend does not carry the same implications for many young people with Down syndrome as it does for typical teenagers and young adults. Many people with Down syndrome do not appear to have a sex drive to the same degree as typical people. Whether this will change with increased education and opportunity is as yet unknown. But at the moment, many do appear to be less interested in sexual activity and sexual intercourse. Even many of those who are sexually active appear to limit this to self-stimulation.

There is a dilemma here for parents and carers. Because of our own fears and inhibitions we are likely to be thankful that these young people are not getting sexually involved. If we believe this is intrinsic to them, and not due to us preventing them learning about sex and restricting their opportunity for sexual experience, we may feel at peace. But we may be denying, for some at least, the right and the joys of sexual experiences and intimate relationships with others. Parents do need to think this through for their own situation and their child. There are books for young people with intellectual disability that deal with issues such as exploitation, contraception, sterilisation and safety (Resources).

There is no reason why people with Down syndrome should all be heterosexual. There is no research on this, but there are descriptions of people with Down syndrome who are sexually active and prefer same-sex relationships. Some of this appears to be part of typical adolescent development.

Society in many countries has developed a more mature understanding of sexuality and the sexual needs of people with disability. The situation is still far from acceptable, and there are many barriers that prevent such needs being met. There is a gradual increase in the number of people with intellectual disability getting married or living together, and there are services focused on encouraging and supporting these relationships. One study found that women with Down syndrome were more likely than men with Down syndrome to get married, and to men who had intellectual disability, but not Down syndrome.

We recently interviewed the young people in our group about their aspirations for marriage or partnership. 30% did not respond – they were the ones functioning at quite young developmental levels and most had little conception of marriage. 14% said they did not want to get married – some of these were like younger children who do not yet want to mix with the opposite sex, but others had higher levels of understanding and explained why they preferred not to be married. 56% said they did want to be married and their understanding ranged from rather simple ideas of being like their parents and siblings, with little apparent understanding of relationships, to several who had mature views about caring for and being cared for by someone special, being in love and having someone to share things with. My rather rough estimate is that a good third of these young adults with Down syndrome had more than just simple or fantasy ideas about marriage or partnership, and aspired to achieve such a relationship one day.

The little information we have, indicates that people with Down syndrome who get into an intimate relationship have the same chances as the rest of us for staying together and being happy. Like typical couples, there are many stories of how finding their partner helped the young person blossom, and brought great happiness. They mostly live together in a supported home often near to their family.

8

Personality and socialisation

- What are people with Down syndrome like?
- Is there a Down syndrome personality?
- How do people with Down syndrome develop socially?
- How do you interact positively with your child?
- How do people with Down syndrome feel about themselves?

This chapter is in three parts. The first is about temperament and personality and the second is about the process of socialisation – how we become the people we are. This includes quite a lot about social interaction and understanding others. The third part is about how society reacts to people who are different, and the awareness of people with Down syndrome of Down syndrome and disability. It is quite long but hopefully can be taken section by section.

What are people with Down syndrome like?

Many people, including professionals, researchers and writers, share a picture of children and adults with Down syndrome as 'affectionate, placid, docile, gentle, having a good sense of fun'. They are also seen as having special talents, such as being 'good mimics' and 'musical'. These ideas can be traced back to Langdon Down, who wrote in 1866:

> 'They have considerable power of imitation, even bordering on being mimics. They are humorous, and a lively sense of the ridiculous often colours their mimicry . . .*

and also,

> 'Several patients who have been under my care have been wont to convert their pillowcases into surplices and to imitate, in tone and gesture, the clergyman or chaplain they have recently heard.'**

Langdon Down was so impressed with these abilities that he built a grand theatre in his institution for the residents. A hundred years later, drama became popular again, both as a therapy and as a recreation for people with Down syndrome.

Langdon Down also noted that people with Down syndrome could be very self-willed and stubborn:

> 'No amount of coercion will induce them to do that which they have made up their minds not to do.'**

A problem with any physically recognizable condition, such as Down syndrome, is that stereotypes are easily attached to it; and we all tend to see what we are looking for. Once Down had attached these behavioural characteristics to the condition, everybody began to see them and report them. There are many descriptions of a 'Down syndrome' stereotype, and these often contradict each other. People with Down syndrome are supposed to be 'pleasant, gentle, outgoing and affectionate' as well as 'mischievous, sullen and stubborn.'

---

*From Down, JHL (1866) 'Observations on an Ethnic Classification of Idiots', *Clinical Lectures and Reports*. London: London Hospital. Reprinted in T E Jordan (Ed), *Perspectives in Mental Retardation*. Carbondale, IL: University of Illinois.
**Quoted in Penrose and Smith, GF (1966) *Down's Anomaly,* London: J. & A. Churchill.

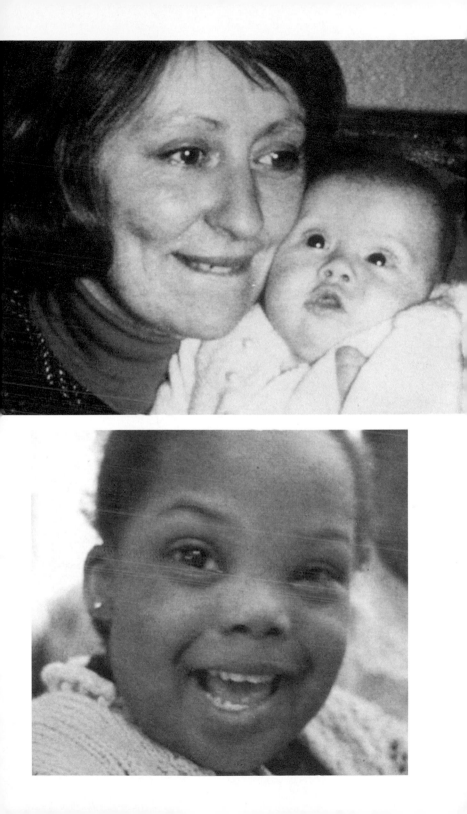

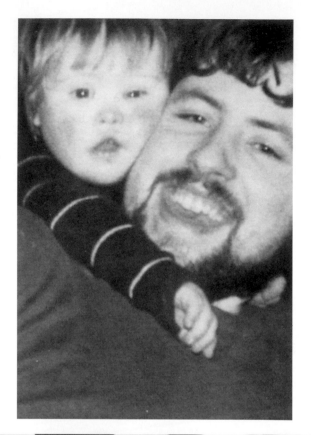

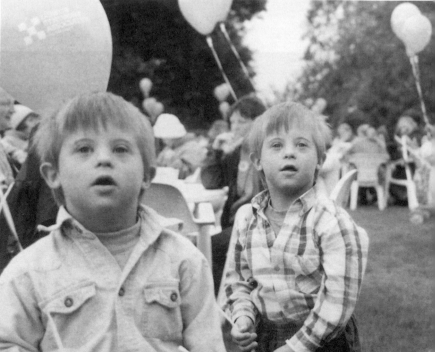

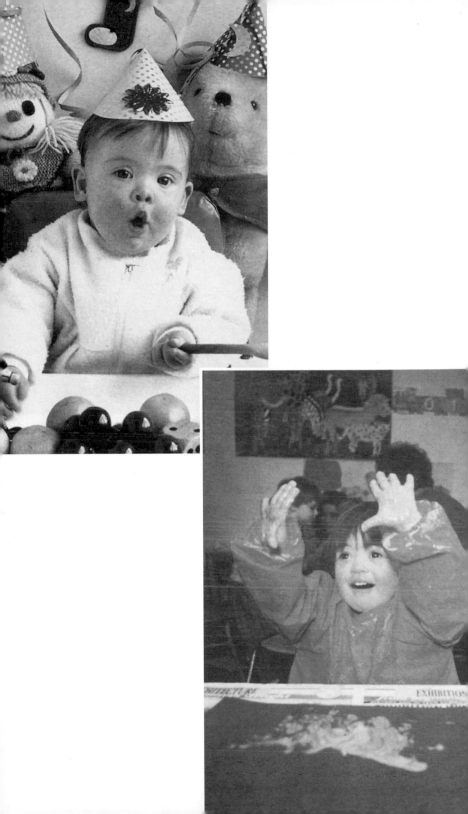

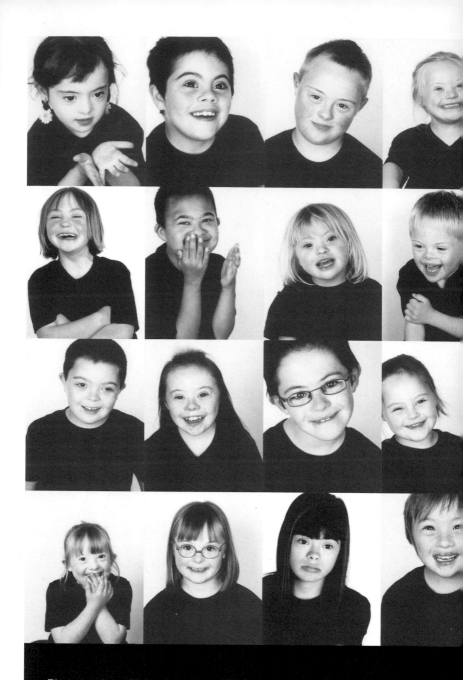

Photographers Richard and Fiona Bailey were inspired by their daughter Billie-Jo to create project '365'. It consists of 365 photographs of children with Down syndrome and represents the fact that between 1 and 2 children born each day in England alone, have Down syndrome.

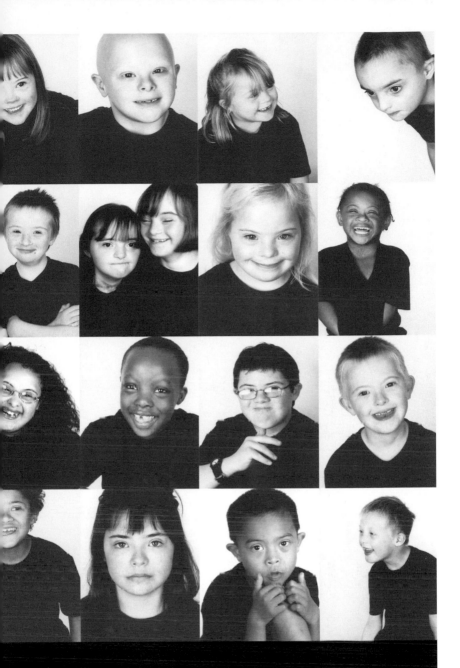

These pictures are a small part of this work, but certainly show the immense individuality between the children. Hopefully it challenges the simple idea that they all look alike. More information and the full range of photographs can be seen at http://www.ds2005.com

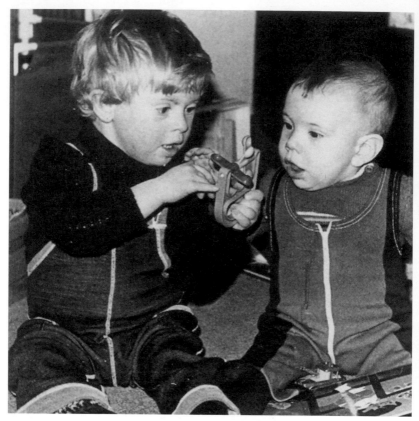

David and his brother Matthew.

With Matthew – David aged 5.

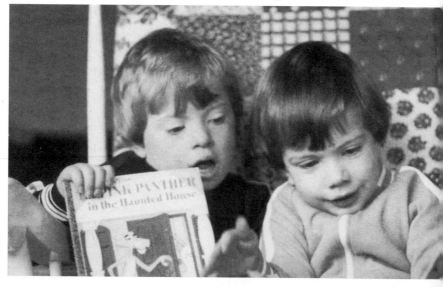

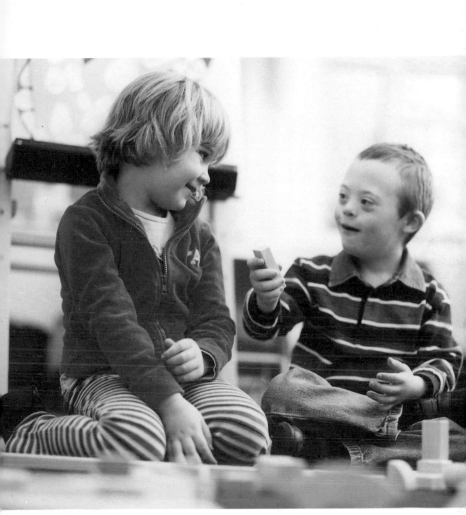

Learning togothor

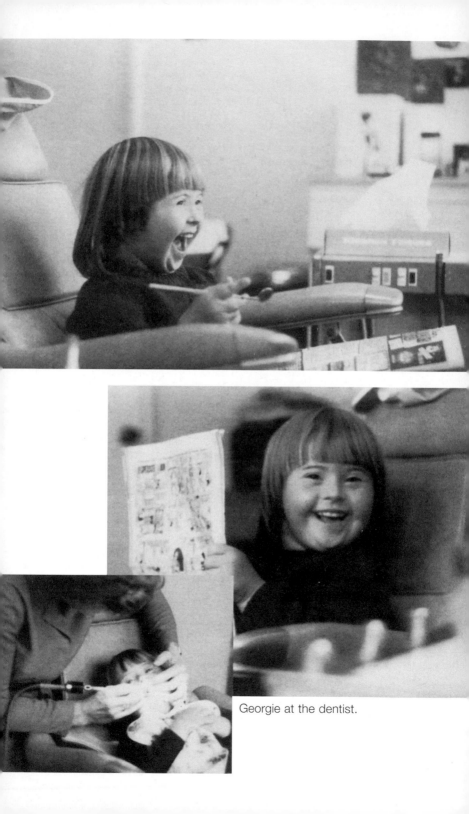

Georgie at the dentist.

Christopher and his family.

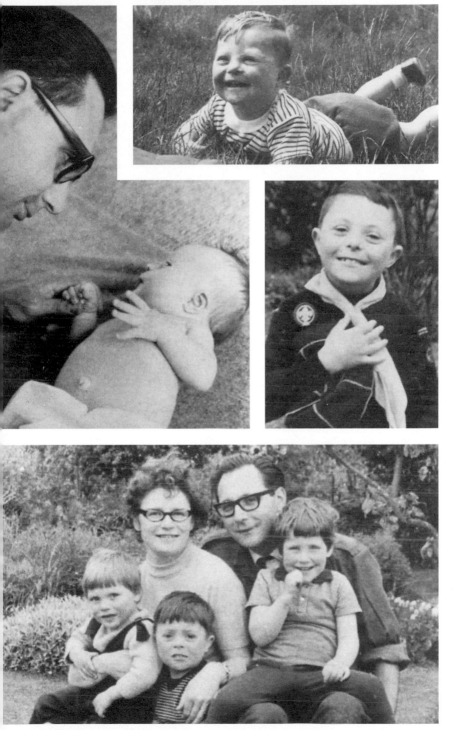

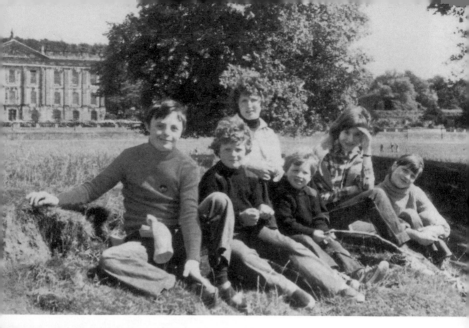

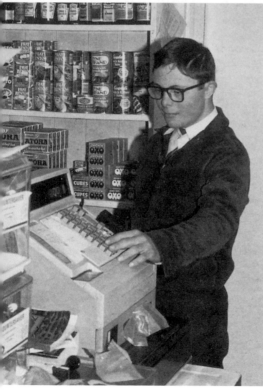

Christopher – 17 years.

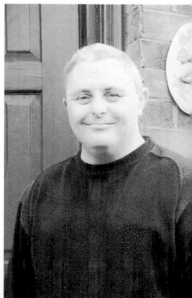

Christopher, 40+, outside his own house.

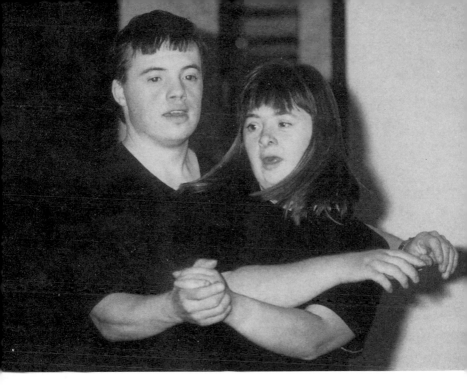

Linda and Gordon, picknicking just after their engagement.

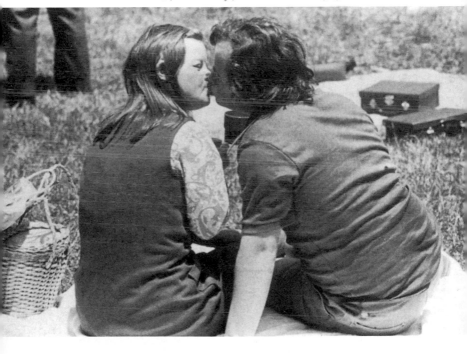

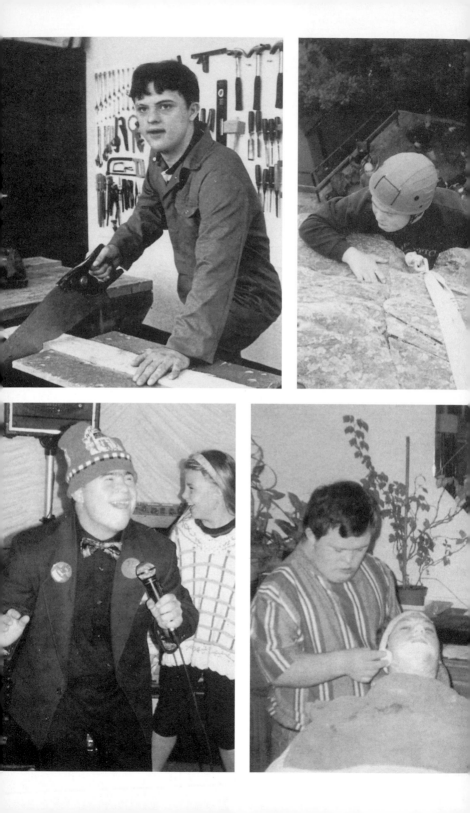

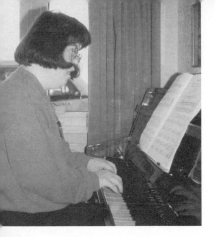

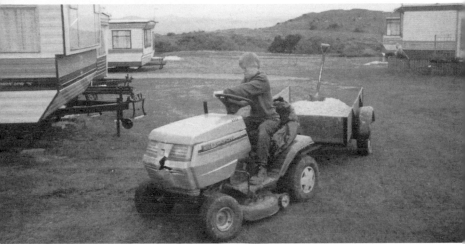

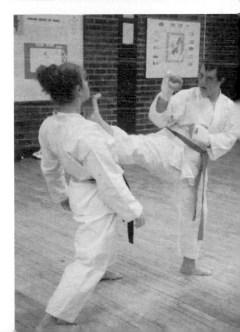

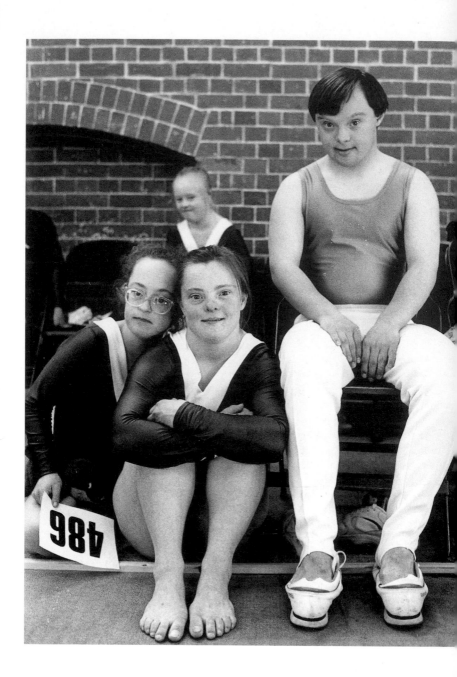

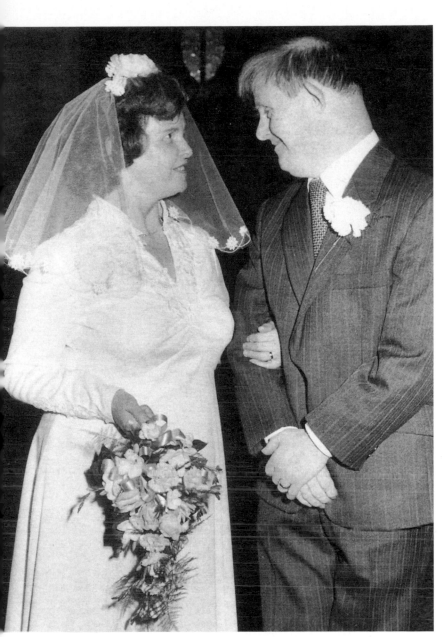

Mr and Mrs Rothwell – November 1981.
They lived very happily together until Mr. Rothwell died in 2000.

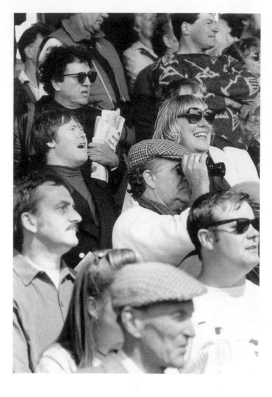

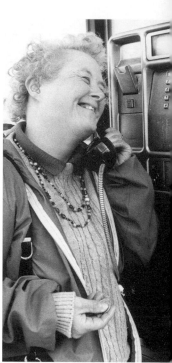

Annual Achievement Award finalist Dennis Cooper behind the camera.

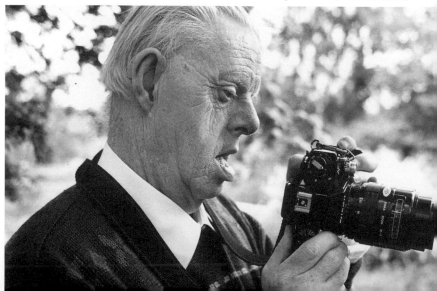

How parents and families 'see' the family member with Down syndrome is also important. We found that 40% of mothers of typical children said the child's temperament was like a close relative, compared to 12% of the mothers of children with Down syndrome. This suggests, that those parents who view the child as different may be more likely to 'see' in them the stereotypes of Down syndrome that they hear and read about. This may then influence how they treat the child.

As we will see, people with Down syndrome are very different to each other; and many studies do not support the idea of a strong or dominant set of behaviours. Before trying to summarize the research, I want to explain some of the difficulties in this area.

Influences on personality, temperament and behaviour

Your temperament and personality governs the manner or style with which you engage with the world. Much of this is seen in our social behaviour, but it also affects how you approach tasks, your persistence and desire to get it right, your need for new experiences and to be creative. Some of us are quiet, reflective and like to think before we act; others are outward going and impulsive. Some people are cautious, others take risks, some are confident and others anxious. The question is how do we get like this; what influences our personality and our temperament. We would all probably agree on the following influences that work together, or sometimes against each other, to produce our personality and temperament:

1   Our environment – this includes our surroundings, the way we are treated by others, our opportunities to express ourselves, and our experiences.
2   Illness, diet, drugs and alcohol – these affect our personality and social behaviour.
3   Our genetic code – innate characteristics can be seen quite early in very young children and can remain throughout life. Parents will often say that one of their children was always impulsive and energetic, whereas another was quiet, observant and cautious, even as a baby. It is this belief that part of our personality and temperament is inherited that leads to the idea that genetic information carried by the extra chromosome 21

in Down syndrome, not only affects physical and mental development, but also behaviour and personality. I find the idea that the extra chromosome produces people who are 'cheerful, pleasant and gentle' very consoling. Why should the effect of this extra material only be seen in a negative way?

4   Our intellectual and physical abilities – these result from genetic and environmental influences. If we are used to successfully tackling problems or engaging with other people, being liked or taking the lead, this influences how we think about ourselves and how we act. Children with intellectual disability often have difficulties with social skills and solving problems; they can grow up experiencing failure, especially if people around them don't expect them to succeed, or tend to direct them instead of encouraging them to make choices and actively participate. It is no wonder that some stop trying and become inactive or frustrated. Perhaps this why some people with Down syndrome are described as sullen and stubborn in later life, or just lethargic.

5   Physical and biochemical changes – though some aspects of personality and temperament are stable, we do change as we mature and develop. The happy, confident child may become a withdrawn and sullen adolescent. The introverted child may later become an entertainer. Our social behaviours and our sense of self change as we grow. Our increasing levels of intellectual ability help us to understand ourselves, and our world.

Is there a Down syndrome Personality?

Most of the early studies of the 'Down syndrome personality' were of children and adults living in large institutions. We now recognise that the results were more about the effects of institutionalisation, lack of stimulation and activities, and not being treated as an individual, than of the Down syndrome itself.

Children brought up with their families have been found to be more developmentally advanced, more outgoing and have wider interests and social skills (Chapter 10). They also have a stronger sense of self. It is not the institution as such that is the problem, but what happens within it. Smaller institutions, such as community or residential schools, which are well staffed and provide educational, recreational and social opportunities, produce positive and more able people. In the same way, families that fail to provide the essentials of care, security, identity, stability and opportunities for development usually have children who are more likely to develop slowly, have poor social skills and emotional problems.

Because so many different influences produce our individual personality and temperament, it is difficult to know whether people with Down syndrome have a characteristic set of behaviours due to the fact of having Down syndrome. I will describe what we know about the 'Down syndrome personality' starting with babyhood, through to adulthood.

Babies and the early months

In the first months, most babies with Down syndrome tend to be quiet and are unlikely to be difficult. Mothers frequently say what good babies they are, and how much easier they are compared to their other children. They are often described as placid, inactive babies who sleep a lot, especially those with heart defects or other complications.

Mothers in our research kept records of how long the baby slept, how often he or she cried and for how long, and how long they spent on activities throughout the day. We found that the babies with Down syndrome cried far less than typical babies – some didn't cry at all in the first weeks – and many slept through the night. Even so, they slept for about the same amount of time as typical babies. Some babies with Down syndrome are very lively and noisy from the beginning. Whether they were quiet and placid or noisy and lively in these first weeks did not predict how they were several months later.

The floppiness of some babies with Down syndrome means their physical movements are less vigorous. This can seem like non-activity and give the idea of a placid, inactive baby. I have found that many parents are a little afraid to handle the baby as robustly as a typical baby in these first weeks. Others are in a state of shock and confusion for some time. Some parents believe that sleep is best and tend to leave the baby in the cot – perpetuating the image of the quiet baby due to lack of normal handling and play. Once parents begin to handle and stimulate the baby, most usually become more active; by three to four months most are lively and responsive. Those who are not well may be quiet and fail to thrive; or may be unsettled and irritable.

My advice to parents is: don't rely on the baby to let you know when he or she wants feeding or needs attention. Instead, establish feeding, bathing and play routines. Give the baby lots of opportunities for stimulation and plenty of handling when awake.

Questionnaire studies of mothers who are asked to rate the temperament of their baby from around three months, report the same range of temperaments for babies with Down syndrome and for typical babies. Most mothers rated the babies with Down syndrome as content, happy and easy. However, when averages are compared for the groups, mothers indicated that the babies with Down syndrome show less positive moods and are more difficult to care for than typical babies. This is because a minority (but more than in the typical group) have difficult temperaments. For some, it is due to illness and anxiety of parents. Others went on to develop additional disorders and were often very slow to develop.

Toddlers and children

Their mothers rate the temperaments of toddlers with Down syndrome as no more difficult than typical children, although as with babies, there is a difficult sub-group. The few studies available show that children with Down syndrome vary as much as typical children at the same level of development, and that there is a lot of overlap between the two groups. This reflects the close link between their development and maturation and their behaviour. Most children with Down syndrome have similar behaviour to that of typical children at the same level of development.

As with the babies, there is a small group who have difficult temperaments. We found these tended to be children who mature and develop slowly or those who have impulsive, energetic and irritable temperaments from early on. As babies they were difficult to calm down if upset, often had strong mood changes and parents found it difficult to establish routines. They were more likely to have quite difficult behaviour problems in later childhood and some were still difficult as young adults. Several had additional disorders (Chapter 9).

We compared the temperaments of 105 children with Down syndrome aged between two and nine years, with 105 typical children aged one to five years old living in the same area. The mothers of the children with Down syndrome rated them as less emotional, less aggressive, less bossy, less moody and more likeable and affectionate. They were also more easily distracted from tasks and less persistent when doing something. This study was done in the early 1980's. A recent large study in the USA found similar results – the children with Down syndrome were rated as more sociable, more positive in mood, less persistent and more distractible. The children in our study are now adults and we are in touch with well over half. We recently compared their early temperament ratings with assessments of behaviour problems as adults. We found no statistical relationship, which may be due to problems in how temperament is measured. It could also be that, in the long-term, early temperament by itself is not that influential on the development of later behaviour problems. As noted above we did find a small number of individuals who had very difficult temperaments as babies and toddlers and continued to cause management difficulties as young adults.

Children, with or without Down syndrome have a great variety of temperaments; they range from quiet and thoughtful to impulsive and active. The overriding impression is that if the child has Down syndrome, she or he is more likely to be happy and sociable, less moody and aggressive, but more easily distracted.

STUBBORNNESS AND TEMPER TANTRUMS, AND MISCHIEF

When the child with Down syndrome is around three to five years of age, parents often start to say he or she is getting stubborn and self-willed. My impressions are that this may be similar to the behaviour of typical two to four year olds who are beginning to develop some independence, initiative and self-will: the 'I know what I want' and 'I can do it myself' stage. It is also linked with their ability to use language to express their concerns. There are fewer temper tantrums and self-willed behaviours in one-and-a-half to two-year-old children with Down syndrome than in typical children. By three to four years, however, children with Down syndrome are producing only slightly fewer temper tantrums than typical two-year-olds. Once the children with Down syndrome become mobile, they begin to 'get into trouble' and 'mischief' like any child. The type of trouble is very similar to that of any other child at the same level of development. As the toddler stage progresses, mothers of children with Down syndrome tend to report more mischief and trouble than those with typical children, and nearly eight out of ten are rated as being disobedient at some time. By three to four years most typical children have grown out of the worst of the 'terrible twos' stage as they learn to express themselves and to reason – this happens much more slowly in children with Down syndrome (Chapter 9).

Around a third of parents find their young children with Down syndrome demand a lot of attention, but for many this reduces dramatically in the teenage years as they develop communicative skills and can amuse themselves for longer periods. Around a fifth are not rated by their parents as showing the typical Down syndrome pattern of sociable, positive mood, less persistence and being easily distracted. This pattern is usually found in the children with less delayed development. They are less likely to be over familiar with strangers, quieter, persistent, and not easily distracted. They were more likely to be moody, fussy and show anxiety.

As children develop mentally, they are more able to understand and anticipate and, like everyone else, they can worry and get upset over ideas and thoughts, rather than just react to immediate events. This was illustrated when we asked parents if their children with Down syndrome had particular fears, phobias or worries. Like typical children, many had fears and in some they had developed into phobias. The few that were described as being 'worriers' were all beyond the three years level of intellectual development.

Older Children and Adults

Several studies of older children and adults have identified three main behaviour patterns in people with Down syndrome. The majority – about two thirds – are classified as being pleasant, outgoing, active, affectionate and sociable with a sense of humour – the classic 'Down syndrome personality'. A minority are described as being less able, and dull and listless, with few or no problems in terms of behaviour and management. The third group are described as aggressive, pugnacious, and sometimes very difficult to control. As our group of children have grown into adults we have found the same – a minority have become inactive, with very low levels of energy, and a few are extremely irritable, restless and difficult to manage.

Most parents report that older teenagers and young adults are easier to manage, as well as less active. Things like being argumentative, oppositional, and demanding attention tend to increase from early childhood and decline in late childhood and the teenage years. Between 20 and 30% of young adults with Down syndrome become somewhat withdrawn, secretive and don't seem to want to talk about things. Over half prefer to be alone, rather than in family company most of the time. Some become depressed (Chapter 9). For many this behaviour is no more than is found in typical adolescence. When we were interviewing young adults, for example, around half did not want their parents to be present during the interview, and several told us that what they were saying was a secret. Others said it was very nice to have a chance to talk about things like being an adult and growing up – implying they did not talk about these things with their parents. These were the more developmentally advanced young people.

It appears that there are quite a few teenagers with Down syndrome – some work has suggested as many as 60% – who become less sociable. They may smile less, are less outgoing and bubbly, and spend more time alone as they move into adulthood. As discussed later, there is no simple explanation of the factors related to becoming more withdrawn.

The other behavioural characteristic that has been repeatedly reported since noted by Langdon Down, is stubbornness. Studies indicate 70 to 80% of children and adults with Down syndrome are described as stubborn by their carers. This is far more than typical children and adults. It is not always clear what people mean by stubbornness. It may just be difficulty to get an individual with Down syndrome to do what you want them to do – 'once she has set her mind against it'. It can also include disobedience; 'not doing what he has been told to do', and oppositional behaviour; 'if you ask him he will do the opposite'. In many cases the child looks stubborn because they do not understand what is being asked of them. The instructions are too complex, or the behaviour of others is too quick for them to follow. So they just freeze or stand and do nothing.

Recent work suggests that a characteristic of Down syndrome is a difficultly in reading the emotional signs on other peoples faces – particularly negative information. A lot more work needs to be done, but if this is the case it would influence their personality and how they engage with others.

In answer to our questions, it would appear that we cannot rule out a 'Down syndrome personality' with the main character traits of being pleasant, good-natured, sociable, less emotional but also stubborn. However, the range of differences between individuals is so great that this group description is not helpful in practice. It is also clear that individual levels of development and experiences play a large part in the developing personality. Early temperament is not very predictive of how the person engages with their social world in later years.

Socialisation – how babies become people

Human beings are social animals. We spend most of our time with other people and engaging with them. To do this we use social skills – speech, language or signing and non-verbal communication skills such as touching, body language and facial expressions. We also spend a lot of our time thinking about what other people do, what we will do with other people and why we do what we do. So we need skills and knowledge about social conventions, rules, how people tend to react, what is acceptable and not acceptable social behaviour. This social knowledge includes having an idea of how other people think; it is impaired in people with autistic disorders.

Early interactions

We learn all this by engaging with other people. Feral children who grow up with animals, do not learn these skills or gain social knowledge. They develop the social skills and knowledge of the animals they live with. Learning starts with the first interactions between mother and baby. The baby arrives with characteristics that ensure a high chance that carers will engage with them and look after them – a wide-eyed innocent look and a reflex for sucking. They quickly develop social signals – cries that communicate hunger, pain, and a need for attention, and then sustained eye-to-eye contact, smiling, laughing, and reaching. By six to twelve weeks they are very responsive and begin to initiate social engagements. The baby will go quiet or look or smile at your voice. Soon the baby and carer are taking-turns in a sequence of communicative behaviours. The timing of pauses is learnt very early and can be found in all our everyday conversation throughout life. At around 6 to 7 months babies show pleasure, displeasure and eagerness in their facial expression and gestures. This helps others to 'read' them and to know how to engage with them. In turn, babies learn to 'read' the expressions or tone of voice of others. Learning about emotional life has started. By 8 or 9 months they are beginning to learn rules, such as stopping if you say 'no'.

Shared communication

Averting or making eye contact is a fundamental communication behaviour we all use throughout life. Young babies will look away from the parent's eye when they want to stop an engagement, probably because they cannot cope with too much stimulation. Mothers follow the eye-gaze of the baby and then respond as though the child had engaged them in a shared act of communication. For example, the baby looks at the cat and mother says, 'Yes, it's the cat, look at him washing his face'. This helps the baby learn about joint attention, sharing, and communication. By the end of the first year of life babies will look at something and back to the carer, to refer to something. This is called 'referential looking'; it is most clear in older children who look at mother to check it is all right to do something, like pull the cat's tail. Babies at this stage have learnt to recognise different people and are beginning to understand familiar words and use sounds and gestures to communicate. Early attempts include reaching for objects too far away. Parents interpret this as a communication, and move the object closer. Soon the baby learns to 'instruct' the parent by using a reach gesture. The baby reaches and then looks at mother to make sure she knows what is wanted. By 12 months the baby can make a clear pointing gesture. Pointing at a toy or some food can be a request, but by 16 months it is also used as a way of directing another's attention to something – like pointing at the cat doing something funny. This means the child has some idea of what other people might think. Studies have shown that during these 'referential' actions, babies look to check they have the other person's attention before they point, during the point and at the end to see how the other reacts. Babies very rarely point when no-body else is around.

These early forms of communication are helping infants learn about being a person as well as social skills. It is not just about making others do things, but about how others might think and feel. You point at something to share your delight, surprise or that it is funny. When you do, you assume the other person thinks the same.

Awareness of the outside world

Children need to learn who other people are, the differences between people and how they react to them, and the structures in social life. They begin with their immediate family – going to mother when they hurt themselves, father when they want to play physically, and brothers or sisters to watch what they are doing. They begin to establish their identity within the family starting with their name, and then learning about how the family 'sees' them; 'he's a very happy boy', 'she's clever at dancing', 'he's my brother and a pest', 'she doesn't like people talking to her'. At the same time, they are beginning to understand kinships such as mum, dad, sister, cousin, granddad, auntie. From this, they extend to other social categories – friends, teachers, postman and eventually nationality. These social roles are often explored in play; 'I'll be the mummy and you can be the boy'.

This process of socialisation continues as the child grows and their ability to learn and understand matures. Their experiences increase as their social world expands from mother and baby to family, family friends and neighbours, to school, and to people and situations in the wider community. These engagements are secure and pleasurable if the child feels loved, valued, capable and competent. How they progress will be influenced by their temperament. Some are more cautious and timid when faced with a new social situation, others pile in with few concerns. A child who lives in a restricted situation without social interactions is unlikely to become skilled in engaging with others and becoming a member of that society. But merely placing a child in a social situation and expecting them to cope is not helpful. We need to find ways to help a child who is less equipped to learn naturally.

The natural process of becoming a socially competent person starts at birth and continues throughout life and for most of every day. It depends upon:
- The ability to learn and use social skills
- Understanding how others think and feel
- Learning the conventions and rules of your society
- Engaging in social situations

Social development in children with Down syndrome

Many studies show that babies and young children with Down syndrome follow the same development pattern as typical babies but at slower rates. The early social signals like sustained eye-gaze, smiling and vocalising appear days or a few weeks later than in typical babies. The slower growth means the differences increase with age. Gestures, like referential pointing, appear around 22 months – six months later than in typical babies.

Emotions

There are several specific problems. For example, many babies with Down syndrome have less intense social-emotional behaviours such as smiling and laughing – it is more difficult to get them to smile and they tend to smile rather than laugh. The same seems to be true for showing displeasure and crying. Carers can have more difficulty 'reading' the emotional expressions of many of these babies than they do with typical babies. This is partly due to the effect of hypotonia on the facial muscles, but also due to slower processing and reactions. There is also emerging evidence that many individuals with Down syndrome may have a problem with reading the emotional signals of others.

Attention

Some children with Down syndrome are passive with low arousal, and parents find they have to work harder to 'wind them up'. Some are more likely to follow and respond to the other person than to initiate an exchange. Although babies with Down syndrome do point, they don't point to request things as much as typical children at the same level of development. They also explore their environment in a different way. We found that over a set period of time they look at their mother's face for the same length of time as typical babies, but typical babies switch their attention from mother to other things and back again far more often. We found the same thing with sound: babies and toddlers with Down syndrome would listen to a selected nursery rhyme for longer than typical babies before switching to the other channel. So it seems that babies with Down syndrome are less likely to switch their attention, I think because they need longer to process information and formulate a response.

Responses

Many studies have reported how you often have to wait quite a long time for children, and many adults with Down syndrome, to respond to an input. But if you prompt them – touch their elbow, point, say the start of a word for example – they will respond. This suggests that they may have the skill or knowledge reasonably well consolidated, but that there is a specific problem in getting it out within the appropriate timeframe. From my observations, familiarity and routines help to trigger responses. Because a routine is a sequence of actions, each action acts like a prompt for the next. It is not just the actions but also the settings that can act as prompts or triggers. We all have to think a bit more when performing a very familiar action in an unfamiliar setting. Often this is because we have to make small adaptations or decide if the response is appropriate in the new setting. Such experiences lead to adaptive behaviour; giving the young child opportunities to experience new places and routines is beneficial, but this needs some planning to ensure the child feels safe (Chapter 3).

Social behaviour

We have noted that many children with Down syndrome are very sociable. They often appear to prefer social things rather than objects, and this continues throughout life. It can become a problem if you are trying to get the child to do a puzzle or look at a book. They seem to get easily distracted and prefer to engage with the person rather than the object. One theory is that they have learned to prefer social stimulation because others compensate for their problem by initiating things. When they try to do something, like reaching and picking up an object, even from an early age, they fail to achieve their intention and become frustrated. Constant failure is likely to lead them to stop trying or to becoming dependent on others.

Protecting babies from 'failure' is a natural reaction of carers (see below), but if the baby shifts into social interaction and away from the object, then they are not getting experience with objects. It is not quite as simple as this. If children with Down syndrome quickly learn to prefer social things, we might expect them to use more pointing and gesture than typical babies to initiate engagements with people, and to get what they want. But they do not; in fact they use less pointing. So it is not just how we engage with them, other things like physical development, arousal and thinking are all implicated.

Even so, studies of two to five year olds have argued that children with Down syndrome avoid learning opportunities and tasks that they see as difficult by getting into social interactions with others and seeking help to solve problems. It could simply be that they are easily distracted and find people more interesting than toys. Or, it could be that they take longer to initiate and react, and life moves too quickly for them. All these explanations may be true to a lesser or greater extent for children with Down syndrome. We met some who refused to do any task, and others who could not wait to get amongst toys and objects. Others happily set up their own games and did not like to be interrupted.

We saw something of this when we examined how infants with Down syndrome develop visually directed reaching. They look at an object, open their mouths showing they want it and intend to put it in their mouths, reach for it, but can't quite co-ordinate the reach. Typical babies show strong intentions around 12 weeks and skilled reaching for suspended objects by 16 weeks. For those with Down syndrome, the intentions appear around 14 to 16 weeks but the skilled reach comes around 22 weeks, with some taking up to 30 weeks. They hit a small plateau with their reaching skill when trying to co-ordinate visual and motor inputs (Chapter 7, the Nervous System). We found that many of the babies quickly gave up trying to reach and shifted to playing with their clothes and looking around and at people, rather than looking at the object. People are delighted if the baby looks or smiles at them and either play with the baby or give them the object.

DEALING WITH FAILURE

Intentions – wanting to make something happen – usually come before the action – doing something to make it happen. If the intention drives the child to new things, but only practice at it helps him or her to become skilled, then babies and young children will naturally experience quite a lot of failure and frustration.

Most mothers are sensitive to the baby's signals and tend not to let them fail too much. But babies also have to learn that there are things out of their control – at one stage they spend quite a lot of time reaching for shadows before learning that they cannot grasp them.

Typical children show different reactions to 'failure' at different ages:

- At 14 to 16 months children show anger and frustration – early temper tantrums
- at 18 to 24 months they show refusal to continue or start, and 'stubbornness'
- From around 22 months they show help-seeking behaviour by asking or getting others to help or do things.

These reactions don't disappear with age – we adults show them all – but generally, we learn self control and what is acceptable or not to others. This requires an ability to inhibit the reaction and regulate our behaviour. Although difficult, we need to find a balance between success and failure because young children with Down syndrome do need to be encouraged to initiate, cope with frustration and try again, and become self-regulating.

Self-determination and motivation

Babies and children learn through their desire and persistence to achieve. We are all born with an internal drive to explore and master our environment. It is an urge towards becoming competent and controlling our own lives. In early childhood, psychologists call it 'mastery motivation'. The child sees a toy or situation, and intentions or questions come into their head; they have a natural desire to test them, for example, 'Can I climb through that tunnel?' "Can I get this object into that box?' This becomes more observable from around two years of age when they begin to insist they can do things for themselves. It is a self-directed activity and relies on the feeling of satisfaction at having achieved something or solved the problem. You can see it in the child's persistence, even when others might give up because it is too difficult. It is a strong force for learning.

It has been suggested that this motivation is not as strong in children with Down syndrome. The main theories as to why are; they have not had the opportunity to learn to succeed; they have a more passive nervous system and don't get aroused; or they have some deficiency in setting up intentions, processing the meaning of their actions and creating a response. Recent studies, however, indicate that the majority of children with Down syndrome are usually as motivated as typical children *once they get involved* in a task that interests them. They are just as persistent, and show satisfaction and pride in their achievements. My thinking is that most children with Down syndrome start out with this built-in drive to become competent, even though they may not show the same amount of energy and range of exploration as typical children. As with most things, they are slower in developing different interests and ideas. For example, most typical children are particular interested in cause and effect toys up to a year or so and then gradually shift to, and persist longer with, toys that have some goal, such as a puzzle. This is because their intellectual abilities have grown; they have the memory and attention span to keep in mind the end goal while trying different solutions. Children with Down syndrome make this shift at a later chronological age, but at about the same level of development as the typical children. However, their drive, motivation, self-competence and control is also influenced by how we engage with them and so we can influence their self-determination.

Positive interactions

We need to ensure that our interactions with the child foster rather than hinder self-regulatory and independent ways of learning.

Early studies of mothers of children with Down syndrome found their interactions with the babies were likely to be more directive and instructional than mothers with typical babies (Chapter 1). It was as if they went into a 'teacher' mode on the assumption that they had to teach the baby everything as quickly as possible to counter the disability. For example, one study found that more mothers of young children with Down syndrome took more control over the child's play by selecting toys and getting the child to use them in certain ways, than similar mothers of typical children. However other mothers of children with Down syndrome tended to focus on the toys selected by their child, and they maintained longer periods of joint attention with the child rather than just directing their play. The children of these mothers showed more understanding of what was being said to them. So the style of interaction helped language development. We also found less mastery behaviour in the children with Down syndrome whose mothers were rated highly for dominance, directiveness and activity. In contrast, mothers who encouraged the child to work independently at a task had children who showed higher levels of mastery behaviour. A recent study from the USA found something similar; mothers of the young children with Down syndrome used more teacher and helper behaviours and less verbal instructions than mothers of typical children at the same developmental levels. Like ourselves, the researchers felt that this reflected the emphasis of parent-training programmes (Chapters 1 and 11). There is now a shift towards advising parents to engage in a less directive and more sensitive style of interaction. I certainly think this is the most helpful way for the child. Fortunately, in my experience, only a minority of parents have a very strong anxious, intrusive and 'teacher' type of interaction with their child.

Positive mother and child interactions

A body of research has shown that the later social and mental development of children, with and without Down syndrome, is more advanced and with fewer behaviour problems when the mother's style of interaction is:

- Warm and positive rather than critical or distanced.

- Relaxed rather than fussy or anxious — children are more likely to show signs of anxiety if their parents also have higher anxiety ratings on psychological scales.
- Responsive and sensitive to what the child is doing — making sure the input is appropriate for the level of ability and interests at the time, and that their actions relate to and respond to the child's actions.
- Subtle rather than intrusive or too instructive approaches — directing the child's attention to different things, then following the child's lead and extending what the child is interested in.

Most research uses mothers as it is convenient —I can't see why the findings should not be applied to all carers.

The idea of early and highly structured training is not just an issue for children with disability. In several countries it has become popular with many parents of typical children, who seek activities soon after the baby is born, driven by a belief that such early interventions are beneficial. Many mothers, even those who don't really believe in such a structured life-style in the early years, can get sucked into it by worrying that they are not doing the best for their child. How much mothers engage in these activities varies between countries and ideologies. For example, a recent Portuguese study found that the mothers of young children with Down syndrome intervened less and were less directive in a play situation, than those of the typical comparison children. This could be because they did not believe these children could be helped, and so did less than normal. As described in Chapters 10 and 11, such beliefs could deprive the child and result in delayed development. The Portuguese researchers felt this style would help the children become more adaptable and self-reliant.

Slow and simple communications

As noted in Chapter 1, I always advise new parents to slow down the natural speed of taking turns in conversations. I also emphasise how important it is to develop sensitivity to the babies' communicative signals and to try and ensure an appropriate response. A characteristic of intellectual disability is a difficulty seeing the important bit of the input – this could be in a picture or when 'reading' the subtle facial expressions of others, which may be impaired in many children with Down syndrome (see earlier). A possible solution is to exaggerate and simplify the inputs – tone of voice and length of utterance, facial expression and touching. We all know that some people can get babies to respond easier than others; they are confident with babies, expect to get a reaction and are not self-conscious. I think the rule is to relax and enjoy and focus on the process of the engagement rather than getting some product or outcome from the baby.

Reduce distractions

Many children with severe intellectual disability become distracted by the social input when they are being taught. This is probably because of their limited attention span and difficultly in monitoring several inputs. Don't put yourself between the task to be learned and the learner. I find it helps to work alongside the child or from behind, and to help as little a possible. This a-social type of teaching may seem a bit strange, and obviously it should be used for some things and not others. If you are teaching a board game you have to be social but not distracting. A-social teaching has received some serious attention over the years by a small number of people in the UK; it is worth exploring when the child seems very distracted by social inputs.

Praise and encourage competence

Another recent study looked at how mothers facilitate pride in their young child with Down syndrome. These researchers found that mothers of children with Down syndrome provided similar levels of direction and were equally as responsive as mothers of typical children, but they praised the child more often. Mothers have been found to gradually fade out their more directive attempts to prevent the baby from 'failing' as described above, and gradually increase behaviour that encourages the child's sense of competence; 'yes, that's good, you can do it if you try that there'.

They shift into a gentle prompt and a light touch rather than an overly instructive style. This is all related to what parents feel is the right way to help babies and young children, and their individual child. They will behave differently depending on the purpose. For example they may want the child to learn to act independently, and to be confident and happy; or they may want him or her to master a skill as quickly as possible. If they think the child can't learn something by him or herself, they are more likely to try to train them.

Matching input to the child's developmental level

How we engage with other people is influenced our understanding of their abilities, by their role or status in the relationship, and by what we think is the purpose of the interaction. Understanding the child's stage of development helps us to work within their zone of development rather than expecting too much or too little. It also helps us select more appropriate toys and activities, and what we might focus in the engagement. Most parents are quite good at judging within a few months the developmental level of their child with Down syndrome. Many find using development checklists helps (Chapter 10). Matching inputs to your child's current abilities and interests is not that easy. Typical toys and games that are used with any child are equally useful for children with Down syndrome, but they will often need some guidance in how they work and more practice than a typical child.

Studies show that helping parents to be more sensitive in the way they engage with the child has a positive effect on the child's development and self-confidence. But parents should not get overly concerned. We should all examine our style of interacting and way of thinking about children and adults with Down syndrome. We should think about the issues raised above, and the chances are that we will find a style that works in individual relationships.

REALISTIC EXPECTATIONS

Expectations of what children with Down syndrome can achieve will influence our behaviour toward them. In the past expectations were low and achievements were low. This has changed in many countries, often through increased publicity and broader changes in out beliefs and attitudes toward disability. The focus in the media is usually on positive stories and more able people with Down syndrome. This can shift the image to the other extreme and result in unrealistic expectations for the majority of children and adults with Down syndrome.

As part of the staff preparation for the inclusion of children with Down syndrome in mainstream schools, I decided to check the teachers' knowledge and expectations of the level of achievements of these children. They were asked to estimate the average age of achievement of developmental milestones and academic skills, and I compared this to the information from our research. To my surprise, most of the teachers in these schools overestimated what the 'average child' with Down syndrome could do, as well as what the children with Down syndrome who were about to be integrated into the school, were likely to achieve a year or two later. Using the same approach, a study of student teachers in Scotland found similar results. A study that recently caught my attention concluded that mothers of children with Down syndrome had unrealistic expectations about the child's capacity to respond to instructions and tasks. In the 1970's we had found the opposite. Another study looking at the quality of communication between a person with Down syndrome and someone else, found it was poorest if both partners had Down syndrome and best if the other partner was a typical student of the same age, but without experience of people with Down syndrome. This pair had better communication than if the parent was the partner. It seemed that the parents used more complex and open questions, whereas the student did more checking that the communications were understood. This is what happens when we try to talk to a stranger in a different language. We use shorter more factual phrases, checking with signs and repeats that it is understood. The students in this study may well have been unsure of their partner's abilities and had no pre-conceived ideas of what to expect. If so, they are likely to adopt the effective strategy of proceeding slowly and finding out how best to fit in with the other person's abilities and knowledge.

Communication

Communication is something we do with other people. It is often seen merely in terms of speech and language, reading and writing. But communication includes facial expressions, gesture, posture, taking turns, keeping on track with the other person, or repairing the conversation if it goes wrong e.g. asking people to re-phrase something or asking a question to be sure you both understand. We all need opportunities to use and develop such skills, by talking with other people.   Unfortunately, there are several barriers for most children with Down syndrome in their development and use of communication. Many will have hearing problems (Chapter 7), as well as specific problems with language development. This is not just slower to develop, but lags behind their general ability, and most find learning grammar and syntax very difficult (Chapter 10). But, as many of us find when trying to communicate in a foreign language, we can do a lot of socialising and communicating with very poor grammar and syntax.

Many people with Down syndrome have major problems with speech and articulation. Most have a prolonged period of unintelligible speech until they are 5 or 6 years old. By the early teenage years, people who know the child well can understand what they say, but strangers find it very difficult for nearly three quarters of the boys and just under half of the girls. Studies have shown that when we cannot control important aspects of our environment, we are likely to develop 'learned helplessness' seen in low motivation, withdrawal, and high dependency. Therefore, encouraging communication from the early months is important.

SIGNING

One way to avoid some of the consequences of poor communication is for the parent, and significant others, to learn and use signing with the child. If you can communicate you can engage socially; it seems reasonable to assume that this helps social development and reduces the risk of unsociable behaviour. Reports from families who have used signing support this, and show that the children who sign are not delayed in developing language. Talking is a far more efficient way of communicating than signing, so children do not choose to take the harder path. Reports indicate that the young children of parents who have used signs as well, have a bigger vocabulary consisting of spoken words and signs.

There is no substantial evidence that early signing reduces the later difficulties with language development, as is sometimes claimed; but it certainly does help functional speech and communication. Many parents start using it when their child is around 6 to 9 months of age. Speech and language therapists can give advice about when to start and which signs to begin with. How well children learn the signs depends on their general development and practice. It helps if all the family, and the pre-school and school, learn and use the signs. Some children with Down syndrome have major speech and language problems and don't use signs very well; there are systems that use symbols instead.

Reading other people's social signals

As noted earlier, recent research highlights that many older children with Down syndrome are less able than typical children at reading the emotional expressions on people's faces. It might be due to a lack of opportunity and experience, but if they live in a typical family then this seems unlikely. It may be they are less able to detect subtle changes in expression.

For some, it may be that their level of development has not advanced to a point when the association between such expressions and their meaning can be made. There is a developmental sequence to recognising and understanding emotions. Children with Down syndrome are generally very attentive to faces and people and by the developmental levels of 3 to 4 years, they can recognise sad, happy, angry and scared facial expressions and will label them and apply them to themselves. If they see someone showing signs of distress, they will usually comfort them by touching and stroking and telling them it will be all right, cheer up and so on. In fact many are described as being very good at cheering people up; as one father told me:

'my son is the best anti-stress therapist I have, after a bad day'.

A recent study has reported that while children with Down syndrome respond to others who are showing emotional distress, they do not actually become distressed in the way typical children do – they do not become distressed when another is distressed. This suggests they have less empathy with the other persons expressed emotion.

It is often reported that many children with Down syndrome do not appear to get very distressed or emotional over things. This raises the possibility of an inherent difference associated with the syndrome. Another recent study has suggested a problem with detecting or processing negative information. It may be that some children and adults with Down syndrome may have problems visually processing some quickly changing facial features, or perhaps they cannot connect the visual input with the appropriate feelings. This is a relatively new area of research and we need to fully document the range of individual differences between people with Down syndrome and how they understand emotion, before making too many conclusions.

But it does suggest that it is worthwhile drawing attention to facial and emotional expressions and helping the child develop some understanding of these.

Society and people who are different

Throughout this chapter, and previous ones, I described how what we do and think is influenced by the society we live in. Therefore, before discussing how people with Down syndrome see themselves, I want to briefly look at the issues of people who are different and society.

Sociological theory argues that most societies try to protect themselves from people that are different because they are often perceived as a threat. The usual reactions when faced with a difference are:

- to eradicate,
- to exclude or
- to remediate or try to make it as 'normal' as possible

I think we see these responses to Down syndrome, and this tells us about our society and may help us examine our own feelings and actions.

Eradication

The main example of eradication is foetal screening and termination. In the past, there was a reluctance to treat life-threatening conditions if the person had Down syndrome, and this remains in some countries today. It is often defended on the grounds that the person with Down syndrome will not have a reasonable quality of life; but considering how happy and contented the majority are, and the fact that they do not 'suffer' from the Down syndrome, this argument does not stand up. The eradication must be for others living in the society. There has also been much pressure to stop people with Down syndrome reproducing. It is argued, with some justification, that women with Down syndrome would put themselves at risk with a pregnancy and would face many difficulties bringing up a child. Another frequent objection is the high risk of producing a child with Down syndrome, implying it is best to avoid a child with Down syndrome being born.

Exclusion

Until recently great efforts were made to exclude children and people with Down syndrome – they were placed in large institutions away from public sight. This policy was supported by arguments that it was for the person's own benefit – to protect them from people in society who would exploit or abuse them. It is ironic that a policy of segregation is defended on the grounds that there are deviant people in the society who cause it. Similar issues relate to segregated schools and leisure activities.

There are lots of examples of protests by people in a neighbourhood against setting up a centre or homes for people with disability. All sorts of arguments against this are raised, including the possibility of threats to the local children from people with intellectual disability. After several years of such housing, there are now very few protests in more enlightened societies. Fortunately, we have shifted from responding to a social category such as intellectual disability or Down syndrome, to looking at individual needs and then matching the solutions to these needs. Hopefully, the days are over, when all children and adults with Down syndrome are seen as the same, and needing the same 'solution'.

Remediation

Trying to remediate and make people with Down syndrome 'normal' is probably the most common reaction. This ranges from facial surgery (Chapter 11) to instructional approaches with an emphasis on conformity rather than choice – 'making them as normal as possible'. Being able to behave in socially acceptable and appropriate ways is important, but we can't produce a homogenous society. Far more of us have a disability or difference than those who fit some mythical 'normal' model. Rather than just focussing on making people socially acceptable, we should question how we might change society to be more tolerant of differences. An inclusive society is one that delights and celebrates variety between people.

Awareness of Down syndrome and disability

The two distinctive characteristics of Down syndrome are physical appearance and intellectual disability. Both are easy to recognise and neither is valued in any culture. When the common reaction of people is not to value those in a different social group, then being a member of that group carries a high risk of feeling unwanted and stigmatised. This can have negative consequences for how people feel about themselves and for their mental health. For others it can be a challenge that brings out their best qualities.

Parents will remember their own feelings and reactions when they learnt that they had become part of a new social group – 'parents of a child with Down syndrome' or 'a family of a handicapped child'. Some years ago well-meaning people used the slogan 'a handicapped child means a handicapped family' as a way of drawing attention to the needs of families with a child with a disability. Unfortunately, many felt stigmatised, and for some it added to the feelings of inadequacy and guilt they already had. It is no wonder many families retreat into small safe and self-supporting groups with other parents of similar children.

Self awareness

Not surprisingly, negative public attitudes trigger reactions and responses in people with disability. Studies have described how many people with mild intellectual disability have low self-esteem and a negative picture of themselves, if they are aware of their status as 'retarded' or 'different'.

Many respond by trying to pass as 'normal'. This can lead to social isolation; their non-disabled peers reject them but they reject those who are similar to themselves. Others try to compensate for their disability by working harder and being more compliant. Quite a lot of people with Down syndrome are described as not coming to terms with their disability, minimising their difficulties and having an unrealistically high sense of competence, self-esteem and expectations.

Of course it is not as simple as this. For many people their disability does not have to be their only identity. We all belong to different groups, we prize and value different things and we can

move in and out of different social identities. If people with
Down syndrome have a range of experiences and opportunities,
they will have a variety of potential identities and reference
groups. A strong family identity and feeling supported, helps the
child and young adult to explore who they are and what they
value.

Developing awareness and social identity

In Chapter 1 (Telling the other children) I described how children
begin to understand themselves, then classify others and put them
into social categories like boys, girls, people with glasses, kind
people, clever people, people with disability and so on. There are
reports that young people with Down syndrome appear to come to
understand disability in the same way, and we recently confirmed
this.

We investigated the issues of awareness with the young people
with Down syndrome in our cohort. We asked them if they had
heard of 'Down syndrome', 'disability', 'handicap' or 'special
needs'? Did they have Down syndrome and disability? Did their
friends have Down syndrome or disability? What was it? We also
asked their parents if and how they told their child they had
Down syndrome and what their reaction was. To see if the young
people recognized the facial features of Down syndrome we used
a set of passport photographs of young men and women with and
without Down syndrome. If they recognised the facial features we
then asked them to place their own photograph on one of the
piles.

Recognition and understanding

We found that about 40 to 50% of young people with a
developmental level of less than 4.5–5 years were rated as having
no recognition and awareness of Down syndrome or disability.
About 10% of these seemed to be gaining some awareness, but it
was not easy to determine and it had no obvious impact on their
lives.

There were a few exceptions where young people were at a
higher level of development but had no apparent awareness. It
seemed their parents might have protected them from learning and

knowing about the disability, by not drawing attention to it. Some of these young people did not have strong features.

Most parents said they talked openly about Down syndrome and did not try to hide it. About a third never tried to explain because they felt their child would not understand; another third took a reactive approach, waiting until something indicated the child might recognise Down syndrome before talking directly with them. The rest were proactive and did try to tell the young person; they were afraid their child might suddenly find out from others in a 'not very nice way'.

'I wanted to make sure he learnt about it from me so that he understood it was OK and no problem'.

Many parents said that their child had not really understood. These young people were usually those at lower developmental levels. Most parents were good at knowing just how much their child would understand.

The group who were aware but whose level of development was below 7 to 8 years, described Down syndrome and disability in terms of physical or sensory characteristics similar to typical children of the same age.

'got glasses, flat head, little nose, little ears'
'there's one boy with disability, he can't do anything, in a wheelchair with his back'
'I'm handicapped 'cos got a bad heart'

Some described disability as not being able to do academic things or learning slowly. This reflected the most common explanation of disability that parents used – needing more time to learn things. Several mentioned positive social aspects; for example that having Down syndrome meant they could go horse riding or swimming:

'handicap means going out with friends to leisure, bowling. Penny comes with her parents'

TRIGGERS OF AWARENESS

Most parents found they could not hide the Down syndrome even if they wanted to, because there were many triggers of awareness. The facial features were frequent early triggers, but so were physical problems such as a heart condition, and social factors like attending a special school. The facial characteristics become identified as distinctive around the 4 to 5 year developmental level and may act to trigger self-identification and discussion within families. But even when the young person recognises that others look similar and form a distinctive group – Down syndrome – they did not appear to automatically place themselves within this group for the purposes of social comparison.

Making comparisons

Like the rest of us, many of the young people readily shifted their reference or comparison group depending on what was being discussed. Some would talk about being disabled because of their heart problem, and then that they were not handicapped because they were good at reading, and having Down syndrome meant they could go to bowling. Some compared themselves to people worse off, or not as good at something as they were, and so felt positive about themselves. In other words they chose what to focus on, which bits to ignore, who to compare themselves to. We all do this as part of ensuring we feel good about ourselves.

There were instances when the young person indicated Down syndrome was not a permanent thing:

'I did have Down syndrome but not now.'

Others suggested they had some limitations like not being very good at writing but that if they just keep trying, they will succeed. Several young people linked Down syndrome with specific things, like not being allowed to drive a car, going to the pub on their own, and getting a boy or girl friend. None of our young people described particularly 'bad' incidents, but their parents did note things like name calling and bullying, or not being chosen to play in the team or asked to a party, which some of the young people associated with the fact they had Down syndrome. Fortunately such incidents are not common and relatively few (less than 20%) of our young people appeared to have been distressed as a result. Many failed to see the implications of the actions of others, while the more able often decided it did not matter. Like any child, such events had only temporary effects if they felt loved and cared for within their family and group of friends, and led interesting and active lives.

As noted in Chapter 1, seven to eight years is the key developmental transition when children begin to make relative social comparisons. They shift from using just physical characteristics and actions, to more social and psychological concepts. They talk about who is better at something than someone else, who is more popular, who is aggressive or does silly things, and how such behaviours affect people's lives. Once children begin to make social comparisons and form social categories they also begin to attach value judgements based on their experience and the attitudes of others. We found the same with our young people with Down syndrome who began to make reference to the effects of Down syndrome on social life, often in comparison to others:

'Mum told me about it. Not really aware, sometimes I am if I think someone is better than me, put myself down a bit – I shouldn't have gone for him, he's brilliant, I'm not brilliant'

'I've got Down syndrome, I'm handicapped. I go to special school for people with handicap'.

And parents' descriptions:

'She says she doesn't see many people with Down syndrome getting married and having children, and asks "can I?"'

The descriptions of Down syndrome become more abstract as young people begin to search for more sophisticated explanations:

'Down syndrome, born ... a kind of disease ... I know four

people who are handicap, three in wheelchairs and one deaf . . .
I have Down syndrome . . . don't know if I'm handicapped . . . I
guess I am but I don't feel handicapped . . . think I might be'.

'A disease you catch it never goes away, have it all your life and
I wore a proper Down syndrome jumper, means I have got
Down syndrome, I'm in the community. Born handicapped all of
us started as a sperm, a little baby, out of your mum's tummy.
I know that everybody has got like, everybody has got genes, if
you have Down syndrome, I have got 26 chromosomes, I was
born Down syndrome and someone added chromosome'.

These descriptions correspond to the explanations the parents said
they had given, except they did not say it was a disease. Disease or
illness is how typical children try to explain the Down syndrome or
intellectual disability, before they have an understanding of the brain
and how it works. It seems the young people with Down syndrome
are doing the same. The idea of illness, disease and suffering was
very common in the past and here we see it as a natural explanation
arrived at by children.

**I think we should try to help the siblings and child with Down
syndrome to understand the differences between illness and
cognitive development or disability as soon as we can.**

When we asked parents to recall how much their child with Down
syndrome made social comparisons compared to their other children, the general response was less often. We also found it quite
difficult to get the young people to make comparisons or tell us
about things they did not like in other people. I think this relates to
their problems with processing facial expressions and emotion
(describe above), but this is speculation. Generally, they focussed on
positive things, which may be why they were seen as very positive
people. This was also found when we measured their self-esteem.

How do people with Down syndrome feel about themselves?

At age 7 to 8, typical children are rapidly developing social comparisons and forming social categories to make sense of their world

and how they fit into it, at this age they change in their understanding of their own self-worth or self-esteem. Up to 7 to 8 years of age they usually feel very positive about themselves and score high on scales of self-esteem. They usually see this in terms of specific things like being competent in running, singing and schoolwork. At around 7 to 8 years they integrate this specific understanding into an overall view of self-worth. Studies of children with a disability at this age (or developmental level) find reduced self-esteem in those who feel they are less competent or in a less valued social group. This is also true for children and adults with Down syndrome. High levels of self-esteem are found up to the 7 to 8 year developmental level; after this, social comparisons about their self-worth lead to some reduction in positive feelings.

I feel that this reduction is less likely for many young people with Down syndrome compared to others with similar levels of intellectual disability. As I noted for personality, it may be that the extra genetic material programmes a higher likelihood of being content and happy, and a protection against negative feelings.

Feelings about having Down syndrome
Some people feel quite positive about having Down syndrome; they associate it with pleasurable activities. Others certainly do not view it in this way. Some young people associate having Down syndrome as the reason why they are not allowed to do things they see others of their age doing. Particular issues related to learning to drive, going to University or on holidays or to the pub without their parents. A few women felt that the Down syndrome caused restrictions on marriage and having children.

Denial and avoidance
Around 20% of the young people showed signs of difficulty. Some, mainly the men, refused to talk about Down syndrome with us; they appeared to deny it, or not apply it to themselves. For example, when sorting the photographs one young man said '*Ugh*' to every picture of a woman with Down syndrome, another shook his head saying, '*she's Down's*', implying he was not having anything to do with people like that, and two others were quite explicit; '*I'm not one of them*', '*definite not me*'. The parents of these young people verified that they refused to talk about it, denied it and avoided any

We asked the young people with Down syndrome, to tell us about themselves. Of the sixty or so who we felt could respond, only one spontaneously mentioned Down syndrome and disability. When we asked the question, 'Is there anything you would like to change about yourself or your life?' most could not think of anything. Of the 22% who could, only two referred to disability; one said *'I want to be normal, so people would be kind'*, and the other *'To be normal like everyone else. Go to University and get a degree. Have a perfect chance to get boyfriend. Get out more, get a better heart, able to do gymnastics. I want a full life'*. Others referred to physical changes such as being taller and changing their hair colour, but none referred to facial features. Some wanted to meet pop-stars, get the local football team started again, or as one young man said; *'win the lottery, be rich, get a car and go on holiday with a beautiful girl'*. (see Chapter 9, on talking to self and fantasy). Some of the young people refused to answer the question; they appeared to have difficulty about knowing they had Down syndrome.

situations where they might meet other people with Down syndrome or disability. The young women were less likely to deny and avoid discussion and more likely to describe practical implications and how they tried to understand them: ' *won't marry a man with Down syndrome because we might have a baby with Down syndrome'*. This comment came from one of the most intellectually able women with Down syndrome I have met, and could be a rationalisation for not liking the idea of Down syndrome.

Many of the parents in our study highlighted a negative experience in mainstream settings, such as staring, bullying, problems getting a particular girlfriend and inappropriate social behaviour. Living in the less protected environment of the mainstream, can increase the likelihood of the person becoming aware and realising the negative aspects of Down syndrome; but we only found this to be true for those who were functioning at the appropriate cognitive level.

Men and women

The men in our study seemed more reluctant than the women to discuss emotional issues – perhaps men and boys with Down syndrome may be just like their brothers and fathers in this regard. The fact that girls and women with Down syndrome develop more quickly and more of them achieve higher levels of development (Chapter 10), might explain why there were mostly women in the group who stated they had Down syndrome and talked about limitations on their life-style.

GROWING AWARENESS – AN INDIVIDUAL EXPERIENCE

The developmental sequence of growing awareness is well illustrated by the comments of an 18 year old woman with Down syndrome. She is among the most able; when she was seven her mother estimated her developmental level was probably around five to six years. The mother recalled the comments of her daughter over the years:

At seven years old: *'All children with Down syndrome have glasses. I don't have glasses, so I don't have Down syndrome'*, and *'that girl is always pushing . . . because she has Down syndrome. I don't push, so I don't have Down syndrome'.*

This illustrates the focus on physical attributes and actions; also that at this time the girl was aware of Down syndrome as different and did not want to be part of the group.

At 14 years old: *'I am finished with Down syndrome. I am a teenager (or young lady) now'.* And also, *'I don't want to talk about it. The subject is closed'.*

Down syndrome was a characteristic of her childhood that she felt she had grown out of and did not want to be associated with.

At 16 years old: Her mother found her making faces in the mirror and asked why. *'I'm practising my expressions so people won't know I have Down syndrome'*

She accepts she has Down syndrome, and probably, that it is permanent. She is attempting to pass as 'normal.'

At 18 years old: she has mainly been with typical children and teenagers in mainstream school, but as part of her vocational training she has to work with a group of people with disabilities, including some in wheelchairs and others with quite severe intellectual disability. She now experiences problems, especially when going out with the group. It seems that by being with the group she feels her Down syndrome will be noticed and she will be stigmatised.

'First the other people (the public in the street) see the wheelchairs and then look at the others in the group too and then they think, ah-ah all handicapped! All stupid! Can't read and write! People stare and eye us with contempt and with low regard'.

Telling and explaining

I think we need to be proactive and openly talk about Down syndrome when appropriate. We need to let the children or young people know they have Down syndrome and that when they want to talk about it we are available. Then we need to be alert and reactive if they have experiences and need some explanations.

The meaning of Down syndrome for one person is not the same as for another – it will vary with their ability, knowledge and situation and life-style. Down syndrome may be an important category for society, but, from our findings, it may not be prominent in the sense of self for many people with Down syndrome. We do not have to force all the information and implications onto them. What matters is the impact of the Down syndrome on the person's life. This should guide us when trying to explain the meaning and implications to people with Down syndrome. We should avoid making it an unnecessary issue or creating worries. Our primary objective is to help them feel competent and to have a positive sense of themselves as adults.

A young person's awareness is growing at a time when they are

**AN ELOQUENT DESCRIPTION OF JANE'S JOURNEY OF
AWARENESS OF DOWN SYNDROME,
RECALLED BY HER MOTHER.**

She has always heard the word (*Down syndrome*) since small. We talked openly in the family . . . about 12 to 13 years old – when she went to secondary special school . . . she was asking if her friends had Down syndrome. She was happy with the idea, would pick out people with Down syndrome. She thought they were the same as ordinary people but with Down syndrome looks. When she was 18, we were in a review with the Social Services. The social worker started to read the school report aloud – 'Jane who has Down syndrome . . .' Jane interrupted, 'excuse me' she said 'I did have Down syndrome but not now'. She was in a special school . . . a cocooned environment . . . she was happy and protected. When she went on a school leavers course at 16, there were many people who looked normal and were more able than her . . . but they had social problems. Some were not nice and one bullied Jane. It was around this time that Jane began to react negatively . . . to feel the stigma . . . she began asking 'what does it mean, what happened, why am I like this?' I explained something went wrong in my tummy before you were born . . . it made it harder for you to learn things . . . but we are very proud of you'. Jane now goes to college and has asked her tutor 'What is handicapped, what is Down syndrome?' . . . she was told 'we don't use words like that' . . . but Jane wants to know why. Soon I'll try to explain chromosomes and problems with jobs and people and having children. But you just have to wait until you feel they are ready and can understand and take it slowly. Now she is fairly happy with the idea, but feels she doesn't really know what Down syndrome is . . . she has started going back through old school photos and finding people with Down syndrome.

becoming independent and are less likely to want to discuss some things with parents. Like many older teenagers and young adults with a chronic illness or problem, they may want to protect their parents from seeing they are distressed. Yet they may not have other people or a peer group they can talk to. Schools and colleges need to make time and space to discuss these sorts of issues, but if the young person is the only one with Down syndrome in a mainstream situation, this may not be possible. They can talk with a teacher or counsellor, but this is not the same as sharing thoughts and feelings with peers. Perhaps this is why parents find that older children attending mainstream school can benefit from meeting up with others who have Down syndrome or other disabilities.

Chapter 3 covers how parents can help the siblings of children with Down syndrome find ways of explaining it to others and dealing with name-calling. Some children with Down syndrome may also have to learn to cope with other children (Chapter 9) and talking, giving them words or acting out scenes may help (Chapter 11).

Summary

1 Most young babies with Down syndrome are rather quiet and placid and less likely to demand attention and feeding. Parents need to establish routines ensure opportunities for stimulation and plenty of handling.

2 Children, with or without Down syndrome have a great variety of temperaments; they range from quiet and thoughtful to impulsive and active. The child with Down syndrome, is more likely to be happy and sociable, less moody and aggressive, but more distractible than a typical child.

3 About 30% are difficult and demanding but many improve by there late teenage years. Most adults have a 'Down syndrome personality' – pleasant, good-natured, sociable, less emotional but also stubborn.

4 There is some suggestion that a characteristic of Down syndrome is an impairment in 'reading' the more subtle signs of emotion in others and possibly having less or different emotional responses.

5 From birth most children with Down syndrome appear
   less equipped to engage with others and learn about
   social life. They largely follow the typical sequence of
   social development. How others engage with them from
   birth has a significant impact on their development of
   their social skills, self-motivation and confidence.

6 Just under half do not recognise they have Down syndrome. Those with developmental levels over 4 to 5
   years show increasing awareness. The sequence is the
   similar to that found for typical children. Those with
   developmental levels above 7 to 8 years make social
   comparisons and many become aware of stigma. Open
   discussion about their Down syndrome appears to help.
   Some deny their differences and this can result in isolation and depression.

9

Behaviour and psychological problems

- **What are the chances of the child having significant behaviour problems?**
- **What sort of problems are they?**
- **What causes them?**
- **How can we manage behaviour problems?**
- **Do they get better or worse as the child grows?**
- **Do people with Down syndrome have mental health problems or developmental disorders?**

This chapter is in two parts. The first is about behaviour problems and how to manage difficult children. The second is about mental health, developmental disorders and psychological problems. Only a minority of children and young people with Down syndrome will experience such problems and parents may wish to skip over the second section. If you make this decision, you may want to look at causes and management of behaviour, talking to self, and routines.

What is a behaviour problem?

It is more than a child's behaviour that makes something a problem or not. For one family, the child getting up at night and coming into their bed is not a big problem, for another it is a catastrophe.

When we asked parents to tell us about any ongoing behaviour problems they were having with their child, around a quarter said there were none. When we gave them a standard checklist of behaviour problems all ticked off something.

> 'There am I saying we don't have any problems and now I've ticked off a dozen or more. But you get used them and sort of live with them'.

From the early days of childhood through to adulthood, we used questionnaires and interviewed parents about the behaviour of their children and how they tried to deal with problems. It is this information that informs most of this section, but I have related it to other studies to try to arrive at an overview.

What sort of problems are they? Are they different to typical children?

Most parents of babies and infants with Down syndrome experience similar problems to those of parents with a typical young child. But as the child gets older, behaviours that are manageable in smaller children become more difficult. Dealing with a large child of six years old who is running away or having a temper tantrum is not the same as dealing with a 2 year old.

For a minority of babies and children, mainly those with severe intellectual disability, the problems are somewhat different, and as we will see later, others may have a development disorder such as autism as well as Down syndrome.

When compared to the typical pre-school child, the children with Down syndrome had more problems going to bed and settling down to sleep (20%); waking up at night (over 40%); sleeping with parents (24%); poor concentration and attention seeking (20%); and fears and worries (15%). However, they are reported by their parents to be more socially engaging and quicker to get involved in and enjoy new activities, compared to their siblings.

Part of this 'out-goingness' is because their ability to inhibit or control their reactions is slower to develop, as is their understanding of social rules. As the children get older, and in extreme forms, these behaviours are seen as impulsive, attention seeking and poor

concentration. They are linked to behaviours that parents find especially difficult including constantly interfering with other peoples'
things, inappropriate behaviour towards strangers, running away in
shops and in the street, and throwing things (discussed in detail
later). We found that over a quarter of the younger children with
Down syndrome had some of these difficult behaviours, though few
had several.

In contrast, the most common problems noted by parents of typical children at the same developmental level were emotional ones:
faddy eating and night wetting, being overactive and restless; high
dependency and clinging to mothers, and having more difficult
relationships with brothers and sisters.

This low occurrence of emotional problems may relate to the
general low emotionality that may be characteristic of many individuals with Down syndrome (Chapter 8). It does change with
development and experience, as illustrated by looking at 'fears and
worries'. Parents noted that around 15% of the young children had
fears and worries, but by adulthood 80% said they had had a fear or
worry during their childhood years and many adults still had fears,
such as of spiders, dogs or loud noises. Fears or phobias are learned
when things happen to you, so as you get older you are more likely
to have them. Worries demand more understanding of experience
and what might happen in certain circumstances. We found worries
were only reported in the children whose mental ability was above
the three-year level of development. Parents reported that only 12%
were worriers or brooders. Most were happy and contented.

What are the chances of the child having serious behaviour problems?

In the early years, 70 to 75% of the mothers in our study felt they
had some behaviour difficulty with the child. This is about the same
as for mothers of typical young children. Many of the mothers were
confident that they were coping, and that the behaviour was not too
distressing or disruptive for the family at this time; 16% felt that they
had no difficulties at all.

About 12 to 15% of families were experiencing a lot of problems
that were distressing and disruptive; this is greater than you would
expect of similar families with typical children. Some of these

problems were part of profound disability and developmental disorders (see later). My overall estimate is that about 5 to 8 % of children with Down syndrome have these additional disorders; they are not 'normal' for children with Down syndrome, but a separate condition.

From mid-childhood through the teenage years, about half the mothers said that coping with behaviour problems was the hardest thing they had to deal with. This compares to about one in five who felt the hardest thing was trying to help the child's development, and one in twenty who felt it was health problems – often a severe heart condition. Behaviour problems and difficulty 'managing' the child reduced in late childhood and adulthood, with far more parents feeling they had no particular difficulties with behaviour.

What causes behaviour problems?

To answer this question we looked for any characteristics of the child, the family or their immediate situation, that occurred more often in children with behaviour problems. We then tried to understand how they might have acted together to cause the problem, keep it going, or make it worse.

Health problems
Younger children with health problems, such as respiratory problems and ear infections, tended to have more behaviour problems. This link was greatly reduced by the teenage years, but parents of adults with Down syndrome and poor health were still more likely to say they had behaviour problems than those in good health. These may lessen because health problems reduce as the child gets older; or it may be that parents are less willing to tolerate certain behaviour in teenagers, even when they are ill. We all tend to be more lenient and indulgent with younger children, and with those who are ill. So we may be more lenient when faced with a combination of Down syndrome, being 'younger' for longer, and having more illness. However, because these children take longer to learn things, they also take longer to 'unlearn' less acceptable behaviour. It is better to be firm and consistent from the beginning than trying to sort things out later.

Intellectual disability

The children most intellectually disabled were more likely to have a range of behaviour problems. These centred around being overly active and attention seeking, taking longer to mature and grow out of 'terrible two's' type-behaviour and temper tantrums, and being slower at reasoning and developing self- control. Some parents said their teenagers with high levels of behaviour problems could not amuse themselves or be left alone for more than 15 minutes, and a few, far less than this.

Family relationships

In Chapter 3 I noted how children in families with poor relation-ships had more behaviour problems. We found a strong association between a mother feeling stressed and behaviour problems in the young child through to adulthood. Although some of the stress might be caused by inherent behaviour difficulties in the child, for many it was related to family problems and the family's resources. In some families we found poor communication and a lack of consis-tency. For example, reprimanding the child for doing something one day, but letting it go when they do the same thing the next day.

Practical resources

Inadequate housing, unemployment and low income interrelate to put stress on families, and in these circumstances we found more behaviour problems for the children with Down syndrome and their siblings. Parents can find it difficult to create a pleasant, con-sistent atmosphere because of the competition for time and space. There may be no garden, or it is too small, or too easy for the child to get out of, there may be no place to store things, so younger children get into everything. There may be no space for other chil-dren to do what they want without interference.

Coping styles and beliefs

We found that mothers who tended to be anxious and who got easily agitated and worried, had children with more problem behaviour. In some cases, they felt they had more problems but in fact, observations of the family showed the child had no more prob-lems than others. Others tended to attribute the problem to the child, and just put up with it. Parents who coped through wishful thinking – hoping it will get better – had children with more problems. Parents who tend towards wishful thinking, need to make the first step to recognise the problem may be with them, and then start to change. It can be done, although some parents may need outside help. We found parents who had a problem solving style had children with more skills and fewer behaviour problems, despite have similar children with Down syndrome and family circumstances.

Adjustment to the disability

In a small number of cases we found that a poor relationship between the parent and the child was linked to behaviour problems (Chapter 3). Many of these parents showed poor adjustment to the disability – they had not really come to terms with it. There was a tension between the parents and the child, and more critical comments were made about the child or the effect of the child on their lives. As above, parents who had a positive view of the child and used an active problem solving strategy had warmer relationships with the child, children with more skills and fewer behaviour problems, even when they were at the same intellectual level and had similar health problems.

The chances of behaviour problems are much reduced if:

- The child's development is not very delayed – the intellectual disability is less severe (Chapter 10).
- The child is in relatively good health.
- The child lives in a family where the father is employed, their house is adequate, they have a car and reasonable finances. Or, in single parent families these resources are available.
- The family has high levels of social support from family, friends and services.
- The mother has low anxiety scores and tends to use an active problem solving approach to problems, not wishful thinking.
- Parents have come to terms with the child and his or her disability.
- The parents and children in the family have a positive relationship.

I use this information when trying to help families who are experiencing major problems. It is like the resource checklist described in Chapter 1. If we identify a lack of resource we can work on that, rather than jumping into a behaviour management programme.

Managing Behaviour

Just under half the parents in our work said that they were less strict with their young child with Down syndrome than with their other children. Less than one in twenty felt they were stricter; these tended to be parents who were concerned that the child would become difficult because of the Down syndrome. Sometimes parents' feelings about the disability and the child prevent them from being firm. As described above, these approaches are linked with more and longer-lasting behavioural problems.

Many parents experience difficulties when their child with Down syndrome is three to four years old. Developmentally, they are in the 'terrible twos' stage, they are 'into' everything, have limited ability to express themselves and reason, they demand attention and have temper tantrums. Many parents said they had to become stricter at this time, and most tended to use the methods of discipline that they would apply to their other children. Some continued to indulge the child, and were less consistent in demanding reasonable behaviour compared to their other children.

The basics of good discipline are sensible rules – but not too many – consistent responses, clear communication and not rewarding behaviour we don't want.

Here are some quotes from parents about the most helpful things they did:

'We refused to treat him differently from his brother and sister or to make excuses for him'.

'We set up rules for how the children would behave and did our best to make sure they kept to them. What would be tolerated and what would not. But we tried to keep them to a minimum –

I think you can overdo it and expect them to be too perfect',

'After reading about the sort of problems that might happen I had this image of a monster. Then I made myself think he'll be OK. Most of them are just like other kids but slower. Same problems. So I made a list of priorities – things I insisted on'.

'We tried everything – shouting, pleading, distracting, bribery and reasoning . . . none of it worked. Eventually we found that just turning away worked, not even looking at him until he ate properly. When he did we quickly got in there and told him how good he was'.

'I realised that he had no idea when I was cross. It was because I spoke to him like my others, firmly and explained things, but he didn't understand. In fact he just laughed and did it more. I learnt to look straight into his eye, and pointing my finger straight at him, up close said NO! Then I would keep looking at him. If he carried on or I didn't see he was upset, I said it again, just the same. I only did this when I was very cross and he soon learnt what it meant'.

'We were told that it is best to ignore temper tantrums. Even the slightest attention is rewarding. So when he did it we just turned and walked away. When he stopped I counted to 10 and went back and told him how nice it was to have a smiley face boy. But I couldn't do that in the shops. If he started I would take him straight outside – leave all the shopping – not speak or look at him until he stopped. Mind you I had to keep the reins on him or he would have run off'.

Controlling Behaviour

The main idea behind behavioural control methods – or behaviour modification – is that behaviour is learned if it is rewarded and it disappears if it is not rewarded, or if it is associated with unpleasant things. You may think that showing the child you are angry, or threatening the child with not watching TV or having a biscuit is a punishment. But if it has no effect, it should be seen as a reward; the child is rewarded by your attention. We have to ensure we do not reward the behaviour we don't want, and that we communicate what is acceptable and not acceptable clearly and consistently. If parents are inconsistent in the way they respond, they are actually teaching the child to persist with the behaviour.

Tackling the problem head on may not always be feasible. Adjustments to the home can often help to reduce tensions and frequent clashes. For example, if the child tends to wander off, then putting bolts on doors and fencing in parts of the garden may be the most sensible solution. Similarly, rather than battle to teach the child not to interfere with people's things, precious objects can be placed in unreachable places and cupboards can be locked. You can gradually introduce more normality as the child matures, for example, allowing one object at a time (not too precious or breakable) that they must learn not to touch.

Avoiding triggers

We all know there are situations that trigger or set off some problems. For example, when the child is overtired and you want him to brush his teeth; when you are rushing to get him dressed for school; when you sit down for a rest. Knowing the context allows you to avoid potential conflict. Often we get caught in these situations but eventually give in. The child then learns he or she can get away with not doing as they are told. The child can take control and produces the behaviour at exactly the time or place he or she has learned that it will have the greatest impact – or reward. Choose your battleground; a time, day, situation and action when you can see the thing through.

Controlling rewards

Controlling rewards is the way most of us try to ensure a child behaves well. In the young child the reward or reprimand must occur very quickly, and within their short memory span. There is no point in telling them off for something when they have already moved on in their thoughts or actions to something else. Delaying a reward or a reprimand weakens the chance that the child will understand that the action and the reward are linked. As they develop you can use more sophisticated methods. Star charts are visual, easy to understand and the child can see his or her 'good behaviour' grow. You can only use one or possibly two at a time and they have to be focussed on specific behaviour.

Seeing the plan through

If you do try a plan of action, be positive and do not give up after a few days. In my experience, such attempts usually fail because the problem was not fully understood and analysed, or because everyone gave up before the child had time to learn what was expected. If the child has established a real habit over many months or years, it is hardly likely to be re-learned in days. Many parents have told me they have tried something and it failed but when they describe what they think they did, it was quite clear they had not understood the problem or had not continued long enough.

Replacing the behaviour

A standard rule when modifying behaviour is to ensure that you replace the behaviour you are trying to stop with another more acceptable behaviour. If the child is doing something for attention or stimulation and you stop it, then they will quickly find something else to meet their needs. Odds are it will be even more problematic. So before stopping a specific behaviour, always work out its replacement and make sure it is incompatible with the unwanted behaviour. For example, the main behaviour for one family was the child grabbing people from behind when they sat down on the settee, or standing in front of the TV or fiddling with the controls and even hiding them. It was clearly a case of attention seeking. Every time one of these behaviours occurred the family would just get up and leave the room. After a minute or two, a member would return and sit at the table and start colouring a book. The child with Down syndrome would soon join in. The rest of the family would return. After a few weeks the child sat colouring and members of the family took turns to give her some attention. Initially they gave her attention at quite short intervals, and then gradually the time lengthened until she actually worked mostly on her own and then asked for someone to look at the final result.

Managing specific behaviour problems

When there is a specific and well-entrenched behaviour you will need to analyse the problem carefully before attempting to modify it. The three stages in this are:

1   Determine what happens that may trigger the behaviour. This could be a particular event or a place.
2   What exactly is the problem? Describe in detail what the child does.
3   What happens immediately after the behaviour that could be acting as a reward.

Only when you have clearly worked out these three aspects, can you begin to plan to control the behaviour and try out ways to get rid of it. Sometimes you try to ensure it is not triggered, other times you change the rewards. Often you need to start this by writing down what you observe – what you think is the trigger, the behaviour and the reward. Sometimes when the parent stops to write these things down, they find the behaviour changes or disappears. The act of writing has broken the link between the behaviour and how the parent responded to it – the reward was the attention.

The Most Common Problems

Constantly interfering with other peoples things
This impulsive attraction to new things can be positive; it is seen in toddlers when they get mobile and start exploring all corners of the house and cupboards, or their siblings' toys or homework. Typical children quickly learn what may and may not be approached, and later, what is yours and what is mine. If the child is out-going, active, impulsive and enjoys getting into things, then the family soon learn to be on constant watch, ready to retrieve or protect their precious objects or avoid a mess. They are likely to jump in when the child starts to approach or touch things. Even the most slowly developing child will soon learn that if he or she wants attention or wants to express their anger, then interfering in this way will do the job. We have all seen this in typical children and siblings who take a favourite object and tease each other.

From the beginning, parents need to use a consistent response when children interfere with things they should not. Consistent means that every time they do it, they are told no in the same clear way, removed from the situation and given an alternative. If the child increases the behaviour – they do it to tease you or get your attention – you need to give the minimal amount of attention, ensuring there is no pleasure or fun in it. Even eye contact can be a sufficient reward, and so avoiding it can be powerful tool in this situation.

Throwing objects

At around six months old, babies explore objects using three skills – sucking, banging and throwing. Some children with Down syndrome seem to get stuck in this, particularly the throwing. I think the reason for this is that throwing, and to a lesser extent banging and making a noise, is most likely to get other people to pay attention to them and engage with them. As described earlier, switching into others may compensate for not being skilled in doing things and entertaining yourself. What at first is a reasonable game of the baby throwing and others retrieving, can become a problem. Try to avoid throwing being used as a way of communicating and getting your attention – mainly by ignoring it and avoiding eye contact. When enough time has passed so the child will not associate the throw with your attention, find some other things for the child to do. You cannot avoid giving attention if the throwing is well established and the child is mobile, running around and causing chaos. But do so with the minimum of interaction.

Running away

Running and chasing is a favourite game for all young mobile children. But over half of all the children with Down syndrome in our study and one in five teenagers still did it. These children tended to be the ones who developed more slowly. It is difficult to make them understand the dangers of getting lost, of traffic or of being accosted. These things are not really learnt until 5 to 7 years in typical children. Most three year-olds can learn that they must not run away; and using reins with younger children is quite effective. Older children look very strange in a restraint and can run faster.

Try to teach them from the very first time it happens. This is a straightforward training exercise focused on the rule that if you run away I am not pleased. It can begin with using reins when the child is small. They pull or run, you give a very clear 'No', not a chase ending with swooping the child up into your arms saying, 'Come here, you little rascal'. Provided it is done regularly at the right stage of development, all that may be needed is walking them through the street with the restraint, and when they get to the park saying 'Now we can run and chase'.

Older children sometimes suddenly start running away. The first time it happens, you may need to retrieve them quickly. But then think of a safe place, and get someone else to keep a watch from a distance. When the child runs, say 'No' and either sit down and ignore them until they come back, or walk away and leave them. If they ignore you and make a bid for freedom, the other person can come to the rescue without setting up a link between the child running away and getting your attention. Some children and young adults just like to wander off. They need to be taught the consequences of doing this as we would with young children.

Inappropriate behaviour with strangers
Being overly friendly and hugging and kissing is very common in younger children with Down syndrome; just under half of teenagers and a quarter of adults also do it, and it causes serious problems. It is also found in other children with special needs and can be a consequence of head injury in typical children.

This over-friendly behaviour is often encouraged in young children, and is seen as a positive characteristic of Down syndrome until they get older. It is difficult to teach children with Down syndrome to control or inhibit their impulses, until they have achieved a three to four year level of understanding. But even at a young age, children can be trained to be less physical. Try to teach them an appropriate behaviour that also stops the unwanted behaviour – shaking hands instead of kissing, for example. When it does happen that they hug the stranger, be consistent in stopping them, and try to prevent the other person rewarding them by making a fuss of them. It is not easy, but being aware of this problem will often prevent such behaviour from becoming established.

Toileting
This is not really a problem with behaviour, but it illustrates slower development. Most children with Down syndrome become toilet trained later than typical children. With some exceptions in families that did not really try to train the child, our calculations suggest that toilet training is largely related to the child's level of

development. In other words, if you are finding that toileting is difficult, ask yourself if the child's general levels of ability are those at which you would expect most typical children to be trained. If not, then keep encouraging the child, but do not expect rapid progress and try not to make it too much of an issue or everybody will start to get stressed.

With the use of disposal nappies, typical children are taking longer to become independent in toilet skills. This is probably because they are comfortable and parents don't insist on training, because they do not have the extra laundry. The same may be the case for children with Down syndrome. I think parents should starting training when they feel the child is ready. In some cases, as with any child, toileting is not 100 percent for some years.

Sleeping problems

We did not find very strong associations between sleep problems and the levels of mental ability in children with Down syndrome. Many who were developmentally advanced had sleep problems and many slower children had none. Some of this was due to physical problems (Chapter 7 – airway obstruction) but we felt the difference was usually due to how the family treated the issue. Current research also shows that the treatment most likely to improve sleep problems is behavioural and not physical or medicinal.

The general rule is to establish a 'going to bed' routine as early possible. It will change over the first year or so, but work towards a routine that you would like for the older child. The routine is a sequence of actions that signal bedtime is approaching. For example; give a warning that it is bedtime in a few minutes, get the pyjamas out so the child sees them, find the soft toy that he or she takes to bed, bath or wash and change into pyjamas, brushing teeth, a cuddle and look at a book to calm down, into bed, a story. This routine will differ depending on the child's age and your family, but the idea is that by a series of small steps you lead into the final act of going to bed. It is not some sudden shock followed by a battle.

Timing is important. If you decide it is bedtime in the middle of a favourite TV programme, it will be difficult. Try to arrange it so that the child goes to bed when they are likely to be tired, but before they become overtired. If you have lost the schedule, then start to readjust it by keeping the child up a bit later or waking them earlier, and ensuring any daytime naps do not go on too long. Planning this with small steps over several days is better than trying to readjust too quickly.

Try to avoid letting your child fall asleep in your arms or on the settee and then putting them to bed. They may prefer this, but it can establish a habit that is difficult to break when they get too big to carry to bed. If you have stayed with the child to help them settle, gradually fade this out by sitting on the side of the bed, then a chair, or replacing yourself with a doll. I recall propping up a pillow and putting my hat on it. If the child wakes at night, have a program of small steps ready, with the first step being the most compatible with the child sleeping, such as stroking his or her head. Do not put the light on, pick the child up, play or take them downstairs to watch TV or have a drink. Most children will soon learn to wake up for this type of entertainment. If children get up and come downstairs, always return them to their bed and then use a programme of resettling.

The difficult one is when they come and get into your bed. Most parents enjoy it until the child gets big and wriggles and keeps them awake. Typical children normally grow out of this behaviour by the time they are five and start school. But for many families of children with Down syndrome, waking during the night and demanding attention is a major issue. It is better to try to resist setting up such habits when they are small, just for the sake of a nights sleep. Of course, as nearly all parents know, it is difficult to remember what you agreed to do at three in the morning, after several disturbed nights.

Here are some other techniques that you might try if you still have problems getting the child to stay in bed and go to sleep. The first is to keep the child up until they are nearly, but not quite asleep. Then do the routine. If they tend to get up, put them into bed, leave the room, wait for a minute and then go back and tell them they are good for staying in bed. Then leave the room wait for 2 minutes and repeat. Gradually you increase the time from putting them into bed and popping back in.

Things can still go wrong after routines are established. The child is ill and wakes coughing. Medication for the infection may help but the routine may have to be suspended. Try to get it re-established as quickly as possible. It is difficult to establish a sleeping through the night routine if a child has sleep apnoea (Chapter 7). A small number of children are hyperactive and have abnormal biological rhythms that make it very difficult to establish sleep routines. In such cases parents should seek out professional help. Many hospitals or clinics have 'sleep clinics' that can help parents who are experiencing problems.

Poor concentration, over activity and attention seeking

Children with lower levels of development are more likely to be rated by mothers as having poor concentration, being restless and attention seeking. Parents of these children have problems keeping up with them and keeping them amused, as most things will only hold their attention for a short time. Families can feel very strained when the child is very active and difficult to control, making noises or throwing things – often because of poor language and communication ability. It is often the unpredictability of the child, and the constant need for parents to supervise and entertain him or her, that causes the problem.

As the mother of a four-year-old boy remarked:

> 'I can't keep up with him, he never stops, he won't play with anything for more than a few moments ... he gets cross because I don't know what he wants ... I dread the holidays ... will he ever grow out of it!'

We found that the families who could share the task of amusing and stimulating the child with relatives and friends, who had access to playgroups, clubs and occasional shared care or respite care, appeared to cope better and experienced less strain. Some children with Down syndrome have attentional deficit disorder (see later) and families need to seek advice from a child psychiatrist or psychologist who specialises in children with such problems and learning disability.

Not all slower developing children are active and difficult:

> 'I know she isn't as bright or advanced as Alan, but at least I'm not run off my feet like Alan's mum, she's a very peaceful, gentle little soul and no trouble at all ...'

Things do improve – as one father said of his twelve-year-old son:

> 'Things are much better in the last year or so. Since his lan-
> guage came on we can have conversations. He is good
> company at times, before he just sat in the car saying yes or no.
> Mind you, I still have to be the organiser and entertainment offi-
> cer, otherwise he would just sit and watch TV all day'.

Other parents comment on the 'what's-he-up-to syndrome'. If
things are peaceful and they have not seen their thirteen-year-old
for over half an hour, they become anxious and usually go to find
out what is going on. This supervisory issue is common for the
majority of parents in the childhood years, and more so in the
slower children. However, the issues are not just about the child and
the disability; they include the support and facilities that are available to the family, and their views of the child.

Professional help

When things are very difficult, a child psychologist or other professional who specialises in child behaviour can be helpful. They not
only help with devising a management programme, but also provide
moral support and are more objective; especially for parents who
feel it just is not worth the effort.

> 'This psychologist came about the sleeping problem. We
> worked out a step-by-step program of what to do to get him to
> bed – a routine, really. We also worked out how I had to send
> him back to bed every time he got up. On his wall we made a
> chart and if he stayed in bed we stuck a star on it in the morn-
> ing. A big ceremony with lots of fuss.'

> 'I thought it was a waste of time at first. I had tried to reward
> him for not getting up before. If the psychologist hadn't
> been coming every week to check up on me, I would have
> given up.'

> 'I kept at it. Sending him back. It was only a few weeks but it
> seemed like months. It made me consistent. And it worked.
> Looking back it made me feel more confident about sorting out

problems. I won't give up so easy now or believe I can't do something to help'

'I had put up with her throwing food for over a year. Once the psychologist worked out the behaviour modification plan I saw an improvement in a few days and it all stopped within the month'.

HOW CAN MY CHILD MANAGE THE BEHAVIOUR OF OTHERS?

So far, we have been concentrating on behaviour problems in the child. Equally important is helping the child cope with the poor behaviour of other people. In Chapter 1 we discussed how parents can help the siblings of children with Down syndrome in ways of explaining it to others and dealing with any name-calling. Some children with Down syndrome also have to learn how to deal with other children who are teasing or provoking them, or daring them to do something. This can also include being approached by strangers. If the child has limited language skills it cannot just be explained. For a child with Down syndrome who has good visual skills and likes to imitate and act things out, drama and play-acting can be very helpful (Chapter 11).

Do behaviour problems get better or worse as the child grows?

Like other studies, overall, we found a steady decline in behaviour problems from late childhood into adulthood. In some families problems persisted whereas in others the same problem did not, and this was associated with the family problems described above. A few children appear to be developing quite well and then showed marked changes in their personality and behaviour (see later).

When the children with Down syndrome reached mid-childhood we found almost the same type of behaviour problems as when they were younger. Parents, however, said they caused more distress or disturbance because the children were bigger and older. During late childhood and the teenage years, fewer parents said these behaviours were a problem. For example, sleeping problems – rated as the most disruptive problem for parents – were reported by 66% of the mothers in mid-childhood and 53% in the teenage years. Running away, an equally difficult problem, was reported by 53% but dropped to 23%; interfering with others' things went from 58% to 36%; inappropriate behaviour with strangers from 52% to 42%; and throwing objects from 37% to 20%. All these behaviours carried on improving well into adulthood for most of the young people. In contrast, some problems were reported as more frequent. Poor concentration was noted as a problem by 20% of mothers in early childhood, 46% in mid-childhood and 42% in the teenage years. Attention seeking was similar, 20%, 42% and 39%. These different rates are part of the issue of what we expect and will put up with in young children, but see as a problem in older ones. By adulthood there were still around 20 to 30% of young people whose parents felt they had short concentration and needed close supervision; because some were less physically active, the problem was less disruptive.

Other behaviour problems that increased in teenage and early adulthood, related to the growing intellectual ability of the child. For example, being 'rude and cheeky' was reported in 63% of younger children but was not too much of a disturbance for parents. However, 66% of the teenagers were also felt to be 'rude and cheeky' and this caused as much difficulty as sleep problems. The child not doing as they were told, stubbornness, and aggressiveness, only dropped slightly from 67 to 63% between mid-childhood and the teenage years, but by the teenage years it was rated very high for the difficulties it caused. Swearing and telling lies increased as children's language skills improved and they became adolescents. Playing with their genitals in public also increased, mostly for boys. However most of these problems reduced, and by the late teenage years and young adulthood, fewer young people showed the behaviour, and even when it was present, parents rated it as less of a disturbance and difficulty.

Of course, knowing this is not helpful for the parents of the small number of children and adults with Down syndrome who are difficult to manage. They may have an additional disorder (see next section). In rare cases, the severity of the disorder – particularly for the very restless, irritable child with poor skills and reasoning ability – may overwhelm the resources of the family and alternative residential care needs to be considered.

THE FUTURE

On several occasions we asked the parents in our research what they think their children with Down syndrome will be like when they are older. About half felt very positive. They felt the child would be sociable, easy to manage, happy and relatively independent. Our assessments and observations of the children when they were adults, showed that these predictions are largely correct. The other half was less sure, but less than 10% had very negative predictions about the future. We found that mothers' fears for their children with Down syndrome were much stronger than for their ordinary children. This was particularly true when the child was difficult to control. As one mother put it, '*He's difficult enough now ... I daren't look that far ahead.*' In many cases, these fears were not really to do with the child, but with the confusion and uncertainty of the parents. Another mother expressed it this way:

> 'I'm dreading the future. He's strong now and might get stronger. I'm worried he might get uncontrollable. But it's other people that put these doubts into your mind, isn't it'.

We found that the chances of this happening are small; most families find the child's behaviour is manageable and improves in later years.

Mental health and psychological problems

For many years, mental health and psychological problems in people with Down syndrome were often ignored. It was seen as strange behaviour related to the syndrome or part of a gradual deterioration. This has now begun to change.

There is general agreement that psychological disorders, especially aggressive and hyperactive behaviour, are found less often in children and adults with Down syndrome than in other conditions associated with intellectual disability. Accurate estimates of the prevalence of these conditions are difficult because of changing definitions and social factors, such as specialists willing to make a diagnosis. But it is thought that between 8–15% of children, and 22 to 29% of adults with Down syndrome will have signs of a psychological problem or disorder that is severe enough to cause concern.

There are several descriptions in the professional literature of individuals with specific problems; including anorexia nervosa, schizophrenia, mania, Tourette syndrome, multiple personality disorders and depression. These cases serve to remind us to be alert and try to recognise that people with Down syndrome, like the rest of us, may have a mental health problem that can be treated.

Signs of mental health problems can include talking to yourself, hallucinations, seeing imaginary people, obsessive behaviour, hearing voices, becoming withdrawn, talking in whispers, loss of energy, enthusiasm and interest in things. If we see such signs we should start with a thorough medical examination to rule out such things as thyroid problems (Chapter 7) then an assessment from a psychiatrist or a clinical psychologist who has knowledge and experience of people with intellectual disability. Possible treatments include drugs and psychotherapy.

Diagnosis of mental health problems can be difficult because a behaviour may be appropriate for the level of intellectual functioning and development of the person, but inappropriate for their age. For example, talking to yourself, having an imaginary friend, being a little obsessive and having rituals, are all normal behaviours of young children but signs of psychological problems in an adult. One of the young people in our group was taken by his concerned parents to a therapist and was placed on medication because he constantly talked to himself, yet he had no psychological problems. I will describe some of our recent work to illustrate the issues.

Talking to self

Typical children usually talk to themselves from the age of 2 or 3 to around 5 or 6 years old. Talking to yourself self offers lots of practice with speaking and language and becomes a way of directing what you are doing. Sometimes it is dramatic, for example, having a conversation with someone not present or going over something that has happened. Children use self-talk in sophisticated imaginary games, taking on different roles and characters, often based on a TV programme. They may invent imaginary friends or animals. This behaviour is seen as functional and developmentally appropriate.

Talking out loud to oneself decreases between 7 to 10 years. There is less of it and the child often talks more and more in whispers and then just shows mouth movements. Eventually the talk is kept just in their heads – silent inner speech. This change reflects both the child's growing understanding that talking out loud is seen as strange by others, and their increasing ability to inhibit and reg-

Recently we asked all the parents in our group about this, and found that 91% of the children had or still did talk to themselves. The few that had never done this were all amongst the slowest to develop, with intellectual abilities under two to three years. The small number (5%) who no longer talked out loud to themselves were amongst the most advanced in terms of their intellectual ability. 53% talked in front of others and 33% only when they were alone; the latter were more intellectually advanced. The content also seemed to be as expected from descriptions of typical children:

'Always has since she was a little girl . . . Still does this talk to self about events or what she will do, but not instructions . . . as if she's trying to make sure she gets things right'.

'She has an imagination beyond belief. You can hear her talking in her room. Working for the big boss, singing. Being on TV, getting paid. We often hear her talking to characters from the 'soaps'.

These young adults with Down syndrome showed the same developmental sequence as typical children and adults. Their behaviour largely corresponded to their level of development.

ulate their behaviours. At this age they have also learnt more about privacy and secrets. Older children and adults do talk to themselves at times, especially if stressed or working on a difficult task. It helps with concentration and releases emotion. We all have conversations in our heads, when we will often mutter or make small mouth movements. The same is found for children and adults with Down syndrome.

Does self-talk indicate a psychiatric problem?

In the absence of other symptoms, self-talk should not be seen as a sign of a psychiatric problem in young people with Down syndrome – it is a useful and normal behaviour. In some of the literature on Down syndrome, it has been assumed that fantasy self talk is sign of loneliness or emotional problems. However, our study found no relationship between self-talk, fantasy and social or behaviour problems. Eleven of our young people had imaginary friends, and while they tended to be in the 'fantasy self-talk' group, only three had behavioural or emotional difficulties.

Self-talk is socially inappropriate and may interfere with an older child's or adult's social life. But, instead of trying to stop the young people talking to themselves, it is probably better to teach them to do it in private. The sequence seen in young children gives a clue. Start with getting them to talk quietly or somewhere private. Some children and adults will have a restricted social life and may compensate with self-talk and fantasy. Observing where and when they do it can give clues and highlight the need to organise a more active and stimulating life-style. Less frequently self-talk and imaginary friends (or hallucinations) will be associated with psychological problems, but there will be other signs. Usually the behaviour suddenly starts or becomes much more intense than previously. Also the content can be quite different. In such cases specialist help is needed.

Routines, ritualistic behaviour and obsessive-compulsive disorder

Many children and adults with Down syndrome like, or need, routines. This may be a personality trait, but it is certainly not an illness. They can appear rigid in their preferences for particular music, food or TV programmes, or activities like sleeping, bathing, walking the dog or swimming. With some planning, these activity routines can make life easier, though perhaps at some cost to family flexibility.

Routines can help people with Down syndrome to feel confident and in control. The first step in the routine triggers the next, and so on. In a similar way, some people like things to be in the same place, and may get anxious when faced with change. If you have some difficulties making sense of the world and thinking quickly and flexibly, it takes less effort and cognitive capacity if things stay much the same. At around the age of 2 to 5 years many typical children have strong preferences for sameness and things in the right place. They can be quite rigid in terms of the food they like and dislike, their play can be very repetitive and ritualised, and others are expected to do things in exactly the right way. These children are often very observant of tiny details in toys and clothes; the slightest imperfection can cause an outburst. Older children have similar ritualistic and 'compulsive' behaviour in their games, such as not stepping on cracks in the pavement and special magical rhymes or actions that protect them. This is all very normal and can be seen in children with Down syndrome.

Adults also have such behaviours, although we think of them as superstitions. Only when they become intense and interfere with our lives, do we think of them as an obsessive-compulsive disorder that requires treatment. Serious problems often appear relatively suddenly or become much more obvious as the child grows and develops.

If a person with Down syndrome is showing a lot of obsessive or ritualistic behaviour, we have the problem of deciding if it is typical development and so appropriate, or due to less mental flexibility and so some form of coping strategy, or a sign of an obsessive-compulsive disorder (see later). The key difference between developmentally appropriate behaviour and a mental health problem is that developmentally appropriate behaviours do not have the same feeling of compulsion; it is easier to divert or distract the person away from the behaviour. It is more that the child or person chooses them, and even if they get upset when the ritual or routine is changed, they soon adapt and calm down.

We recently investigated this with children and adults with Down syndrome and typical children. The 'routine' behaviour fell into those that were 'repetitive', such as repeating the same action over and over again, and those that were 'just right' such as wanting things done in a particular way, wearing particular clothes and having specific routines. The children and adults with Down syndrome had higher levels of these routine types of behaviour than the typical children at all ages. This suggests that such behaviour is characteristic of Down syndrome or of people with slower mental processing. For typical children the levels of such behaviours reduce as they get older – suggesting that the need for external routines to help feel in control reduces as their ability increases (see executive functioning – Chapter 10). Older typical children who maintain quite high levels of routine behaviour are more likely to have other problems of behaviour. It seems that if these demands for order and routines continue, they may signal psychological or personality problems.

We found the same pattern with the children and adults with Down syndrome. Those with higher 'just-right' and repetitive scores under 5 years mental age had higher social adaptation scores. This suggests these behaviours have a positive function in early development. However, high repetitive scores in the adults and more developmentally advance children with Down syndrome were associated with behaviour problems. Some of these had other symptoms, which indicated they had additional developmental disorders such as autistic spectrum disorder (see later).

As with self-talk certain levels of routinised behaviour would seem to be developmentally appropriate for many children and adults with Down syndrome. Certainly one needs to think about its function before trying to change it. However adaptability and flexibility in thinking is far more useful and so needs to be encouraged. Part of this is about having choices and making decisions.

Giving choices

From early on children with Down syndrome can experience making choices and decisions relating to food, clothes, toothpaste, decoration of their room and so on. If they have made a choice or been part of the decision-making process, they will be more committed to it. It is not easy waiting for the child to make choices and then trying to persuade them their choice is possibly not the best, but in the long term this investment in decision-making is worthwhile. If you share what the implications of certain actions are with the child, and let them help with making decisions, 'stubbornness' may be avoided. I recall a conversation with a parent of a teenager with Down syndrome who had also been diagnosed as having autism and who does not use speech to communicate:

> 'People underestimate him and when they tell him to do something or assume to know what he is interested in, they get no-where. He switches them out. But if you take your time and follow his interests and then introduce little extensions or reasons why you feel this might be better, you don't get the blank switch-out.'

Mental Health and Developmental Disorders

In this last section I will describe some of the more likely disorders found in children and adults with Down syndrome. But I must emphasise they are relatively uncommon and most individuals with Down syndrome will never experience them.

Obsessive-Compulsive Disorder (OCD)

OCD is when a person feels driven to carry out a particular behaviour due to fear that something dreadful will happen if they don't. It usually causes great distress and disturbance to the person's lifestyle. OCD affects between 1 to 4% of people with Down syndrome – about the same as in the general population. It appears earlier in boys with Down syndrome than in girls – around 7 to 12 years – and is mostly compulsive actions rather than obsessive thoughts. Examples include ripping paper, shaving so frequently the skin became raw, repeated washing of hands, insisting on wearing the same clothes, having to go to the toilet at the same time each day, going in and out of doors, opening and closing cupboard doors in sequence and looking in the same drawer at frequent intervals. This behaviour can appear gradually or suddenly after some event, like a change of residence or an accident causing post-traumatic stress disorder.

As described above it needs to be distinguished from routine or ritualistic type bevaviour seen in many people with Down syndrome.

Depression

This is the only mental health problem that is more common in people with Down syndrome than in other people with intellectual disability. Current figures indicate that between 10 and 14% – mainly young adults with Down syndrome – have depressive episodes. This is less than in the general population, and supports my earlier point that people with Down syndrome have a higher chance of being happy and stress free than most people.

Depression can start in late childhood and adolescence, but the peak age is the late 20's. We all experience mild depression at times, often as a reaction to some event or situation, or following an illness, but the episode is usually short-lived. As described in Chapter 2 learning that your baby has Down syndrome can trigger depression in many people. Most move through a period of adaptation – taking in and accepting the event, reacting to it, and then learning to deal with it –getting over the depressive feelings. This is easier if our life-style and situation is active, supportive and familiar. Some people are more susceptible to depression, which can be an inherited condition, and medical treatment is needed.

The symptoms of depression in people with Down syndrome are similar to those seen in typical people – withdrawal, lack of interest, irritablility, sadness, weight loss or gain, sleep disturbance and occasionally hallucinations have been reported. Women's periods may stop. Symptoms that may be more frequent in people with Down syndrome are talking in whispers, withdrawal into a fantasy world and talking to self and imaginary friends. But these are also part of typical development (see above). A group of symptoms is required to diagnose depression.

Causes of Depression

Symptoms of depression can also arise from medical problems, particularly hearing, vision and thyroid dysfunction (Chapter 7); these must be ruled out first. For many, depression is a reaction to an event, such as bereavement, or a close friend, relative or carer moving away. Sometimes there is no obvious cause of the depression. Problems can be precipitated by relatively sudden changes in the daily routine such as moving school or residence, a longish stay in hospital, illness in a parent or an accident. The problem can be worse if the person with Down syndrome cannot understand why the change has occurred. It is easy to assume they are not feeling disturbed and to exclude them from talking about the event or activity because they may not show signs of distress at the time. Parents may do this to shield the child from pain, but this approach does not prepare them for life-events.

Sometimes the event causing the depression is something that we would not even think of. For example, I knew one teenage boy who became quite distressed when the family car – an object he was very fond of — was damaged and then towed away. Over several months he became withdrawn, constantly looked out of the window, started to refuse to go out, and just wandered about the house. He refused to go near the new car, and when out walking he kept staring at cars. One day he saw a similar model and refused to leave it. This was the first real clue as to the problem – a sense of loss and reaction to the loss of the car. It was decided to take him to a scrap-yard to help him understand about what happens to cars when they get old or don't work. He played with toy-models of the old car and new cars; taking them to the scrap-yard and changing them for a new car with his father. At the same time, a step-by-step program, without pressure, was started. This involved looking at the new car, approaching it, touching it, washing and cleaning it, sitting in it with the door open, sitting in it with the door closed and playing, being strapped in and starting the engine, and eventually going for a short ride in the familiar neighbourhood. Soon after, all his symptoms disappeared. This was a mixture of bereavement and post-traumatic stress, plus a lack of knowledge and understanding. The child's 'symptoms' did not appear all at once when the car was damaged, but gradually emerged over weeks, which was why it was difficult to pin down the event that caused the behaviour.

In some cases, withdrawn behaviour and depression coincide with advances in intellectual ability, and developing awareness. The young person suddenly gains new insights into his or her life that can be unsettling. For example, some years ago, a young woman with Down syndrome who had always said that one day she would marry Prince Charles, became upset and withdrawn at the time of his wedding. This event appeared to trigger her realisation that she would not marry him, and then gradually, an understanding that she was unlikely ever to get married. This insight proved to be very upsetting, and she needed a lot of supportive counselling to develop new ideas for her future and a new way of life. The family had seen the fantasy about marrying prince Charles as typical of Down syndrome (see Self Talk above) and not very serious – like the games of younger children. They had missed the fact that many people with Down syndrome continue to develop their intellectual ability well into their early twenties; beyond the age that typical people reach their optimum level (Chapter 10). This young women was able, not just to react to the disappointment of Prince Charles getting married, but to reflect on this and on its' wider implications. Again, this process took much longer than one would normally expect and the very gradual onset of changes can make it difficult to see what may have triggered depression.

As with typical people, depression can be treated in those with Down syndrome using medication and counselling. In many cases organising a more interesting and active life-style is of great help.

Anxiety

Children can show anxiety – becoming fearful, worried or withdrawn. Usually there is something that is causing stress for the child and it is important to determine what this may be. For example, it can be feeling pressure at school, bullying and teasing or feeling left out. Removing the source of stress can result in dramatic improvement. I have known children with Down syndrome attending mainstream schools and showing such signs. These disappeared once they moved to a special school with a simpler regime, more individual attention and, I think, where they felt more competent. There are similar problems with young adults in work situations who feel they are not coping or don't fit in. Any marked change in behaviour should not be seen as a physical aspect of Down syndrome, like ageing or deterioration and ignored. It should be fully investigated and treated.

Fears and Phobias

As we saw earlier around three-quarters of children and adults have fears of something. For many, these are usual childhood fears. When such fears become so strong they have a major impact on the person's life-style they are phobias.

Sometimes, a childhood fear of dogs, for example, can gradually grow into a phobia where the person has a panic attack just seeing a dog. The main behavioural approach used is to use a stimulus with a bit of a threat such as a picture of a dog and help the person to learn to relax. Gradually the stimulus becomes more and more real and the person learns to tolerate it. Dealing with the fear early can help.

Sometimes, the onset of the fear or phobia is sudden. One young man refused to sleep in his bedroom, believing someone was hiding in his cupboard. At first, his parents, who were used to him having fantasies, thought it was part of some new game. Over weeks it grew strong and he became withdrawn and very agitated. He stopped talking about it and refused to go near the bedroom. His parents then thought it might be due to deterioration, which they had read about in books on Down syndrome. Eventually, he saw a psychologist for counselling and, although it was never discovered where the fear came from, he was able to get back to a normal life. The solution was a mix of talking about things, making his life more active and stimulating and involving him in designing, decorating and fitting out his bedroom – including removing the cupboard.

Developmental Disorders

I will describe the two developmental disorders that are most often found in children with Down syndrome.

Autistic spectrum disorder (ASD)

This is commonly called autism. It is called a 'spectrum disorder' because it includes a range of behaviours from mild to severe.

Children within the spectrum can be very different. It is a developmental disorder, not a psychiatric illness or a psychological disorder. ASD is more likely to be found in the small group of children with Down syndrome functioning at the severe and profound range of intellectual ability (Chapter 10). But some able children with Down syndrome also have ASD.

There are probably several causes of ASD, but none are fully understood as yet. It probably results from some underlying disorder in the brain. There is some evidence suggesting a higher risk if the child with Down syndrome has a first or second degree relative with autism, has suffered from infantile spasms, or had early hypothyroidism or further brain injury.

People with autism have differences in the brain; this affects the limbic system, which controls emotion and mood and the corpus callosum, which joins the hemispheres. There are also some differences in brain chemistry involving the neurotransmitters dopomine and serotonin. Other conditions such as attentional deficit disorders (ADD and ADHD – see below) have similar differences and share some of the symptoms of autism. The signs of the disorder vary with age and the developmental level of the child. Many of the symptoms used to diagnose ASD overlap with other conditions like ADHD and obsessive-compulsive disorder (OCD), and are similar to ritualistic behaviour described above. This makes diagnosis difficult.

Until recently it was felt that children with Down syndrome could not have ASD. This was partly because of the belief that their strength was in social interactions; one of the main signs of autism is disturbed social interaction. This view has changed to the extent that ASD may now be over-diagnosed in children with Down syndrome. This may be because of the increased knowledge and recognition of ASD and the number of specialists making the diagnosis. It may also be that as more children with Down syndrome attend mainstream schools, parents of more severely affected children with Down syndrome find it difficult to get special help and special schooling. Having the additional ASD label opens up the choice of schools.

There is often disagreement between specialists about diagnosing ASD. This only matters if the parent needs the diagnosis to ensure the child gets appropriate treatment. Often the specialists will advise on the same treatment, in terms of special schooling or medication, whether ASD is diagnosed or not. Due to problems with diagnosis, the demands of parents and the perceptions of specialists, it is difficult to estimate how many children with Down syndrome are likely to have autism. Current figures indicate between 5 and 9%.

Parents of children with severe behavioural problems often withdraw from Down syndrome support groups. Sometimes they become isolated or feel they must be doing something wrong as a parent for their child with Down syndrome to act in these strange ways. They often find more help and support from a group for children with ASD or ADHD than a Down syndrome group.

Signs of ASD

Some children who are very slow to develop show 'strange' behaviours from the first months. Parents find it difficult to deal with or understand their baby. It is difficult to establish routines and they tend to be over-active. They can get upset and be difficult to calm down. They are also more likely to have seizures or infantile spasms and severe hypotonia (Chapter 7). These children frequently repeat behaviour like hand flapping, finger sucking, and shaking a toy, sometimes to the extent that it is the only thing they will do. Parents may get a very slow response or no response when they call the child's name, even though they know their name and have no hearing problems.

As they get older, a range of behavioural signs can be seen. As described earlier, many are normal at certain times in development and more common in children with Down syndrome. What makes them signs of future ASD is when one or two behaviours become predictable, extreme and resistant to change. Other signs are when the child:

- stops learning new signs and words
- stops using, or is using less often, speech or signs they used before

- seems to be happy playing by themselves and needs no one else
- shows little interest in what others are doing
- has very repetitive play or actions
- tends to line things up and need things 'just right'
- shows more interest in objects than people
- eats only a small selection of foods – and suggesting new foods can result in a tantrum
- stares at things like lights or fans or changing numbers and gets angry or distressed if you try to take them away or make them look at something else
- likes things such as furniture, in order and in the same place – often they will not move until it is replaced in the 'correct' position

Sometimes, a child with Down syndrome who has been developing 'normally' regresses or changes. This usually happens between three and seven years of age, but has been seen in some adolescents. In older children it is difficult to decide if they are just becoming very withdrawn, or if they fall into the autistic spectrum disorder. Until we have specific treatments for the different disorders this issue is mainly of academic interest. The signs are a sharp and very obvious loss of communication skills – signs, language and looking at people and responding to conversation. Also, changes in emotion and personality – irritability, signs of anxiety and withdrawal, and the onset of repetitive behaviours as described above.

GLUTEN AND CASEIN-FREE DIET

There is some debate about whether children with autism can be helped with a gluten and casein-free diet. Casein is a protein found in milk and cheese. The evidence for positive effects is very mixed; sometimes the structure and attention imposed by a strict diet can help as much as the diet itself. There is no danger in this diet, but it demands a lot of work. Until there is more evidence, and a good scientific theory for why it might work, parents could probably use their time and energy in more useful ways.

Attentional Deficit Disorder (ADD) and Attentional Deficit Hyperactive Disorder (ADHD.

Like ASD, these developmental disorders are more common in children with severe intellectual disability, and no more frequent in children with Down syndrome. Children with slow development may show signs of ADD, but this may just be just typical behaviour seen in an older and more mobile child. As the child matures, the behaviour changes and they become more manageable. The main signs of ADD and ADHD are fidgeting, being easily distracted, being unable to stay with a task or game for long, being overactive, impulsive, excitable and impatient, and not very good at listening and following instructions. Only when these behaviours increase with age or become more and more disruptive to the child and family, is the possibility of ADD or ADHD considered. The diagnosis needs to be made by a specialist child psychiatrist or psychologist in intellectual disability. The usual treatment is a behaviour management programme used alongside careful management of things that may over-stimulate the child or young adult. In severe cases, psycho-stimulant drugs are sometimes prescribed. The idea is that they excite the nervous system and so trigger the bodies own 'dampening down' or inhibiting reactions. As far as I can determine, there is no known physical reason why children with Down syndrome should not be treated with these drugs but this has to be done under close medical supervision and there is much dispute about how effective the treatment is for children with intellectual disability.

Summary

1   Only a minority of parents of pre-school children with Down syndrome experience significant problems of behaviour. Whereas typical children show quite high levels of emotional problems these are rare for those with Down syndrome. More common than typical children (around a quarter), are problems with going to bed, waking at night, concentration and fears. They are also more likely to have problems such as running off, throw-

ing things, interfering with others belongings and showing inappropriate behaviour to strangers and for much
longer. Establishing early management systems can help.

2 As the child matures, behaviour difficulties reduce in the
   teenage years. However some problems are related to
   family problems and how the child is managed. In these
   situations behaviour problems often continue into later
   years. Professional help is often required and can reduce
   the impact of such behaviours to the benefit of the child
   and family.

3 A minority of children and adults with Down syndrome
   have additional mental health problems or developmental disorders. Carers need to understand the signs and
   seek up-to-date information, help and support. Diagnosis
   by a professional is needed and treatments are available.

10

Intelligence, development and attainments

- What is the range of intellectual abilities in Down syndrome?
- Is development just slower or is it different to typical development
- What factors influence development and attainments?
- What can we expect children with Down syndrome to achieve?

I believe that understanding the past can help us to understand the present. For this reason, I begin with a look at the past for Down syndrome, then the changing 'models' of intellectual disability and society and what this has done for people with Down syndrome. Some of this was noted in previous chapters. After that there is a section about the nature and use of intelligence and attainment tests. If you want immediate answers to questions about the range of intellectual ability and attainments of children and adults with Down syndrome you may want to skip the first sections.

A Look at the Past

There have been babies born with Down syndrome throughout human history. As we saw in Chapter 4 chromosomal errors are part of the system that reproduces human beings, but ensures each one is unique. Brian Stratford (see Resources) describes a skull from Saxon times and several paintings from medieval times onwards of people with the distinctive features of Down syndrome. One is of a well-to-do man who has clearly survived childhood and is quite able, but certainly looks to have all the features of Down syndrome. Others are from 16th Century Flemish paintings and some from Italy and England. Last year two more papers were published about old paintings that appear to show children with the facial features of Down syndrome. Of course only the rich members of society could afford portraits and only the more able and healthy children would survive. Down syndrome had not been classified at this time and so if the child's development and behaviour was within reasonable normal ranges they would not be labelled or segregated.

Figure 14 shows a photograph from the early part of the 20th Century. It was published in 1930, in a memorial edition of a book by Margaret MacDowall (see Resources), who is one of my 'heroes' in the education of people with intellectual disability. She founded a pioneering school in England in1895 specifically for 'idiots and imbeciles' (see 'Terminology' below), which included many children with Down syndrome, but 'mainly the more defective of this type'. So we might assume the boy depicted in this photograph was not more able – but he still looks quite capable. There were people who recognised that teaching and training could help. At the time Langdon Down published his work classifying the syndrome in 1866, he also wrote that people with Down syndrome:

'. . . are usually able to speak; the speech is thick and indistinct, but may be improved very greatly by a well-directed scheme of tongue gymnastics. The coordinating faculty is abnormal, but not so defective that it cannot be greatly strengthened. By systematic training, considerable manipulation power may be obtained'.

The message for me is that that Down syndrome has been

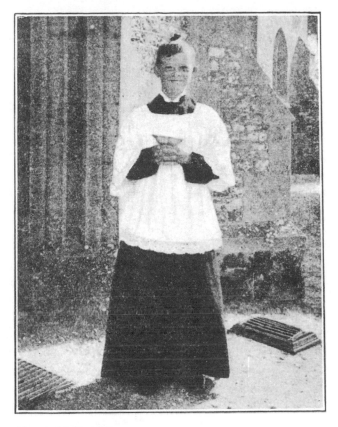

Figure 14 Chorister

around for a long time. There has always been a range of ability, with some quite able people and not all were locked away
from society, as is often depicted in some modern descriptions.
This history throws doubt on the suggestion that recent 'treatments' have resulted in wide ranging advances in the
intellectual capabilities and skills of persons with Down syndrome. People have been 'treating' and 'training' those with
Down syndrome for many years. What has changed is the survival of more people with Down syndrome and the
opportunities offered to them to develop skills and varied life-
styles. The latter is largely due to changing our 'model' of
intellectual disability, and of broader values in society.

Different views or 'models' of Down syndrome

We each have our own 'model' of Down syndrome formed by our experience and knowledge of the condition. If we do not have direct experience our model is likely to be based on the general understanding and attitudes of our society, or the sub-group of the society we live in. The way people with Down syndrome are treated at one point in history or in any particular society reflects the ideology or shared model of that society at the time.

Even within any general shared understanding there are usually opposing views. We may all agree that people with Down syndrome benefit from stimulation, opportunities to learn, and should live as normal a life as possible within the community. But parents, relatives and professionals will often disagree as to how this is best achieved.

Professionals also learn about Down syndrome from the perspective of their profession through formal training; different professional groups will have quite different models of Down syndrome. This can lead to conflicting advice to parents, and add to their frustration and stress. A common example comes from the social work profession, whose members may have what is thought of as a 'political model' with strong beliefs about the rights of people with disability, and the aim to treat those over 18 as adults. Other professionals and parents may subscribe to a model that places more emphasis on the person's limitations, saying they may not be able to make certain choices and decisions for themselves. I frequently hear parents and professionals from other disciplines complaining about 'political correctness' driving decisions rather than an understanding of the reality of the person's ability:

'they see her as an adult, but they don't understand she has a sophisticated veneer of competence . . . but underneath she is very much a young girl',

'I know it's right to treat him as an adult and give him choice, but they don't know him. If I let him do what he wants it would be a disaster. He thinks he can just go up to any young woman, preferably a blond, and they will be his girl friend. He can read and write pretty well and cope with small amounts of money and shopping, but if we are in a shop he would buy anything someone told him too'.

Finding the balance is not easy. Studies and personal histories have shown how many young people with Down syndrome blossom in terms of new skills and taking more control over their lives, when they leave the protective environment of the parental home.

MY MODEL OF DOWN SYNDROME

I should state what has influenced my model of Down syndrome. It comes from my training as a teacher; a biology teacher initially, and then children with learning difficulties. Afterwards, I studied psychology and sociology, specialising in developmental psychology. My work has mainly been as a researcher with a focus on applied rather than theoretical issues. My experience of children and adults with Down syndrome has been through what parents tell me and through my research. I am not a parent of someone with Down syndrome, and have not spent large amounts of each day over many years in close contact with children or people with Down syndrome. It is these influences, as well as my upbringing, my views on life and how the world works, that have formed my model of Down syndrome. For example, I want to live in a society that treats all its citizens equally and provides them with the necessary support and opportunities to run their own lives – my political perspective. My influences are apparent in the ideas expressed and the references to research studies in this book. Some things are missing, for example discussions of religious beliefs and disability. Others will disagree with my interpretations and points of emphasis. My model emphasises developmental delay and how 'normal' development can help us understand children and adults with Down syndrome. Others would see this as less important or too negative, too much emphasis on differences and deficits. In a sense, what I am doing is offering my model of Down syndrome and disability for the reader to react to, and so look at, and develop their own model.

In real life, we all have a mix of ideas and more emphasis to one aspect than another depending on situations. Describing 'models', therefore, is a like a caricature; it is an academic approach and a way of examining ideas and implications.

The 'medical model' of Down syndrome

The dominant model in the past is called the 'medical' model. This is not to suggest it is predominate in the medical profession. It was held by society at large. The name refers to the fact that intellectual disability was seen as a medical condition arising from biological factors and not social or environmental factors. People with Down syndrome were so intellectually impaired that they could not profit from stimulating environments or education. Low intelligence was equated with low everything, including emotion and feelings. Some felt that people with severe intellectual disability did not have emotions, feelings and needs like the rest of us. This belief may have been supported by reduced expression of emotion seen in some people with Down syndrome (Chapter 8).

The danger in such a model is that it becomes a self-fulfilling prophecy – you think nothing can be done, so nothing is done and hence nothing changes. It follows that a medical problem should be the responsibility of the medical profession. Until the 1960's for example, it was the role of the community medical officer in the UK to do developmental and intelligence tests on the young children in order to decide if they were 'educable', and so go to a school, or 'ineducable', and go to a centre whose staff were often nurses rather than qualified teachers. As noted later IQ tests were actually devised in order to identify young children who would not benefit from education.

Langdon Down was exceptional and had much direct experience. His model did not reflect the popular model of society at that time, which may explain how his writing sparked off many studies of classification, and searching for syndrome characteristics, but few about education and training. Margaret MacDowall captures the essence of the prevailing attitude (model) at beginning of the 19th Century in the UK. She quotes typical questions and reactions to her attempts to provide education for these children:

'Why teach them? They are happier left alone; the result is so small, and these children are not chargeable for their own actions . . . why make them suffer . . .?' (p1).

This again is part of the medical or pathological model. One consequence of this view was that those 'afflicted' were usually placed in 'safe havens' or large institutions for their own and societies protection (see Chapter 8 – society and deviance). They were seen as patients and not distinguished from people with mental health problems. Parents were advised to put their babies with Down syndrome in institutions because taking them home would be of little benefit to the child and could damage the family (Chapter 3).

There was a strong movement – Eugenics – to ensure people with disability would not reproduce 'more of the same,' and programmes of sterilisation were common. Well into the last century, people with intellectual disability were considered as potentially dangerous and as menace to society. The same ideas are still found in some countries.

Most large institutions tended to be run on very low costs. Many developed ways of generating money from their own initiatives through crafts, gardens and farms. This was probably therapeutic for those who could be 'useful'. There are stories of how particularly able 'inmates' were highly prized for their work, and how any suggestion that they might live elsewhere was resisted.

Life for the people who were more severely disabled was not as fulfilled. Most of these large institutions were un-stimulating and both infants and adults received minimal attention. The residents tended to be herded together and treated collectively. They lacked personal possessions, even their own clothes, and had no identifiable space to call their own.

Changing societies

Following the huge social upheavals brought about by the second world war, the late 1940's was a period of rapid and major change. The post-war shifts were not just about views of people with intellectual disability, but about major changes in society as a whole. There was a spirit of optimism and the belief that ordinary people could take more control over their lives. People could see the evidence of science in everyday life, and there was a growing belief that science could solve all our ills. For example, the introduction of vaccinations had a considerably impact of reduced infant mortality and childhood illnesses, which effected every family.

There was a shift away from the belief that your abilities were largely biologically determined (nature), towards a belief that, given the right opportunity, most people could achieve what they set their minds to (nurture). This is a picture of the changes in the UK and similar countries. Other countries have different histories and views of their world that effect their treatment of children with Down syndrome.

These changes in society had spin-offs for intellectual disability. Parents began to form voluntary groups for support and as a pressure group to influence society. A first issue was the demand for respite care while they took a break or a holiday – the shortage of this type of care is still top of the needs list for many families of children with a severe disability. The idea that children with intellectual disability might benefit from more help and education was gaining momentum.

Theories of 'Institutionalisation'

Large institutions began to be seen as depriving children of the stimulation necessary for good development, and that the behaviour of residents might be due to the style of life in the institution – institutionalisation – not just their inherent impairments. It became clear that one could not predict the potential of people with Down syndrome from those who had been brought up in large institutions or deprived circumstances. Environment did matter.

From the 1930's, and increasingly in the 40's and 50's, studies began to appear showing that if more stimulation, attention and opportunities for learning were provided in these institutions, the residents showed quite marked changes in their behaviour and skills. Later studies showed that children with Down syndrome who were brought up at home were more developmentally advanced, and had better social skills and fewer behaviour problems than those who lived in institutions. Studies also showed that children with Down syndrome cared for at home for the first three to four years of life before being placed in an institution, were not only more developmentally advanced, but maintained their advanced level for several years. Those cared for within a family, were also described as being more emotionally mature and having a wider range of interests compared to those in institutions. Similar studies of typical babies in orphanages also showed that by increasing the amount of individual attention, the babies developed more quickly. All this evidence is about depriving children of the levels and type of care and stimulation they need to thrive and make the best of their inherent abilities. It does not show, as sometimes argued, that more intensive and early training has additional benefits (Chapter 11).

Theories of Early Child Development

During this time there was a rapid increase in studies of typical child development that showed very rapid development in the first five years of life. As noted above, others showed the effects of early deprivation. It was suggested that deprivations in these early years would have long lasting effects on both intellectual and emotional functioning. These studies also showed that by two to three years of age the social background of children had a significant influence on how well they scored on tests of intelligence and academic achievements. Others documented the effects of separation from parents and problems of attachment to later emotional problems. This led to the idea that children from disadvantaged backgrounds needed something to compensate for not having the same levels of care and stimulation as those from less deprived homes.

Other studies began to change our views of young babies by showing how they responded to stimulation from the first days of life. They were no longer seen as passive recipients of parental care but as active learners who could benefit from stimulation. Mothers were encouraged to talk to and stimulate their babies from birth.

A shift occurred in society, resulting in a popular belief about the benefit of stimulating babies. By the mid-1970's business people had caught onto this shift in thinking, and were producing a wide range of 'educational' toys and equipment for babies and young children. Nowadays, we may think a baby without such toys and equipment is deprived.

By the 1960's there was a growing emphasis on early education for all children. For those at risk because of social or biological factors, intervention programmes started shortly after birth. In the

USA this was called the Head Start programme and had considerable political backing. The current Sure Start initiative in the UK is a continuation of these developments.

The programmes were targeted at socially disadvantaged children, in the belief they could break the cycle of disadvantage seen in deprived communities. There is much evidence that they did change attitudes and the parenting practices of many, which then had a beneficial effect for the child. Except in cases of sever deprivation, including poor diet and medical care, the gains made in developmental test scores (see later) of the children in the first year or two were small. However the impact of early education and parental support programmes was seen from three years of age.

The ideas for early stimulation filtered down to children with disabilities resulting from biological and not just social factors. In the late 1960's the law changed, and all children in the UK, no matter what level of disability, were included in education. There was an expansion of special schools, and teachers were trained in special education.

There was considerable optimism about these programmes in the 1960 and 70's – the time I started working with parents and infants with Down syndrome. As described later, and in Chapter 11, these were often overly optimistic in what they expected to achieve in terms of improved intelligence. However they certainly had a positive impact on the lives of families and the children with Down syndrome.

Social changes usually swing from one extreme to another. I think the swing towards a strong emphasis on nurture and environment in our development has reached its highest point. Everyday, advances in genetics and the bio-chemistry of the body are showing influences, previously thought to be environmental. Techniques for looking at human growth and development even before birth are illustrating individual behavioural differences. I have noticed an increasing number of articles and comments questioning the assumptions and beliefs about very early 'educational' activities for typical children, and the pressure (and guilt) many mothers feel about providing such activities for their children. Play, as opposed to more formal training of skills and achievements, is once again being given prominence in some settings. Evidence from many sources where young children have experienced quite major deprivation suggest they are more resilient than we think. The issue in intellectual disability is whether these children are more vulnerable to deprivations because of their problems with learning. I will return to this point in Chapter 11, 'Early Interventions'.

Disability issues enter the mainstream

The shift from providing care in large institutions to care at home, and the idea that children with intellectual disability benefit from education and therapy, brought demands for services and for qualified staff across a range of professions. Voluntary associations were the first to respond. Soon after, mainstream institutions set up training programmes; specialists in intellectual disability appeared in all the major professions. Disability began to compete with other areas of need for limited resources. Research into issues around intellectual disability increased, and Universities and Colleges of Higher Education developed special departments. By the 1970-80's, intellectual disability was no longer some minor sub-division of life, but had become 'respectable' and recognised as an important part of society. People became specialists and made careers in the area. Disability was represented at the top level of government.

Social Models of disability

By the 1980's and 90's, we began to see the limits of intervention and education; the majority of people with Down syndrome still required varying levels of support throughout their lives. We also saw improvements brought about through social change and the opening up of opportunities and expectations. Disability was seen as a consequence of society failing to meet the needs of its citizens with impairment. Instead of aiming to reduce or remedy the person's disability (Chapter 8), the focus moved towards recognising that people are different, and that providing resources and support for these differences will improve their quality of life. It recognised the importance of working *with* people with a disability rather than *on* them; that they should be active participants in their lives rather than passive recipients of societies benevolence.

The impact of these shifts in how society views disability is discussed more later and in Chapters 11, 12 and 13.

Terminology

The way we name and define something often highlights our 'model' of it. This is clearly seen in the changing terminology in the field of intellectual disability.

The World Health Organisation defined 'impairment' as some sort of damage to any part of the body, and 'disability' as the effect of impairment on the person's quality of life. 'Handicap' is seen as being disadvantaged in a particular situation – in this sense we are all handicapped in some circumstances. The term handicapped has been largely dropped. In the late 1990's, the Disability Discrimination Act in the UK defined disability as: the result of an impairment that has a substantial and long-term adverse affect on a persons ability to carry out normal day-to-day activities. Many people with disability do not like this simple causal link between impairment and disability, in the sense that it is about functioning in normal situations. They define disability as restrictions put on people with impairment because of social factors that exclude them from engaging in normal day-to-day social activities. In other words, I may be unable to walk but I am not disabled if I have easy wheelchair access. This is part of the social model of disability.

Although many of us object to labels and terms, they represent social categories and we all use them to help us make sense of others. Terms are needed to classify levels of disability for administrative purposes; to count how many people are affected and what services they might need. As our understanding changes and new models are formed, so we change the terms. If the term is associated with something less desirable, it often becomes used in a derogatory way. In these situations, changes are a reaction to the stigma that becomes attached to the terms.

Because family members of children with Down syndrome will meet many of these terms in one form or another, I think a brief overview might be helpful.

The old scientific terms of intellectual disability were **'idiots'**, **'imbeciles'** and **'morons'**. All are now used as abusive and they fail to convey any meaning as to the condition. The term **'mongol'** changed to Down syndrome for the reasons I described in earlier chapters. Similarly, **'mental deficiency'** – the official UK term between 1913 and 1959 – changed to **'mental subnormality'**. This was felt to be less prejudicial and more accurate. It reflected developments in psychological testing and statistical analysis, which showed a normal distribution of measured intelligence. Those with scores below the normal range were sub-normal – an objective term that soon became used in a derogatory way.

'**Mental handicap**' became a common term. It emphasised that handicap is not impairment or a deficiency, but the difficulties experienced by somebody with an impairment in certain situations. A person who is blind in one eye will only experience handicap in situations requiring binocular vision such as catching balls or pouring drinks into glasses. Children who find it difficult to sort complex information and learn new things will be less 'handicapped' in their learning if the information is presented in simple ways to help them learn it step by step.

'**Learning disability**' and '**learning difficulty**' are popular terms. They are easy to understand, and capture the main issue – that the child learns more slowly and needs more help to learn things. Learning difficulty is also used to describe children who have specific problems, such as learning to read, but are of normal intelligence. These terms do not encompass the fact the person may be developing slowly. They terms are used differently in different countries, leading to confusion.

When the 'slow development model' became popular, the term '**mental retardation**' emerged and is still widely used in some countries. But 'retard' has taken its place alongside 'idiot' as a derogative word of abuse. The term 'children with **development delay**' is also used. It does state clearly how children with Down syndrome are seen and is not easy to turn into a derogative name. Others object to 'developmental delay' because it fails to indicate impairment and problems with learning and other intellectual functions.

The term '**intellectual disability**' is preferred in some countries and is becoming more widespread. I use it because I think it reflects the main characteristic of a difference in intellectual functioning, which includes slow learning and slow development. I also see disability as a result of impairment and a less than supportive social environment; but as yet we do not seem able to find a term that encompasses all this without detailed explanation. Figure 15 illustrates some of these terms in relation to intelligence test scores.

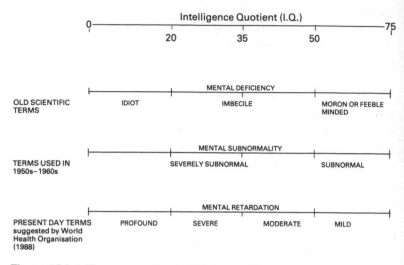

Figure 15 Intelligence quotients (IQ), terminology and categorisation in mental handicap

Adapted from Clarke, ADB and Clarke AM, 1974,
British Medical Bulletin Vol. 30, p179.

Intelligence Quotients (IQ scores)

Tests of intellectual ability were invented in the early 1900's and soon afterwards classification of intellectual disability was based on these test scores. Figure 15 shows the early official terms and the main categories according to IQ. What I find interesting is that while the names have changed, the cut-off points, in terms of IQ, have remained much the same. So it was mainly the names that changed.

In educational circles in the UK, the category of 'severe' refers to IQ's below 50, and 'moderate' refers to 50 to 70/75. However, the worldwide categories as shown in figure 15 are still used by other professional groups, and have different levels of IQ and terms. It is easy to get confused.

These classifications and test results had a major impact on the lives of children with Down syndrome. Until the late 1960's children with IQ's below 50 were classified as severely subnormal and unable to be educated. They attended Occupation Centres, later called Junior Training Centres. When they were included in the education system, these centres became schools for the Severely Sub-Normal (SSN). Those with IQ's between 50 and 70/75 went to schools for the Educationally Sub-Normal (ESN). Sub-normal was replaced by learning difficulties, and they became Schools for Severe or for Moderate Learning Difficulties (SLD or MLD). With the emphasis on community living, attending mainstream schools, and assessing individual needs, the use of intelligence tests and categorising people has diminished. Most typical people progress through life without having an intelligence test. It is far more important to assess quality of life and what is needed to improve or maintain it.

Social Functioning

With the shift away from medical models, the groupings were broadened to include social functioning. People in the profound category are described as requiring constant supervision, having limited mobility, no literacy skills and basic levels of understanding and communication. In developmental terms they tend to function within the sensorimotor stage of development typical of children up to 2 years, and never above the mental or development age of three years (see later sections). People in the mild category usually have good understanding of language, good communication skills, and are fully independent in self-care skills such as dressing, washing, and toileting. They have functional levels of reading and writing, can manage simple money, are fully mobile and able to travel reasonably independently. In developmental terms, this roughly corresponds to mental ages over 7 years. These children or young people require some supervision and do not lead fully independent lives.

Special needs

In the UK, children began to be classified according to their needs, rather than an IQ score or a condition. It was not sufficient to say a child had Down syndrome and then decide on the school. A statement of their level of functioning and additional needs was required (Chapter 13). The term 'special needs' became widespread. The aim was to integrate or include as many children as possible into mainstream services. A place in a special school was to be provided only if their special needs exceeded the resources of the mainstream school.

Other terms
Terms like 'exceptional children', 'atypical children' or the 'uncommon child' are also used, although not officially. Recently, I have noted that some people are talking about children with 'additional needs' rather than special needs. I like it, because it gets around the negative connotations that have emerged for 'special', and at some time in our lives we will all have needs that require extra or additional resources.

People First
Running alongside these changes is the **'People First'** movement. We do not talk about 'the disabled' or 'Down's babies', but about 'people with a disability' or 'children with Down syndrome'. The idea is to emphasise that we are all people with a difference or condition. To see us as a condition first denies this, and can categorise us so that we may be denied the same rights, respect and opportunities as others.

Psychological and Attainment Tests

Psychological and attainment tests are still used in some administrations. Some parents want their child to be tested, so they can see how they compare with others, make plans and have some idea of their child's future. They are used in research studies to demonstrate the effectiveness or otherwise of treatments. But they have their limitations and can be misleading.

The first 'mental functioning' test recorded in the UK, is from the 14th Century when people wanted to distinguish between a 'lunatic' (mental illness) and a 'born fool' (permanent intellectual disability). They would be asked questions or observed to see if they performed in accordance with some 'normal' expectation. If the person was a 'lunatic' the Crown took possession of the property only during the illness; if they were a 'born fool' all the person's possessions were taken permanently, with the crown providing for their needs.

Psychological testing did not really take off until the turn of the 20th Century. They were devised to find out which children could profit from education and which could not. Current tests include many that measure specific aspects of intellectual functioning, personality, skills and aptitudes, even some about levels of masculinity-femininity.

Normative Tests

Normative tests compare an individual's performance to a score derived from a sample of 'normal' people of the same age. They are at the heart of deciding if a child is 'abnormal'. There are tests for different aspects of intelligence or ability. In the area of language, for example, there are tests for understanding words (receptive language), saying words (expressive language), both of which can measure vocabulary (number of words known or used), tests of grammar and tests that assess reasoning using language. There are also normative tests for academic subjects such as reading, arithmetic and spelling.

There are different models of intelligence, and so tests differ in their emphasis and task selection. Most intelligence tests are divided into items related to use of language (verbal intelligence) and those that are non-verbal and require manipulation of objects and visual patterns (non-verbal intelligence). The items are selected because it is thought they indicate various aspects of mental ability such as verbal and non-verbal memory, attention, conceptual reasoning and problem solving. The tasks usually involve spotting the odd one out of a series, matching similar pictures, naming pictures, defining the meaning of words, identifying missing parts of a picture, or solving a logical problem.

These tests usually cover a specific age range, although some range from young to quite old children. The items in the tasks are ordered from easy to difficult. The tester starts at a level that s/he thinks the child can do (usually based on the child's age) and continues until the child fails a specific number of items. This signals the limit of their performance.

Standardisation

Since the purpose of the test is to be able to compare the person being tested to a set of norms, it is important to ensure the test is reliable and valid for that person. It needs to be standardised. To do this, large numbers of children of different ages are given the test using a standard procedure. The items are then put into order according to the numbers passed or failed at different ages. If tasks are passed by about half the children in a specific age range, they are felt to represent the ability expected on that task for the average child at this age. Tables are constructed showing these normal levels of performance by age, and the ranges of scores.

The words normal, norms and normative are statistical descriptions and 'abnormal' merely means outside of the normal range. Each child's performance can be compared with this set of norms. If the child is five and scores above the five-year level, we can say the child is above average on this test at this time in his or her life. We can say a child achieved the level of a six year-old on the visual memory task, or that when the scores on all the tasks were added together and averaged, their overall level was equivalent to seven years. This is called the **mental age** or **age equivalent score**. One can also have age scores for reading, spelling, and arithmetic or social functioning. **The score does not mean that the child is like a three, five or eight year old; it merely shows the level achieved at the time on that test.**

It can be frustrating for parents to watch their child do these tests, especially if they feel it is unfair to ask the child to do more difficult tasks, knowing they will fail, or when they feel the child could do the task if it was presented slightly differently. But, to get a valid result, a trained person must present the test in a standard way. This person then interprets the results and whether they felt confident the child performed as well as expected.

These 'norms' are only correct if the child being tested is similar to the group of children used in the standardisation. If the child tested is from a different cultural background to this group, it will affect the result. The pictures and words used will be different and children with have different experiences and levels of familiarity with the test. This is a big issue when using these tests with children who are different. For example, they may use a task to test reasoning that requires good fine motor coordination. This means the test is not valid for children with physical disability. Similar issues arise for children with language or vision problems.

ENVIRONMENTAL INFLUENCES

Environmental factors influence the scores even for children who are typical (normal) and from the same cultures. Studies have shown that children of later generations score higher on intelligence tests. This does not mean they are more intelligent, in the sense of synthesising information, reasoning, solving problems or coping with complex cognitive tasks at a higher level. All psychological tests are influenced by environmental factors and familiarity with tasks. Babies today sit in special chairs; have baby walkers, and a whole range of cause and effect toys. Young children watch educational TV programmes, attend pre-school facilities, and play games that depend on memory and fine motor skills. Therefore they have more experience with the sort of tasks used in the tests and score at a higher level. Normative tests have to be modernised and re-standardised after several years to keep the 'norms' up to date.

Intelligence Quotients (IQ)

By comparing the mental age (MA) to the chronological age (CA) we can see the rate of development of the child. This is the idea behind the **Intelligent Quotient or IQ**. In its simple form, the mental age is divided by the chronological age and then multiplied by 100. If a child has a MA of 5 years and is five years old, his or her IQ will be 100. The average IQ is therefore always 100. IQ scores can vary from day to day; they can be influenced by how the person feels at the time, their motivation or how the test is presented. This why the IQ score should always be given with a statement of the **confidence interval** that shows the range of score likely if the person was to be tested on another day. For example, you may have achieved an IQ of 120 and there is a 90 to 95% chance of scoring between 117–127 if tested on another day. This shows that IQ

Recently we tested children with Down syndrome on an old version of a developmental test from the 1970's with the new re-standardised version. They scored a month or two higher in developmental age on the older version, just like typical children. So they too have become more skilled earlier with some tasks on these tests. But in terms of the norms there was little difference. Like typical children they had to score higher on the new version to attain the same mental age, because all children were doing the items earlier.

The actual difference we found was of a month or so which is not that important. Recent studies show that the ages of attaining skills have remained fairly similar for children with Down syndrome over the last twenty or so years, provided they have a good quality of care and stimulation. But even small differences between tests can affect the categories that individual children are placed in and the services they receive, especially if they are on the borderline.

We have also used re-standardised normative tests of intelligence with young adults with Down syndrome, and compared these to other studies that used older standardisations. We found the same as with the developmental tests. Their derived normative score (MA and IQ) were lower, yet their scores on functional measures and vocabulary were higher. This suggests their intellectual disability as defined by IQ is more severe yet their social functioning is more advanced! This is a good example of why we need to understand these tests, especially their limitations, and how to use them or not, in classifying people.

scores are estimates and again the point is that problems occur when the score falls around borderlines between categories.

Depending on the test, 50% of children have an IQ score of between 90 and 110, classified as average. Those with scores of 110 to 120 are high average, 120 to 130 are high and those with over 130 are exceptionally high. Scores of 80 to 90 are low average, 70 to 80 are low and below 70 are exceptionally low. These fall into the category of intellectual disability. Around 1 in 10 children will score over 120 and a similar percentage will score below 75. Depending on definitions and cut-offs the average range is 20 points and most people fall within a range of 40 to 50. Beyond this they fall into the categories of exceptionally low (intellectual disability) or high (gifted).

Although the average is lower for children and adults with Down syndrome, the range of 40 to 50 points is also found. Like the range for height (see Chapter 7) this indicates that there is as much variation of intellectual ability in Down syndrome as in the 'normal' population.

Developmental tests

Developmental tests assess the sequences and rate of development of children under two to three years old. The results are usually given as a mental or developmental age but can be turned into a quotient as shown above.

The aim of early developmental tests was to measure the child's intelligence, but it was soon found that the scores did not predict later IQ scores very accurately. In fact it is not until typical children (those falling into the normal range on the tests) are over three to four years that their results on intelligence tests start to predict later results. This indicates that the activities and skills measured by the tests are not tapping into the abilities that make up later intelligence. For example, much of the development we observe in the first two years is about physical and sensory development and coordination; it is called the sensorimotor period. After two years of age there is a rapid development of language, classification and problem solving. These are more involved in later intellectual functioning (see stage model of development later).

A number of mechanisms of intellectual or cognitive functioning also predict later levels of measured intelligence. Testing children in their first year of life on things like speed of responding, memory and attention, can predict later IQ scores better than a developmental age. Even so, it is not that accurate. For practical purposes, social measures and things like parental education are just as useful as developmental tests at predicting the future scores of typical young children.

The picture is different for children with intellectual disability. The rate of their development in the first years is much more predictive. For most infants who eventually fall in the profound category, scores on these developmental tests usually fall two to three months below the average by 6 to 12 months of age, and there is a very obvious slowing down in development at around 4 to 6 months developmental age. Other reasons for the delay, such as medical or health problems must be taken into account, but if the child is showing very observable slower than average development during these first years, then this is predictive of their later levels of intellectual functioning. This is what the DQ or IQ does. It compares the rate of development (DA or MA) to the chronological age. Therefore in the early years a low IQ means slower development.

Limitations of intelligence tests

- They only test what they are designed to test. This does not include special practical aptitudes, initiative and creativity, emotional maturity nor social ability. Low IQ does not mean low everything. Many people with low or lower IQs live fulfilled, meaningful and happy lives.
- Two children can get the same IQ score in very different ways because intelligence and mental ability is not a single entity. They may have very different needs, skills and areas of strength and weakness. Some will do better on language items and others on non-verbal items.
- Normative tests may not be suitable for children with a disability; because they assume many normal functions, they may actually be misleading.
- They are not very useful when it comes to deciding what a person can do, can't do and might need to learn next, because their main purpose is to allow comparison to the norm.

Because of these concerns, behavioural and functional tests are preferred.

Behavioural and Functional Assessments

These tests are about how the child functions now, and what they need to do and learn next in order to function as independently as possible. They depend upon observing the child as they go about everyday things or testing their skills. Functional behaviour is about walking, counting, reading, drawing, writing, using money, using the rules in a game, following an instruction, flushing the toilet, putting shoes on the correct feet, or any skill. It also includes life-skills like being able to entertain themselves and explore, having interests, making decisions, and understanding family relationships.

This behavioural approach makes no assumptions about the child from general labels. The danger of labels, and IQ or MA assessments, is that they may indicate the child is not ready, and so he or she is not taught or given opportunities to learn. For example, you may think a six-month-old child with Down syndrome is not ready to learn to drink from a feeding cup, because that is when the average typical infant achieves this skill. But if the child can sit up reasonably well with support, hold his head steady, grasp the cup in two hands, lift it to his lips and tip it, then he has all the skills required to learn to use a feeding cup.

Functional behaviour is also called adaptive behaviour; there are several checklists that put skills in developmental order ranging from what the young child does to what an adult could be expected to do. This behaviour is organised into groups, and the skills are in an order where they build upon each other:

- **Self-help or daily living skills:** such as washing, eating and toileting, understanding danger, keeping things tidy, taking care of clothes, using a telephone.
- **Communication skills:** including gesture, speech, language, reading and writing, from a practical point of view.
- **Social skills:** engaging with others, turn-taking, understanding rules, kinship relationships, friendships, sharing, manners, appreciating feelings and so on.

Parents and teachers who know the child, tick off what they see the child can do and then look at the next item. This gives some idea of what things to encourage or teach next. A judgement has to be made to decide if the child has truly attained the skill or behaviour. For example, the criterion may be that he can do it 9 times out of 10, or most of the time, with help. For this reason, some of these checklists are called criterion-referenced tests.

Because most children with Down syndrome follow the typical developmental steps and sequences, having an idea of their developmental level can be helpful in understanding what to expect next, and so what to look out for, encourage and teach. It is the actual skills the child has and is using, that tell us about what they can do and what the next step might be – not their mental age.

Intelligence and Development in Down syndrome

In this section I describe the range and level of development and intelligence found on tests, and factors related to mental ability. Understanding the wide range of ability in children and adults with Down syndrome is necessary when investigating questions about the benefits of treatments and predictions about the future.

The wide range of ability and variation between people with Down syndrome means that you can have two groups – all with Down syndrome – but quite different in terms of ability. To counter this, an unselected sample is needed that represents the range of differences found in Down syndrome. This usually means a large sample, which can be difficult to establish and co-ordinate, especially if individuals are living in the community and attending a range of schools, centres, colleges and work places. Always carefully check the sample used when being given information about useful treatments or ranges of ability.

Early studies

Research was easier when many people with Down syndrome lived in large institutions; but these are not representative of people with Down syndrome today. Up to the early 1900s, most people with Down syndrome were classified in the 'idiot' range – the profound mental retardation category in current terms – but these were not based on IQ tests, and there were no chromosome tests to confirm the diagnosis.

With the development of IQ tests there were numerous surveys of children and adults living in the large institutions. Most reported that half to three-quarters had an IQ in the 20 to 50 range – with the average score between 20 to 35. This classified them in the severe mental retardation category, and most textbooks of the time described Down syndrome as being associated with severe sub-normality. There has been much debate about a possible selection bias towards the less able being admitted to institutions. Hence these results may not be representative.

Since then, children have the advantage of being raised at home and educated; health has improved and life expectancy increased for people with Down syndrome. There may be more girls in to-days groups of people with Down syndrome because the infant girls are more likely to die than the boys (Chapter 5), but, as a group, are more advanced than boys.

Environmental influences

These changes can be illustrated by looking at the results of a small number of studies around that time, including ours. These studies measured the mental abilities of groups of children with Down syndrome at regular intervals from their first months of life to five or more years of age. In Table 4 I have separated the studies into two categories: those that provided limited or no educational advice, and those that included the family in an early education and support programme. The Ludlow group received this through visits to developmental centres, and our group through home visits. The de Coriat study from South America is the earliest study to my knowledge that has published such data. I must emphasise that this table is meant to give a global picture based on early studies, and not what can be expected from individual children today. I have averaged the scores around yearly intervals and calculated simple ratio IQ's. This is not very precise.

What is striking is that despite the studies being done by different people, at different times, in different countries and often using different developmental and intelligence tests, the yearly averages are consistent. There are other studies including several later ones, with similar findings. Some even indicate that these averages might be conservative but there are technical problems with the sample and testing. However I have not found a recent study showing lower levels.

Table 4 Progression of average IQ as reported by various studies

	Age in years					No of children
	1	2	3	4	5	
Children living at home but with limited help						
Share et al. (1964)	68	58	51	46	49	45
Loeffler & Smith (1964)	65	51	46	43	43	47–54
Carr (1970)	67	56	48	48	–	45
de Coriat et al. (1967)	66	54	48	44	43	9–189
Ludlow & Allen (1979)	69	61	53	49	44	23–71
Children living at home and enrolled in an early education program and then attending school						
de Coriat et al. (1967)	83	70	66	61	61	9–189
Ludlow & Allen (1979)	80	70	63	58	56	9–63
Cunningham	75	67	59	60	59	59–60

The range of intellectual ability in recent studies

The three UK studies in Table 4 (Carr, Ludlow and Cunningham) have followed the children into adulthood. Our study (Cunningham) found a mean IQ of around 40 for the children between 7 and 14 years of age and, using a different non-verbal test, the same average at 20 years. Carr, using a different test, reported an average IQ of 37 when her sample was 11 years, and, using a different non-verbal test, an IQ of around 40 when they were in their twenties and thirties. Ludlow, with yet another different test, found an average IQ of around 45 at 10 years and 40 at 20 years. Average IQ's, therefore, appear to be fairly stable from around 4 to 6 years of age.

The tests used by Ludlow and Carr for the adults, and by us with the children were not recent and so may give slightly higher IQs than recent tests would (see earlier section – Psychological and Attainment tests). Ludlow also had slightly more parents with higher levels of education and Carr had more children falling into the profound range of disability.

A similar compilation of studies in the USA for the same period reported average IQ's of 45 to 55 over the childhood and teenage years. My interpretation is that the differences in the means mainly reflect the use of different tests, problems of establishing representative samples and accounting for families who drop-out over the years.

Despite such problems, the averages are higher than earlier studies but the range of scores are similar. Given the considerable changes in survival, care and education it is difficult to draw conclusions about improved levels of intelligence. But taken together the picture is not of steadily declining IQs. There is a suggested of higher levels of intellectual functioning and most people with Down syndrome fall into the moderate and mild range of intellectual disability (see Terminology above).

Mental age ranges in adults

The studies produced mental ages for the late teenage and early adult years. We found mental ages ranged from less than two years – they could not be assessed on tests – to 9 years. We used a recently standardised non-verbal test of mental ability. Around 6% of the young adults had a mental age of under three years, around 50% scored at 5 years or under, and 85% at 6 years or under. Around 10% had scores of over 7 years. These levels are somewhat lower than data from Ludlow's group but this may be due to issues noted above. However, she found the same mental age range of less than two to nine years; and about 17% had a mental age over 7 years and 40% under six years.

On balance, the more recent the study and the more the participants lived with their families and in the community, the higher the percentage of children and adults classified in the moderate and mild categories. The range of ability for young adults expressed in mental ages is from unmeasurable to around 9 years. The average appears to fall between 5 and 6 years.

Factors associated with intelligence and development in children with Down syndrome

Studies of typical children have found that parental education and socio-economic class is associated with early development, educational achievements, self-esteem and motivation. Innate intellect is part of this – people with higher IQs tend to get more educational qualifications, more highly paid jobs, and are more likely to be in higher socio-economic categories; around 20 to 25% of the IQ of typical children relates to their parents IQ. Siblings, especially identical twins also have IQ's that are more likely to be similar than between non-genetically related people. Few studies have looked at this relationship in Down syndrome, but a similar effect is suggested.

As for typical children, we found, along with several other studies, that parental education is associated with the levels of development of those with Down syndrome. Similarly, compared to males, females with Down syndrome develop quicker and score at higher levels on mental ability and attainment tests. Again this is a group score and there is a lot of overlap.

Recently we re-analysed the Ludlow and Alan data used in Table 4 to include parental education and gender and found similar relationships. When we put this in the equation to look at the effects of early intervention the differences between the groups with and without the additional help reduced. This is a good example of the sort of problems found with many studies – not all the factors that might effect development are accounted for (see box). Carr found no effect for parental education or social class with IQ scores, but children from families classed as non-manual had an advantage for various attainment and language scores. This advantage was still present at 35 years of age for those raised at home and those from non-manual families.

The picture for children with Down syndrome is the same as for any child; gender, socio-economic factors and parental education are associated with mental ability test scores.

This is group data, and some children with Down syndrome have high scores on intelligence tests and come from families with little education and from low socio–economic backgrounds whilst others whose parents are highly educated are profoundly disabled. Some parents appear to do little extra with their child but have children with high scores and attainments; the children of other parents who worked extremely hard from the birth to encourage the child's developments and abilities remained in the lower levels of ability. As with typical children, innate capacities do set limits on some things and this is reflected in tests of intelligence and early development.

The possible influence of early intervention is indicated in Table 4 and is discussed in detail in Chapter 11. By early, I mean in the first two to three years of life. The evidence to support the benefits of these programmes and long-term outcomes is not that strong. This may seem to contradict the studies shown in Table 4, but the benefits in those studies may reflect the changing attitudes about infants and disability and a reduction in deprivation. Not all deprivation is obvious. When we started work we felt there was **hidden deprivation**; the child lived in very capable and caring families but the 'medical' model prevailed and they felt there was little they could do. The early intervention programmes helped to change this.

COMMON PROBLEMS WITH EARLY INTERVENTION STUDIES

Many early intervention studies have problems with biased samples. In some, the parents are those able and interested enough to attend a centre. In others, parents whose children made little progress drop out. In several, the person responsible for the training also did the testing and can bias the results. These education programmes involve activities very similar to the tasks in developmental and IQ tests, such as making towers with bricks and naming toy objects and pictures. Thus the higher test scores may partly reflect this training effect, and not enhanced intellectual ability.

Children with Down syndrome brought up in positive and stimulating homes are advantaged and score higher on mental ability and functional tests. It may be that many families may not need the high input from a formal early intervention programme.

Child Development

I have the impression that some people – parents and professionals alike – see early child development as a ladder of equal steps, and their job as encouraging, pushing or cajoling the child upwards, step by step.

Developmental checklists can certainly push parents and carers in that direction. For specific behaviours, we can produce ladder-like programmes of attainments. There are also developmental sequences in different areas such as motor development and language. Although development in young children is similar and is organised by innate factors, there are still many different pathways a child can take. This is the essence of variance and uniqueness that I keep mentioning. For example, about 1 in 10 babies do not crawl before they walk; they get around on their bottoms. There was a long debate about whether all babies, and especially those with development problems, should be made to crawl first, but there is no evidence that 'bottom-shufflers' have problems of any kind in physical, emotional or mental development. Some children are slower in walking but quicker in talking, but will learn both skills equally well, and when they are older you can't tell who walked sooner or talked earliest.

I like the analogy of child development as an upside-down Christmas tree with the baby as the star and the tree full of exciting discoveries. There are a series of stages representing levels of intellectual understanding, rather than specific behaviours. As you get older and go up the tree, the stages or zones of development get bigger, your experiences and your environment have more influence. While typical progress is up through the main trunk, there is plenty of room for branching out sideways and applying the abilities gained to different interests in an individual way.

Children with developmental delay may move up through the

stages more slowly. This gives them more opportunities to work and explore sideways. As we will see later, they may reach a stage typical of 4 to 6 years, but they have had several years to explore and develop many skills at this level. We often find they attain higher levels of skills than one would expect of typical children within that level of ability. As I will emphasise throughout this section, they may be adults with measured age equivalent scores (or mental ages) of 5 years, but they are certainly not like typical five-year old children, and should not be treated or thought of as such. The mental age should only be used as some index of potential intellectual competence.

Stages of intellectual development

This way of looking at mental growth or intellectual development was put forward by the eminent French psychologist Jean Piaget and has been an important model in developmental psychology for many years. In my opinion, it is a good starting point in trying to understand development. The main stages are:

Birth to two years – the sensorimotor period
The child explores the immediate world, discovering how to act, what things are and what can be done with them. They learn to co-ordinate senses and actions, and to organise their perceptions of the world. They will also try to set up goals and find various ways of achieving them. Most children who are profoundly disabled tend to function within this stage of development. Piaget breaks this period down into three sub-groups that reflect rapid changes in how children engage with their world around the ages of six, twelve and eighteen months.

Two years – symbolic representations
Children begin to use symbols to help them classify and organise their perceptions. They can use one thing to represent another, such as a stick for a gun. Words are the most useful symbols to use to organise the world, and language develops quite quickly at this stage.

Four years – the intuitive stage

The child is good at using symbols, and at ordering and classifying. But they will normally use intuition when reasoning out cause and effect. For example, if a child is asked 'What makes it rain?' they may answer, 'because it is thundering'. Their explanation is based on the fact that things happen at the same time. This stage lasts up to about seven years of age and covers mental ages two to seven years (corresponding with the categories of severe and moderate intellectual disability).

Seven to eleven years – the concrete –operational stage;

The child is concerned with finding out and knowing about the reality of the world. They learn that some things are constant and their reasoning is increasingly based on knowledge about the laws and physical properties of events. Monday is always followed by Tuesday, a piece of clay can be made into many shapes but it is still the same size and weight, $5 + 2 = 7 = 2 + 5 = 8 - 1 = 7$, and so on. This stage corresponds to the mild intellectual disability category.

Eleven years – abstract reasoning

The child can reason in formal and abstract terms. They begin to think in terms of propositions, can evaluate a range of information, set up possible explanations and reason out which ones may be appropriate. People who are intellectually disabled seldom reach this stage.

Stages and plateaus

A number of studies have reported that development in children with Down syndrome is marked by periods of little observable progress or plateaus. Some of these correspond to the stages above with many children taking longer to move up into the next stage.

The categories of mental disability (see Figure 15) have approximated these mental ages and stages since the first intelligence tests. Of course, the cut-off points between the stages are not precise, and the ages given are very approximate and variable, especially as the child gets older. For example, some children at the concrete-operational stage may show advanced formal reasoning.

Trying to understand what might be causing these plateaus gives an insight into how children with Down syndrome learn. They could be caused by problems with the mechanisms of learning like memory, attention and information processing, and/or slower growth and maturation.

SLOWER LEARNING AND SLOWER DEVELOPMENT

I like to think of this in terms of two children walking along a fairly broad path with different gradients, things to look at, and some obstacles. One is slower than the other, and so the further they walk, the greater the distance between them. To complicate things, the slower person might get more behind if they stop, trip or meander, or can't jump across a barrier as easily, but have to find ways of climbing over it. The faster walker might have sections of slower progress, but these are less noticeable because s/he is walking quite quickly and is better equipped to cope with obstacles. Because less energy and attention are being used in walking, they are more able to take in things of interest.

Differences in brain structure, cognitive abilities and patterns of development for children with Down syndrome

Information from neuro-anatomy studies of the structure of the brain, neuro-imaging, and neuro-psychology (relating behaviour to brain functioning), all show that between 6 to 12 months of life there is an important change or step-up in the structure and function of the pre-frontal lobes of the brain. These are the areas dealing with functions like selective attention, anticipation and inhibition.

Chapter 8 looked at how young babies with Down syndrome switch their attention from one thing to another. Chapter 7 discussed how delays in accurate reaching might relate to problems in pre-planning or anticipating effects and preparing the response. Inhibition is about stopping something and exerting control. These very important mechanisms are the first signs of what are called

executive functions. They also appear at the 'six-month' sub-stage when Piaget described very observable changes in babies' behaviours; and they coincide with the first marked differences or plateaus between babies with Down syndrome and typical babies.

From our developmental tests on over 120 babies with Down syndrome, we calculated how much development had occurred between each of our six-weekly assessments. If the baby's developmental age went up one month in line with their chronological age, their rate of developmental would be one. If it only went up two weeks in a month it would be 0.5. Figure 16 shows our results – if you turn it sideways and use some imagination, you might just see half of an up-side-down Christmas tree. There were slow and fast periods in development.

The first slow period appears to start around the three months typical development age. This is when babies learn to reach and then pick up and explore all sorts of objects. This corresponds to problems with sensory coordination – Chapter 7) With careful observation you can see other differences between the majority of babies with Down syndrome and typical babies, for example, they are less responsive and slower to react. The differences are there, but the developmental test is not sensitive enough to detect them.

The slowest rate or plateau falls around the five to six month period – the expected transition to a new stage of development. In

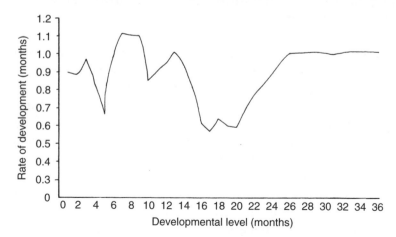

Figure 16 Changes in mean developmental rate: mental age

this second period 'mastery play' is dominant; strategies are used to explore and learn about objects. It includes exploring objects by sucking, banging and throwing, putting in and taking things out of containers, realising an object is still there even when out of sight. It is partly about having an intention or goal and developing sustained attention from one action to two in a sequence, for example, picking up, sucking and then put in a container. It is also about processing information and building up memories and consolidating learning through lots of repetition and practice. This is the when we see a rapid decline in IQ (discussed later).

This first barrier or plateau also corresponds to the rapid physical development of the pre-frontal area of the brain noted above. As we saw in Chapter 7, the nervous system is different in children with Down syndrome; there are fewer nerve cells and slower growth of interconnections. If this area functions differently, it is no wonder we find problems with attention and self-regulation, and analysis and synthesis of incoming information.

Figure 16 shows another very slow period around the developmental levels of 14 to 26 months, and particularly 16 to 20 months. This again is an area of transition between stages in typical children. This stage is seen in much use of gestures and some first words. There is a lot of imitation of actions, like kissing dolls, and increasing vocal imitation. There is a lot of problem solving and more complex play like hiding and finding things. The ability to keep several things in mind, plan things and engage with people in teasing type games is emerging. A child may put several things in boxes, then turn it up side down, anticipating that anyone observing might react by laughing. This suggests they are beginning to understand other peoples' thinking. Symbols (words and gestures) and advanced memory, planning and attention are all being used.

By two years the rapid expansion of vocabulary is starting and with it more social interactions, playing alongside others, watching and initiating, then trying things out, setting up goals and getting cross if they do not achieve them or have their own way. These are the 'terrible two's' when the child knows what they want but can't inhibit or control their desires and impulses, or be reasoned with. Again, inhibition and control are part of the growing executive function sub-system. By three to four years, this part of the system has matured in typical children.

Our observations suggested that at this 18-month stage, many children with Down syndrome showed problems linking a sequence of actions, and we saw lots of repetition of simple behaviour. When someone – often a sibling – prompted them, they would complete the task. It is as though they had lost the plan, but not the goal. When playing, the child with Down syndrome progresses more slowly through the same stages as typical children, and within each stage, they show difficulty in devising new variations and setting up sequences. They will perform with prompts and by imitation; with practice, they will learn the skill and perform it with pleasure. What many fail to do is initiate new ideas and to expand their play in a creative way.

Executive functions are involved in planning and focussing attention on different aspects and strategies relating to a task. This involves memory, and controlling the processes by which incoming information is stored while decisions are made.

Working memory

This is a particular weakness in many people with Down syndrome. 'Working memory' relates to the maturation and development of the brain structure. Short-term auditory memory can be measured by asking people to repeat back a series of random numbers. Most adults can recall 7 numbers with a range from 5 to 9 numbers. The average span for children aged two to three years is 2 numbers; for those aged three to four years it is 3 numbers, and five to six year olds recall 4 numbers. Many children and adults with Down syndrome hit a plateau of about 3 to 4 numbers, indicating that the necessary growth in the nervous system has not occurred. This is probably one of the main reasons for their slow development of language, and a barrier in developing grammatical language and reading. It will also influence many aspects of intellectual functioning and learning.

So, we have evidence that, in typical children, executive functions and memory may develop in stages, which approximate the stages and sub-stages identified by Piaget and described above. It seems sensible therefore to view the intellectual functioning and differences in children with Down syndrome from a neurological perspective in terms of executive functioning and working memory. Neuro-imaging can help to see the structure of the brain and which parts are working during specific activities. As these techniques become more widespread and less expensive, we may be able to directly test the effect of early stimulation or medication of the areas of the brain that we think are impaired in children with Down syndrome.

Inconsistency

Many studies report that children and adults with Down syndrome are inconsistent in their responses and their behaviour. As one father said, '95% of the time she is very safe and competent in the kitchen . . . makes hot drinks, cooks an egg, and then she gets it wrong'.

I have mentioned problems with consolidation and skills becoming automatic in Chapter 7. But even when skills are consolidated, they can still be inconsistent. A good example is in articulation and phonological errors. Unlike errors with some typical children, these errors do not have the same pattern; it as though each time the child with Down syndrome says a word it is for the first time. Similar lack of consistency has been described for errors in sentence structure and in perceptual processing. This could be related to executive functioning problems, the selection and retrieval of information, pre-planning, maintaining strategies and so on. A simple way to understand this is that many children with Down syndrome are less able to impose structure on information, and this interferes with their learning. If this structure is imposed for them, they can learn. Parents and teachers can do this by breaking down complex tasks into small steps and using prompts to focus the child's attention on the key points (Chapter 13).

Inhibition, control and impulses

A problem often noted with children with Down syndrome is a lack of inhibition. They will hug and kiss strangers or say embarrassing things. This is a stage seen in many typical young children before the full maturation of executive functions.

Children and adults who have experienced a serious head injury that has damaged the pre-frontal areas have similar problems with inhibition. They are more impulsive, behave inappropriately or speak to themselves. In more serious cases, it can lead to obsessive-compulsive disorder because the person cannot inhibit their thoughts or actions (Chapter 9).

Sometimes, very young children who have suffered brain injury seem to recover well, but problems appear later. The explanation is that there was damage to the brain structure that was not needed at the time of the accident and so no problems were seen. When later in the developmental process this area is needed, the child's behaviour appears more atypical and becomes a problem.

This is similar to the development of children with Down syndrome. Any difficulties may not appear until later in development. This may also explain the emergence of attentional deficit disorders and autistic type behaviours, as the child gets older (Chapter 9).

Language and communication problems

In the pre-school years the weakness of auditory processing and auditory short-term memory becomes more observable. This particularly influences the development of language and communication. By three years, there is an indication that receptive language (understanding what is said) is relatively stronger than expressive language (speech). This suggests that receptive abilities may be less impaired than expressive ones, which is along the lines noted earlier of problems sorting out information and planning. Articulation is a major problem and is thought to relate to difficulties in planning and coordinating across different systems. It is not just about motor problems making sounds.

Some recent estimates suggest that by 12 years, the average child with Down syndrome may have a vocabulary of about 2000 words. The typical 4 to 5 year-old will have around 4000 words. Although vocabulary continues to develop well into adulthood, syntax and grammar is a major problem for nearly all people with Down syndrome. As usual, there are some with exceptionally good linguistic skills.

The continuing expansion of vocabulary in later years, indicates again that when a certain level of maturation or stage of intellectual development is reached, children and adults can learn and expand their skills within that level. This is the idea of side-ways learning in the Christmas tree analogy above.

We tried several intensive training programmes with a group of infants with Down syndrome in the first and second year of life to see if we could improve attention span and memory, and so move the children through the plateau. Compared to matched children they did pass the items sooner but there was no significant benefit in their general developmental progress (as measured by the DQ), and the difference between the two groups quickly disappeared. We also found that some of the children disliked being pushed along and, sensibly in hindsight, began to refuse to cooperate. I concluded that much of delay causing the plateau at this time was due to the slowness of the maturation process, and problems with growth and reconstruction of the nervous system. Pressurising an immature system with intense practice is not helpful for parent or child. Frequent practice is beneficial once the system is more mature and will help consolidation of the skill.

The declining IQ and rate of development

In typical children the average developmental age (DA), or mental age (MA) should increase at the same rate as the chronological age because that is how MA is calculated (see above). This would produce a straight line when one is plotted against the other.

If you are developing more slowly the IQ will decline because, as noted earlier, it is computed by dividing the mental age by the chronological age. You can see the declining IQ of children with Down syndrome in table 4. The IQ score is high in the first year, but then drops quite quickly and begins to steady out at around three years, when it still declines, but more slowly. The levelling out indicates that this decline is not just about slower development and the method of calculation. If it were it should be relatively even and continue for longer. As noted above, part of the probably is the insensitivity of developmental tests in the first year, giving a higher score and not picking up the innate problems with intellectual function. This accentuates later decline. Several studies evaluating the effects of early intervention have concluded that the decline in IQ score is not found. However there is some dispute over the samples used and frequency of testing as described in the earlier section. But as we have seen children with Down syndrome will develop more slowly if deprived of the necessary inputs to encourage and facilitate their progress, and so early reports showed greater decline. Also training the children will help to maintain higher schools, but this is not the same as preventing a decline in functioning.

Many studies have shown that the average developmental age of children with Down syndrome rises just above half the rate of their chronological age. Therefore if the child's age is divided by two one can get a quick idea if they are average for young children with Down syndrome. Based on our data and assuming the child has had plenty of experience, is in good health, and lives in a positive and active family, I divide their age by three fifths in the preschool years, and in half by ten years of age. This is because the rate of development slows down over the childhood years. I also take into account that the girls generally develop quicker than the boys.

Issues of deterioration

For many years the apparent decline in IQ and slowing rate of development indicated by the mental ages, was often interpreted as mental deterioration. We have seen above that some of the apparent decline was an artefact of the tests, and low levels of stimulation.

We all know that we lose some mental functioning with age, although this is less likely if we remain active and use our mental skills. The same is true for people with Down syndrome (Chapter 7). Mental functioning is also lost with conditions like Alzheimer's disease, which is more likely in Down syndrome (see Chapters 4 and 7).

This has prompted theories that the process of deterioration is related to whatever is causing the ageing, and that it starts much earlier in people with Down syndrome. It may be related to the problems associated with anti-oxidants (Chapter 4 – superoxide dismutase). However, more recent work, is reporting that the IQ of most people with Down syndrome is stable well into adulthood and probably up to 40 or 50 years of age. Other studies have shown the same pattern for social competence; including self-help skills, independence and the ability to engage with others. There is a steady climb through childhood that gradually slows down, levelling out or reaching a plateau in middle age, before declining.

Therefore, at this time, the observations and data do not support the idea of deterioration as a general characteristic in Down syndrome. But the possibility of deterioration due to organic factors cannot be totally ruled; it needs direct evaluation with controlled studies. There are a small number of individuals with Down syndrome who show serious changes, very long plateaus, or a decline and loss of function, well before middle age. This indicates possible deterioration. Others seem to show early onset of ageing. I described some of the related health issues in Chapter 7, and in chapter 9 looked at the late onset of autism in some children.

Does the mental growth of people with Down syndrome continue for longer?

The evidence for this is limited, but the answer is probably 'yes', especially for those in the moderate and mild categories of intellectual disability. Less able children reach plateaus much earlier and appear to be less likely to move through them in terms of mental age. However, we have found that slower children may make relatively more progress on basic skills, such as reading at later ages, whilst the faster ones stick at another plateau. In typical people IQ scores level out at around 16 to 18 years, although some studies indicate a slight rise with further education. Studies of adults with Down syndrome indicate that their IQ scores may become stable, but mental ages continue to rise in early adulthood and many move into higher levels of intellectual functioning, or the next developmental stage. There is ample evidence that many adults learn new skills often to the surprise of parents.

The old idea that people with Down syndrome levelled out earlier, deteriorated and so did not profit from further education is false. They continue to learn and most go on to further education.

Are there differences between areas of development, like mental and social abilities?

Early studies found that social quotients (SQ) and social ages were usually higher than IQs and mental ages in children and adults with Down syndrome. Some studies reported as much as three years difference in late childhood. There were issues about whether the two were comparable because many of the social skills tested were self-help skills, which probably receive more attention and can be taught more easily than some of the mental ability and language tasks. Recent studies of younger children have found that the faster attainment of social skills does not emerge until the second or third year of life.

We found self-help and social skills are highly correlated with mental ability in the first years, but that after the mental age of 4 or 5, this relationship gets weaker. This suggests that the mental ability of four to five years plus physical growth is sufficient to learn most of the self-help and social competence skills measured in the tests. This is a good example of achieving stages or levels in intellectual ability and then learning other things in that zone of ability. In other words learning sideways rather than just advancing upwards.

Like most studies, we found a pattern in Down syndrome where social age is highest, then mental age and then language age. This pattern appears to be stronger in children with Down syndrome than in other children with similar levels of intellectual disability. This suggests it is specific to the syndrome and the extra genetic material from chromosome 21.

Another consistent finding is that the visual perceptual system is usually stronger than the auditory perceptual system, particular in terms of aspects of memory and processing. So we find task involving visual imitation or matching pictures are passed sooner than those involving auditory input and words.

When and how can you predict future levels of ability?

After taking into account the quality of care and stimulation a child receives, any health or medical conditions and the parents' education, the slower the child is in their overall development, (excluding motor development) the more likely that they will achieve lower IQ scores. A child with profound difficulties can be recognised in the first year of life. Children who eventually fall in the upper end of the mild range of intellectual disability may not be recognised until they start school. This is in terms of their behaviour and skills. If they have a label or look different people will be looking for signs. For other children this recognition is when they reach the 7-year old level, and the school curriculum shifts to higher demands on intellectual functioning. Of course there are individual children, typical and with intellectual disability, who seem rather slow and then blossom, and others who start very brightly and then level out.

Many studies have looked at predicting later IQ scores from earlier tests. This is done by correlating the scores; showing how well one set of scores, say at three years of age, relates to another set at five years on the same children. For groups of children with Down syndrome, these correlations begin to rise from the second year of life, and become quite strongly related by 18 months to 2 years. This is when we found the first major plateau, and the children were moving out of the sensorimotor stage. We found scores around the 2 to 3 year level predicted around 80% of the IQ scores in later childhood. The problems in the transition from this stage to the next, which includes much symbolic functioning and language, were indicative of later development and levels of intellectual functioning.

Specific behaviours and predicting future ability

We also compared the actual test items or tasks in the early assessments to mental ages at five years. We selected out those items which did not consolidate quickly; these were items that were passed initially, then failed six weeks later, then passed after another six weeks, then failed and so on. Consolidation was when the infant passed the item every time for three assessments or more. We then looked at how these items correlated with mental age at five years.

The main item in the first three months was 'showing excitement in anticipation to be picked up'. The 11% of our group who passed and then failed this item developed more slowly – at 5 years of age they were 10 months behind the average for the rest of group. From the 3 to 6 month period, the two most predictive items were 'looks at a small pellet' such as a raisin and 'smiles at themselves in a mirror'. The infants who were slow consolidating these compared to the rest, had mental ages around 7 to 8 months lower than the rest at 5 years. For the 6 to 12 month period 'looking at pictures in a book' was the main predictive item and at a slightly lower level 'co-operates in games,' 'listens to familiar words,' says 'Da-Da' or 'Ma-Ma' and 'reaches for a third cube while holding one in each hand'. The children who showed a lack of consolidation with these items also showed longer plateaus at this age; at five years of age all their mental ages fell into the lower third of our sample.

Looking at what these items have in common, my conclusion is that they highlight difficulties with emotional reactivity and arousal, attention and auditory monitoring of the environment. All of these have been noted as areas of weakness in other studies and in previous sections of this book. Even though the overall scores of mental age may not be that predictive, these items seem to tap into major problems and indicate the probability of slower or faster development and later levels of intellectual ability. Of course no single item can be used to make judgements about future ability.

Percentiles and future prediction

We looked at predicting future development in another way. We divided the mental age scores of the children into five percentage groups of: 0–20, 21–40, 41–60, 61–80, 81–100. Those with a score of less than 20 percent of the whole group went into the 0–20 category and so on. We then asked how many stayed in that category at some later test age. From 12 months of age, about half the children were in the same category three months later, but at four years of age over 80% remained in the same category on later tests. After the first year no child moved more than three groups during childhood and this remained much the same through to adulthood.

By the second year of life the scores are fairly stable, and the probability is high for the children remaining in or about the same level. Therefore if a child with Down syndrome is developing above the average for the group at two to three years, you can be fairly sure they are unlikely to drop into the 0–20% category unless they have a serious illness, accident or are one of the few that deteriorate. Equally it is unlikely that a child in the lower group will suddenly develop rapidly and achieve what we find in the upper group. But these are probabilities and there are always individuals who surprise us. What really matters is what the child is doing day-to-day and giving them opportunities to develop.

Using mental ages for prediction

In Figure 17, I have plotted the mental ages of our sample over the first five years to give an idea of the range and development. The scores are organised as percentiles, and show the percentage of the children who attained the score at different chronological ages. The fastest are the 100% line and the slowest the 1% line.

If you have a mental age for a child with Down syndrome, find their age on the chronological age line at the bottom, and draw a straight line upwards. Then find their mental age on the other axis and draw a horizontal line. Where they cross will give you an idea of how the child compares to our sample. If the child is 40 months old and has a mental age of 25 months for example, s/he would be falling around the 50% percentile and in the average range for children with Down syndrome. You then take into account gender and

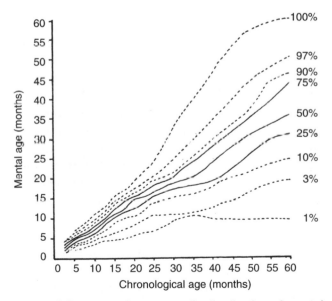

Figure 17 Down syndrome: centile distribution of mental ages

health – long period of illness could slow development. Having taken this into account you may feel the child is doing as well as expected. You can then make some informed guesses about the future needs.

What can we expect children and adults with Down syndrome to be able to do?

I hope the previous sections have helped parents understand why there are plateaus and why some people with Down syndrome advance more quickly than others, despite both having the same amount of help and support. In this section I will give an overview of what children and adults achieve.

Early Developmental Attainments

I have listed the major developmental milestones used in developmental tests in table 5, and the average age range when children with Down syndrome achieve them. Much of this information is based on our group of children, but I have incorporated results from other studies.

Since first compiling these tables, I have compared them with every report on similar data that I have found. I have also compared them to development tests on young children with Down syndrome in our recent studies. Taking into account sample and test differences, I have not found the age and range of achievement of most items to be that different. I have not found any indication that recent generations of young children with Down syndrome are attaining the milestones at much younger ages. I think these data show what might be reasonably expected for children with Down syndrome. This reinforces my belief that the big breakthrough came when we got rid of the things that deprived children with Down syndrome of opportunities to learn and to be loved and cared for like any child.

All the results in table 5 are based on children whose parents have received some help and guidance on how to stimulate the babies. I have not included the very small number of children who have severe complications, resulting in late achievement of these milestones. For example, out of 150 babies in our study who survived to five years of age, only two did not learn to walk. One had very severe motor difficulties, possibly due to damage at birth, resulting in Cerebral Palsy. The other developed leukaemia at two years, and this set his walking back considerably. However, his treatment was successful and he did walk by six years of age. I have included children with serious heart problems in the data, although they were slower in their gross motor development.

It is important to note that Table 5 provides a general guide that does not reflect the individuality of the children. Some will achieve one milestone later than average but another earlier; girls are more likely to develop quicker than boys, but of course, some girls will be slower than some boys. Because many parents of young children with Down syndrome feel the need to make comparisons I have put in averages for typical children, which may need to be adjusted slightly for new generations. But making such comparisons is not helping the child. It can help parents judge the degree of disability and make prepare for the future.

Table 5 Developmental milestones for children with Down syndrome

1. Gross motor activities (ages in months)

Activity	Children with Down syndrome Average		Typical children Average	
	Age	Range	Age	Range
Holds head steady and balanced	5m	3m to 5m	3m	1m to 4m
Rolls over	8m	4m to 12m	5m	2m to 10m
Sits without support for one minute or more	9m	6m to 16m	7m	5m to 9m
Pulls to stand using furniture	15m	8m to 26m	8m	7m to 12m
Walks with support	16m	6m to 30m	10m	7m to 12m
Stands alone	18m	12m to 38m	11m	9m to 16m
Walks alone	23m	13m to 48m	12m	9m to 17m
Walks upstairs with help	30m	20m to 48m	17m	12m to 24m
Walks down stairs with help	36m	24m to 60m+	17m	13m to 24m
Runs	around 4 years		—	
Jumps on the spot	around 4 to 5 years			

2. Personal/social/self help activities (ages in months)

Activity	Children with Down syndrome Average Age	Range	Typical children Average Age	Range
Smiles when touched and talked to	2m	1¹/₂m to 4m	1m	1m to 2m
Smiles spontaneously	3m	2m to 6m	2m	1¹/₂m to 5m
Recognises mother/father	3¹/₂m	3m to 6m	2m	1m to 5m
Takes solids well	8m	5m to 18m	7m	4m to 12m
Feeds self with biscuit	10m	6m to 14m	5m	4m to 10m
Plays pat-a-cake, peek-a-boo games	11m	9m to 16m	8m	5m to 13m
Drinks from cup	20m	12m to 30m	12m	9m to 17m
Uses spoon or fork	20m	12m to 36m	13m	8m to 20m
Undresses	38m	24m to 60m+	30m	20m to 40m
Feeds self fully	30m	20m to 48m	24m	18m to 36m
Urine control during day	36m	18m to 50m+	24m	14m to 36m
Plays social/interacting games	3¹/₂ to 4¹/₂ years		—	
Bowel control	36m	20m to 60m+	24m	16m to 48m
Dress self partially (not buttons or laces)	4 to 5 years			
Uses toilet or potty without help (often too small to get up onto a toilet unless a special step is available)	4 to 5 years			

3. Fine motor and adaptive activities (ages in months)

Follows objects with eyes, in circle	3m	1¹/₂m to 6m	1¹/₂m	1m to 3m
Grasps dangling ring	6m	4m to 11m	4m	2m to 6m
Passes objects from hand to hand	8m	6m to 12m	5¹/₂m	4m to 8m
Pulls string to attain toy	11¹/₂m	7m to 17m	7m	5m to 10m
Finds objects hidden under cloth	13m	9m to 21m	8m	6m to 12m
Puts 3 or more objects into cup or box	19m	12m to 34m	12m	9m to 18m
Builds a tower of two 1" cubes	20m	14m to 32m	14m	10m to 19m
Completes a simple three-shape jigsaw puzzle	33m	20m to 48m	22m	16m to 30m+
Copies a circle	48m	36m to 60m+	30m	24m to 40m
Matches shapes/colours	4 to 5 years			
Plays games with simple rules	4 to 5 years			

4. Communication activities (Ages in Months)

Activity	Children with Down syndrome Average		Typical children Average	
	Age	Range	Age	Range
Reacts to sounds	1m	½m to 1½m	0 to 1m	
Turns to sound of voice	7m	4m to 8m	4m	2m to 6m
Says da-da, ma-ma	11m	7m to 18m	8m	5m to 14m
Responds to familiar words	13m	10m to 18m	8m	5m to 14m
Responds to simple verbal instructions	16m	12m to 24m	10m	6m to 14m
Jabbers expressively	18m	12m to 30m	12m	9m to 18m
Says first word(s)	18m	13m to 36m	14m	10m to 23m
Shows needs by gestures	22m	14m to 30m	14½m	11m to 19m
A few two word sentences	30m	18m to 60m+		
Uses words spontaneously and to communicate	1½ to 6 years			

Overview of children's developmental milestones

I shall describe very broadly what we can expect for 50 to 75 per cent of the children with Down syndrome at each age in the main areas of development. About one half will be slower than the descriptions, and another quarter will be well in advance.

One Year

By the end of the first year, the babies will be able to sit with reasonably good balance, and pick up and play with toys. Most will be able to roll over and can be pulled to a standing position and support their own weight. They will be able to take solids from a spoon, feed themselves with a biscuit and will have begun to hold a cup and drink from it – with some mess, of course! They will be able to reach and pick up objects, even grasp small objects such as raisins, though not with a neat finger–thumb pincer movement. They will hold an object in each hand, bang them together, bang one object on another (like a drum), suck things and shake them. They will transfer objects from one hand to the other and spend much time examining them. If they make a noise they will enjoy trying to make the noise over and over again, and listening to it. They will try to get toys out of their reach, and some will pull a string to get them.

They will enjoy rough and tumble games and will laugh and giggle spontaneously. They will be beginning to laugh at 'tug-of-war' and 'teasing' games, but not as often or with the same gusto as typical babies. They will listen to voices and will recognise familiar voices and people, some will be shy of strangers. Around the first birthday many will enjoy peak-a-boo and clapping-hands games, and will be saying 'da-da', 'ga-ga' and 'ma-ma'.

Two years

By the end of their second year they will be able to get up on their feet, stand alone and take several steps, if a little unsteadily. Many will be able to crawl, but quite a number of children with Down syndrome do not crawl but learn to walk first. They will use 'da-da' or 'ma-ma' with meaning, and may have a few words. They will be jabbering with expression and using gestures to tell you what they want. They will be beginning to follow simple instructions and to imitate words. They will enjoy 'conversations' with people and listening. They will be able to use a cup by themselves, and will be trying to use a spoon to feed themselves, with varying success! They will try to help in dressing and undressing; pulling vests or sweaters off once they are over their head, stepping into pants, if holding on to something for support.

They will be putting objects in and taking them out of cups and boxes. They will scribble with a pencil or crayon and look at pictures in books, turning the pages for themselves. They will usually be able to push or roll a ball and play rolling games. They will play with simple post boxes and pegboards, use jack-in-the box type toys with a switch or catch to release the toy, and know how to make them work. They will be interested in boxes with lids, opening cupboards and emptying handbags! They will also imitate the things they see you and other children do. Many will have fun switching on the TV and changing channels!

Three years

As children get older the range of achievement gets wider, and it is difficult to be precise and confident in describing what they can do. At three years they will start to trot, pull a toy behind them, walk backwards, climb up and often downstairs with support such as a hand- or rail. They will throw a ball and make attempts at kicking. They usually manage to feed themselves, with varying degrees of mess. The majority will have bowel control and be clean. Over half will be dry during the day. They will be able to help put on and take off simple clothing with varying degrees of help. They will do simple jigsaws, draw lines rather than scribble, match simple pictures and enjoy picture dominoes or snap games, even if not very concerned with the rules. They will have favourite books and recognise pictures in stories. They will be beginning to name a few familiar pictures, and understand instructions such as 'go and get your teddy'. They will engage in simple play sequences, which will include much make-believe, such as putting dolls to bed, feeding teddy bears. Their play sequences are noticeably short and often repetitive when compared with those of typical children; they may not develop unless another child or adult is present who can extend the activities.

The greatest variations from the typical development will be found in language. Whilst most will understand many words and instructions, only a small number will use language extensively. This is more likely in girls than in boys.

Four years

By four years of age they will be able to ask or indicate to use the toilet, and manage it by themselves or with a little help. Over half will be clean and dry by day and night, with the odd accident. Some may have bouts of wetting when ill, over-excited, or far too busy doing things to 'go'. The majority will be able to feed themselves without difficulty but not necessarily without mess. They will be able to clean their teeth, wash their hands and face, dry themselves, dress and un-dress with varying amounts of assistance. Buttons and zips are usually a problem, for some even as adults.

This does not mean they will do it, only that they can do it.

Many have a strong sense of independence and demand to do their own thing; temper tantrums are likely, as with typical children. They will enjoy games with children and other people, and often seek out company, getting cross when it is not available. There is quite a lot of imaginary play, but it does not compare in the range and spontaneity to that of typical children. When they are with other children they will engage in quite complex play by imitating what they see. They will be exploratory and want new and varied experiences and to be doing things like any toddler.

Because they are often unable to develop their play without the help of an adult or child, many give up quickly and demand frequent attention and changes of activities. This can be demanding for parents and teachers, and a high level of resources is needed to cope. Help from grandparents, brothers and sisters, playmates and playgroups are all very welcome.

Four to five years

Around four to five years language will be developing. Vocabulary will increase and two or three words will begin to be linked together. Articulation is likely to be poor, so the child can become frustrated in trying to make him or her-self understood. Access to speech therapy is particularly useful at this time. By the age of **five to six years** the differences among the children are so great that an overview is difficult. I feel the fact they have Down syndrome in common is often of little consequence in understanding their future development.

Academic Attainments of people with Down syndrome

As late as 1978, and after a thorough review of studies and reports, Gibson (see Resources) concluded:

> 'The orthodox position has been that Down's syndrome individuals do not profit much from academic study, although a few are observed to develop reading and writing skills'

**BEWARE OF OUT OF DATE AND INACCURATE
CHARACTERISATION OF DOWN SYNDROME**

*e.g. Black's Medical Dictionary 39th Edition – page 15.
Published in 1999 by A&C Black: London*

'It has been estimated that 6% of Down's children are
probably capable of profiting appreciably from attendance at
schools for the educationally handicapped. Practically all who
survive to school age gain some benefit. Most eventually
acquire some degree of speech, and about 5% learn to read.
They practically never learn to write.'

---

and the outcome for those exposed to academic training:

'is frequently an increase in stress levels . . . and a decline in
self-regard without any useful educational gain'

This view of Down syndrome appears to have dominated the education of these children for many years with the result that few
attempts to teach them basic skills were tried in special schools.

However the picture is not that clear. Margaret McDowall (see
earlier) included reading and writing skills as a major part of the
curriculum in her pioneering school in 1900's. She wrote:

'The reading lesson is of manifold value: it helps speech and
memory; it presents an opportunity for teaching the *meaning* of
words and sentences; and also the imagination may be developed. Even if the children should never get far with reading, the
channel is not closed to them. When they see printed words
they realise what they are'. (p.51)

McDowall also notes that the children with Down syndrome are
more receptive to reading than other groups of children with severe
learning disability, and descriptions of her step-by-step teaching
programme suggests that many were reading single words and
simple sentences.

There are reports, dating back to the 1940's, of children with Down syndrome who can read to proficient levels. However, the average IQ of these children places them in the mild range for people with intellectual disability, and we would expect them to learn to read and write to some degree if taught.

This is another example of the need to understand the considerable differences in ability between children with Down syndrome and not get stuck on the label, and then assume all are the same.

Factors associated with developing academic attainments

By basic academic attainments I mean reading, spelling, arithmetic and writing. Like many studies, we found attainment scores increased throughout childhood. The rate of increase slowed down in the late teenage and early adult years, and the difference widened between the less able and the more able. Those adults in the lowest ranges of intellectual functioning made no progress on basic skills after their early teenage years. However those in the next level, but still lower than average for the whole group continued to improve skills, if taught. Unlike some other studies, we found a possible plateau in basic attainment skills in the later teenage and early adult years, and felt that it was partly because attempts to teach them had stopped. A few young adults had received little encouragement or opportunity to develop basic skills, yet on other measures such as their mental age, they were similar to those who were reading. Many reports on attainments make the same point and suggest that the information we have may underestimate what is possible.

Several reports have described adults with Down syndrome learning to read and write, and recently developed adult literacy programmes for people with Down syndrome say that many make good progress.

Like other studies (Carr, for example,) we found that IQ and mental age scores, plus earlier scores on tests of basic academic skills attainments recorded when they were children, were strong predictors of academic attainments for young adults with Down syndrome. We found that the child's IQ predicted 35% and mental age around 65% of the achievements during the teenage years. Mental age is made up of both ability and age, hence experience. I think this all part of the sideways and continuous learning idea (the Christmas tree model) described earlier.

We found higher academic scores are also more likely for girls and children attending mainstream schools; each predicted about 5% of the academic scores. We also found a similar level of family influence, highlighted by higher attainments of children whose fathers felt they were in control of their lives, as compared to those who felt life generally controlled them, reflecting active coping and positive expectations. Although most of the child's attainments relate to their intellectual ability, these others factors do add up and in many individual cases make a great difference. Carr also found that young people with Down syndrome from non-manual families were more likely to have higher achievements in basic skills.

The benefit of attending a mainstream school probably reflects the greater emphasis on basic skills, probably more than in special schools. However, many of the young people who attended a special school that taught basic skills, and whose levels of intellectual ability were the same as those in mainstream schools, had similar levels of achievement in basic skills.

Levels and range of attainment in people with Down syndrome

Reading

The first section of this chapter discussed problems and issues with using standardised normative tests or functional tests and checklists (see box below). These also apply in attainments. In terms of reading, normative tests provide reading ages, and functional tests show achievement of reading skills, such as reading signs and newspapers. Normative tests of reading start around the reading age of 5 years. This means that many people with Down syndrome who have some reading skills do not score on the test. We found that only 17% of our cohort could be tested on a normative reading test in the mid-childhood and early teenage years, but teacher and parent reports using a functional checklist showed many could read some words and write their name. Therefore, studies using standardised normative tests do not give an idea of the range of achievements for the Down syndrome population.

Another problem is that to obtain a reading age of 5 years on some tests the child has only to read five to 10 basic common words. This is supposed to be a sample of words, but quite young children can be taught to recognize a number of simple words. If you teach children with Down syndrome the words on the test then they will obtain a reading age; most people would not think of this as reading in the functional sense or similar to that expected from a typical child at that age. It can be misleading when people report reading ages at such low levels; in practical terms, functional measures are more useful than reading ages.

NORMATIVE READING TESTS

There are two main types of normative reading tests. One has lists of words starting with simple, high frequency words such as 'and', 'the', 'on', 'go' and ending with complex unfamiliar words. They test the ability to recognise and say the word. The other type of test involves sentences or short stories from simple to complex. These can be used to test word recognition and pronunciation, accuracy when reading sentences, and most importantly, comprehension.

FUNCTIONAL TESTS OR MEASURES

These use parent and teacher observations of what the children and young people can and do read. Parents tend to give higher ratings than teachers but generally there is close correspondence between these results and those on standardised reading tests.

Normative tests have provided some insights. Like Carr, we found that people with Down syndrome with a reading age of over seven and half to eight years, were reported to read simple books for pleasure by parents. This is the same as in typical children; and by the time the reading age is nine years they can read popular newspapers, menus, and time-tables. Around a reading age of 7 or so, most are breaking words down into sound (phonetics).

We used both types of normative tests on the young adults who were all described as readers by their parents. Their word recognition scores ranged from the lowest reading age of 5 years to the highest reading age on the test of 14.5 years. On the test with stories, several of the individuals with lower word reading ages could not score, and the reading accuracy level was some months lower. This is expected, and is found in typical children. Not found in typical children, but found in those with Down syndrome, were comprehension scores one to three years lower than their word reading scores.

Like other studies, we found older children with Down syndrome have larger vocabularies and reading skills than is expected from their mental age, when compared to typical children at the same age. Recent studies have also shown that those people with Down syndrome who are given early reading experience appear to develop their vocabulary more rapidly. This may be because they spend more time and effort learning words. They also appear to develop more awareness of the speech sounds (phonemes), which may then help vocabulary development, and possibly articulation. We need more research to answer this issue.

This again supports the idea, voiced by many parents, that the reading and communication skills of some young people with Down syndrome can give a false appearance of their levels of reasoning and understanding.

In typical children, progress with reading is closely associated with the maturing capacity of auditory short-term memory, as seen in their gradual increase in digit span; and the same relationship is found in children with Down syndrome. A span of 3, typically found around four years of age, is achieved by the majority of individuals with Down syndrome, and seems sufficient for continual vocabulary expansion and word recognition skills. However, increased short and long term memory capacity is needed for the large vocabularies and language skills that typically develop between 4 to 6 years. This does not happen for some people with Down syndrome and places a limitation on their progress.

People with Down syndrome have good skills at visually recognising the words but still have problems with memory processes and understanding meaning of what is read. The

limited evidence does not support the idea that teaching reading, early or later, has direct benefits on memory or more complex language development, such as grammar, but like signing, it does appear to help vocabulary.

Number skills

Number and mathematical skills can be assessed using both normative and functional tests. There are few studies using normative tests, and the problems are as described above for reading. Most IQ tests include items on number and mathematical skills. These skills are usually reported as being weak in children and adults with Down syndrome, particularly compared to vocabulary and visual tasks.

Functional attainments

I have used data from all the studies I could find using functional tests for older teenagers and young adults. There are not many, and you may find other sources give different percentages because of different samples, different questions and ways of summing up the responses. Some only count definite 'can do it' responses, others add in those who 'can do it most of the time' or 'usually'. Parents seem happier with the last two categories. I think this is because many people with Down syndrome are less consistent in their responses and behaviour than typical people. There is little information on this and many explanations for why it might happen. I have tried to take this into account in the tables to give a representative result in terms of 'can do it most of the time'. The percentages show how many were rated on the item. There is very little information about spelling in people with Down syndrome.

Reading

Reads 10 words	65–80%
Reads at least three common signs	60–80%
Reads simple sentences	55–60%
Reads simple stories 6 to 7 year level	45–50%
Reads books around 9 to 10 year level	40–45%
Reads adult newspapers for interest and Information (though not complex reports)	30–40%

Between a half and three-quarters of people with Down syndrome can learn a good range of words. Recognising major signs such as toilet, exit, danger, push, bank etc. will help their independence. There are a number of programs containing these words; it is worth looking at them closely to see how they fit into the young person's every day environment.

Writing

Writes first and last name	65–75%
Writes a simple sentence of at least four words	40–50%
Writes ten words from memory and short notes	40–45%
Writes simple letters and postcards	25–30%
Addresses envelopes	20–25%
Writes understandable compositions and stories	20–25%
Writes adult-type letters to friends	16–20%
Write business-type letters	3–8%

Some people with Down syndrome have additional motor coordination problems that affect their ability to write legibly. Using computer keyboards can help children with such problems. I certainly expect far more children with Down syndrome to engage in writing using computers, spelling programmes and e-mail. As yet, I have no information on what might be achieved, and suspect the current percentages may be on the low side. Judging from the magazines published by young people for others with Down syndrome, there are certainly many who enjoy writing and write well. Several of the young people in our sample are particularly keen on writing poetry, stories and dramas. I know some with an extensive circle of e-mail friends.

Number, money and time

These percentages are for young adults around 18 to 25 years of age.

Basic arithmetic

Names and matches numbers up to 10	70–75%
Adds numbers up to 10 with materials	45–55%
and adds in head, using fingers if needed	35–45%
Adds up to 20 in head	20–25%
Subtracts numbers up to 10 with materials	15–25%
Simple division	3–7%

Time

Understanding the function of clock	75–80%
Tells time accurately to five minute intervals (non-digital)	25–30%

(I have found no data on telling time from digital clocks but my impression is more children with Down syndrome can do this)

Money

Knows values of low value coins	45%–55%
Knows values of all coins	25–35%
Copes with change for small amounts	20–25%
Copes with change more than £1	10–15%

(up to 25–30% depending on how complex the purchase price and change is)

Saves money for something special	30–40%
Uses a current account independently	4–7%

Investing effort in attaining basic literacy and numeracy skills

The above figures may be an underestimation because they include children and adults who may not have been given all opportunities and encouragement to attain basic skills. There is no doubt that for many the effort to attain the skills is well worthwhile.

Others fail to achieve significant levels of numeracy and literacy, despite coming from very supportive and educationally oriented families, and attending schools that taught such skills. This raises the issue we started with, as to how much effort should be made by the child, the parents and teachers to achieve such skills. I know of some children who have become very stressed because of the pressure to achieve these skills, but this seems rare.

However, the figures above indicate that by emphasising achievement in academic skills, there is a real danger of undervaluing a large group of children with Down syndrome. It is the same as comparing the development and achievements of people with intellectual ability with typical people and then making value judgements about their general worth.

Inherent levels of intellectual ability are the main predictors of attainment and while there may be useful spin-offs in teaching reading for example, we should take into account when the child is likely to have matured sufficiently to make learning the skills a relatively happy and successful event. A balanced view is needed, that looks at other skills that may be more useful and achievable for the child at different times in their development. For many we need to make some judgement about their future levels of functioning, the implications for their life, and then address the question about the part basic academic skills will play in their lives.

Attainments of Self-sufficiency and Social skills

As with academic skills, we found that the child's mental age predicted how quickly he or she attained self-help and social skills, and the eventual levels achieved in adulthood. However, as noted earlier, the IQ predicted less and less of the scores as the child grew older. There is no strong evidence that health, gender, social class, or parental education is related to the levels achieved in life skills. This suggests that once the child or young adult has reached the 4 to 6 years developmental stage, they are intellectually equipped to learn most self-help and basic social skills. How they use them is determined by practice and the expectations of others.

Once we took mental age into account we found that the children of mother's who generally used practical coping strategies in dealing with problems, as opposed to wishful thinking, were more advanced in this area of development. It only related to 4% of the scores compared to 50% for mental age, but is still significant. We also found that if the child had an excitable and impulsive temperament and/or behaviour problems, the scores were lower. Together this had a 6% influence. It seems reasonable that children with behaviour problems are difficult to teach, but at the same time, parents who take on the issue and try to deal with it, get a measurable result.

Levels of attainment

Again the actual percentage of people acquiring specific skills varies between studies. There is some indication that more recent samples have more skills than earlier ones. These percentages show the wide range of ability and achievement within the Down syndrome population, but that the probability of full independence and living in their own home without help and supervision is small. I think we will see a shift towards the higher levels in new generations, but that most adults with Down syndrome will always require some level of supervision and support. Even so, well over half do achieve good levels of competence in their basic self-help and social skills; certainly sufficient to create their own space and life-style and lead varied and interesting lives.

In the following table I have used our data and other studies to give an approximation of the ranges achieved by current samples of young adults with Down syndrome at 18 to 25 years of age. It is based on the response, 'does it independently most of the time'

Personal Skills

	% competent
Uses knife, fork, spoon and drink from cup etc.	over 90
Reasonable table manners	over 90
Cope with all foods	70 to 80
Eating out, ordering a complete meal from menu	45 to 50
Washes hands and face	80 to 90
Brushes teeth	75 to 85
– regularly	65 to 75
Baths or showers	75 to 85
– and dries thoroughly	60 to 70
Washes hair	70 to 75
– and dries thoroughly	40 to 60
Keeps nose clean	75 to 85
Fully toilet-trained	70 to 95

(this figure varies depending on what is considered an occasional mishap, and judgements about competence in wiping the bottom. Many cope well except for this. Our mean was 80% and included no accidents, reasonable wiping and washing hands).

Undresses except for difficult fasteners	over 90
Undresses with no help	80 to 90

Dresses self except for difficult fasteners and tying shoelaces	80 to 90
Dresses self with no help	65 to 70
Coping with menstruation	60 to 65
Coping with shaving	40 to 65
Selecting appropriate clothes for the weather, work, school etc.	60 to 70
Keeps clothes tidy, folds, hangs them up etc. (women more than men)	40 to 50
Takes complete care of own clothes, washing, ironing, etc. (depends on age and the extent the parent does it for them)	less than 10
Understands danger in the home – hot etc.	over 90
Looks both ways crossing road	50 to 55
Aware of potential dangers accepting things from strangers	50 to 55

Domestic Skills

These are influenced by whether the person is given the opportunity and training. I believe the higher levels are for those that have been encouraged and are indicative of what is possible.

Sets a simple table	over 90
Clears away the table	80 to 90
Washes dishes	70 to 80
Washes everything and cleans kitchen	40 to 60
Can use a stove or microwave	35 to 45
Prepares simple meal , cold	40 to 60
– requires mixing and cooking	20 to 25
Keeps own room tidy	65 to 80
Cleans own room	30 to 60
Regularly cleans other room, like kitchen or bathroom without being asked	20 to 25

Social Skills – Out and About

Listens to and copes with simple spoken instructions	80 to 90
Will listen to a story/conversation for at least 5 minutes	80 to 85
– to a lecture or talk for at least 15 minutes	60 to 75
Tells a story, lengthy joke or about some experience	60 to 65
Gives complete address	65 to 70
Initiates telephone calls to others	60 to 65
Can make emergency calls	60 to 65
Uses telephone for all kinds of calls	20 to 25
Can go out and travel with family and responsible friends (depends on how far, mobility, who the friends are and willingness of parent)	60 to 80
Can move about the neighbourhood independently (again depends on were family live)	30 to 50
Can travel independently on public transport	less than 25

Social life of people with Down syndrome

This is related to social skills, communicative abilities and behaviour, and therefore mental ability. Our own and other studies have found that most of the young people in the profound and lower end of the severe range had no friends and very limited social contacts. Those in the upper end had quite extensive social lives, except for the very few with mental health problems or autistic symptoms. As for any of us, the number and range of contacts for an individual depended on lots of factors other than their skills and personality. They had more contacts and were more likely to have friends if they lived within a safe community; if their parents had the resources to take them to and from clubs and friends; if there were good local resources for people with intellectual disabilities like clubs, drama groups, swimming and so on. Some refused to take part in these 'special' activities (see 'awareness' in Chapter 8).

Overall, there was a steady decline in social contacts from late childhood onwards, and social isolation becomes an issue for many teenagers and adults with Down syndrome. A constant problem is that their contact with typical children in school and the community gradually reduces. Children and adults tend to select friends of similar interests and abilities (see Chapter 13). Many parents describe how the local children of the same age 'outgrew' the child with Down syndrome. If there are other children in the neighbourhood with intellectual disability, then they usually become friends. Also the siblings and their group of friends often include the child with Down syndrome. We found the decline in the number of social contacts partly occurred when siblings became more independent or left home. It is the resources available, and not just the characteristics of the child or young person with Down syndrome, that affects their social life. These findings are based on people living at home with their parents. My impression is that social contacts and social life for many improve when they move into accommodation with other people with intellectual disability. Improvements have been seen as services become more focussed on life-styles and person centred planning (Chapter 12).

We should be aware that with increasing age, people with Down syndrome are vulnerable to social isolation, but it is not inevitable.

Further Education and people with Down syndrome

In many countries further education is now provided for people with intellectual disability. Eighty five percent of the young people in our group had been or were attending further education courses. Three-quarters of these courses were in local mainstream Colleges of Further Education. A small number attended residential colleges. They were studying a variety of subjects, depending on ability. For the less able these are often a continuation of life-skills to improve basic levels of independence. For the more able they include vocational training. Skills that improve the young adults use of their leisure time are valuable, such as photography, art and drama. In some locations there are gym and drama groups for people with intellectual disability. Several also use mainstream facilities and further education evening classes. Some colleges are more successful than others at forming links into the community to help with the transition from college.

Unfortunately, at the present time many parents find that once their child leaves college there is little for them. Hopefully the shift to person-centred planning will have an impact on this for future generations.

Employment of people with Down syndrome

Accurate figures on employment of people with Down syndrome are very difficult to obtain as they depend on were people live, jobs available, ability and skills, support available and so on. There are many people with Down syndrome who are in employment and coping well, and it is not just those of the highest intellectual ability.

In many countries there has been a shift in thinking from merely occupying adults with Down syndrome or employing them in highly supervised training centres, to seeking wider opportunities and employment in the community. Supported employment schemes have been operating in some places. These seek out potentially suitable employment and employers and carefully prepare the workplace and people. A designated person from the workplace or the agency works alongside the young person, until they have mastered the necessary skills and understanding. Schools and colleges do arrange work experience.

We found that two thirds of the young adults in our group wanted a job. Nearly all the parents wanted the young person to have some purposeful and meaningful activity, and over half felt this should be some form of employment, paid or voluntary. Some parents had found part-time work for their child whilst still at school.

Many of the young people had little idea of the actual work they wanted to do, how to go about finding work or the implications of work. Some had very fanciful ideas. I think this will improve with the introduction of person centred planning and targeted resources on the aspirations of the young people themselves (Chapter 12).

Many who had started in some form of employment failed to continue. Often this was due to problems with controlling emotions and behaving appropriately, rather than ability to do the job.

About 15 to 20% were unlikely to ever work in any meaningful way because of their disability, and several able young people did not want to work. Some had come to this conclusion after having work experience.

Those in employment were more likely to be in part-time than full time work, and in some cases this was related to the problem of losing benefits. My current very rough estimates are that around 10 to 25% could be in some form of sustained employment, but more are able to engage in meaningful occupation often through some voluntary agency.

Leaving Home and Place of Residence

Living in the parental home depends upon family circumstance and local services. A very small number of children with Down syndrome leave the parental home in their teenage years because they have behavioural difficulties beyond the coping resources of their families. Most continue to live at home well into adulthood. In areas that provide supported homes in the community, more adults with Down syndrome live in them than with their parents. Such moves of course depend upon the wishes of the young people and/or their parents. Some parents have made separate accommodation within their own homes in order to provide independent living, but maintaining a watchful eye and giving support.

In the older London sample, Carr reported that 60% of people with Down syndrome were living with their parents at 30 years of age and 51% at 35 years. We found corresponding rates in our younger sample, with about 20% leaving home in late teenage to early adult years, often to go to residential college and then into their own accommodation. This gradually rises with age; many of the young people and their parents seemed to think that by around 30 years they would be living elsewhere. Most of those who do leave home and live with other people with disability, or in their own homes, do not appear to regret it. They do seem to enjoy more freedom and more friends.

Summary

How we view Down syndrome and disability has a considerable impact on their lives. The current social model has focussed on barriers in society rather than the person's impairment. This has opened up many possibilities for people with Down syndrome.

Although IQ becomes stable in early childhood, over 90% of children with Down syndrome can be expected to continue to develop their intellectual functioning well into their teenage years, and many into early adulthood. They also continue to acquire new skills into their middle age. Only a few show deterioration during this time. From middle age, they do begin to lose skills, but like typical people this is related to life-style and levels of activity.

Childhood development is marked by periods of plateau. These relate to specific problems and to transitions between different levels of intellectual functioning. The majority of children fall into the categories of moderate and mild intellectual disability. About 10 to 15% fall into the profound category and require considerable levels of care and supervision, although many achieve quite good basic self-help skills compared with other conditions causing profound and severe intellectual disability.

The majority of people with Down syndrome attain levels of personal self-help skills and communication skills to be reasonably independent and not require close supervision. They also have a range of interests, hobbies and activities. The majority are able to live meaningfully in the community, either with parents or relatives, in shared houses, their own accommodation or sheltered communities. It is a matter of what is available, the preference of the young person and the feelings of the parent. Very few achieve the levels of independence of typical people; most require varying levels of support and supervision.

There have always been some people with Down syndrome who show exceptional abilities and skills. They have written books, become artists, photographers, actors, athletes and gymnasts, weight-lifters, mechanics and so on. As expectations and opportunities have increased more and more engage in such activities and increasing numbers are achieving higher levels of independence and control over their lives.

Although a minority, many have mature and caring relationships with others, some within marriage. Many more would like this, but finding someone is difficult unless they have opportunities to meet people with similar interests and abilities. Some find employment and like it. Others choose not to. More and more people with Down syndrome are joining in advocacy groups and making their voices heard. Some are members of committees and advise or make decisions about needs and service provision. Many more are making decisions about their own lives.

Whether or not they amaze us by their achievements will depend upon our understanding of Down syndrome and our expectations. But although the majority will be dependent on understanding and attitude of others, there is no doubt that far more people with Down syndrome will lead happy, fulfilled and more independent lives than Langdon Down could ever possibly have imagined when he first recognised and described the condition in 1866.

11

Treatments, early interventions, teaching and learning

- What medical treatments are available?
- Can alternative treatments or therapies be beneficial?
- Is cosmetic surgery useful for people with Down syndrome?
- Can early intervention and stimulation programmes help?

How can we help our child learn? In this chapter I describe some of the main attempts to remedy problems connected with Down syndrome. These are not standard therapies or medication that you would give to any child, such as physiotherapy for displaced hip, or medication for thyroid disorders.

There have been many 'treatments' and every few years a new one emerges with the usual claims to improve the physical features behaviour or intellectual abilities of children with Down syndrome. Usually professionals examine the evidence and say it is not very scientific. There may have been small numbers of children used, poor controls for comparison of treated and non-treated children or poor measures and statistical analysis. More scientifically credible studies are then carried out and fail to find evidence to support the original claims. This is publicised and the treatment falls out of favour, but the next generation of parents are faced with some new treatment. Sometimes, parents get caught up in 'treatments' because of their need to do the best for their child. As the hoped for benefits fail to emerge they give up and tell other parents.

I discuss these treatments in the first section and then early interventions and stimulation programmes. In the third section I discuss practical ways that you can help your child with Down syndrome learn.

Remember that children with Down syndrome are all very different and that having Down syndrome is not a reason for any treatment. Before you agree to any treatment for your child, refer to the checklist of questions below.

QUESTIONS PARENTS SHOULD ASK BEFORE PROCEEDING WITH TREATMENTS OR THERAPIES FOR THEIR CHILD WITH DOWN SYNDROME

1 Is this treatment being advised just because the child has Down syndrome?
   YES: since they are all very different it is unlikely to be effective. Leave alone.
   NO: find out more.

2 Have you been given, or found, a theory or set of reasons why the treatment should work for your child?
   NO: Ask for more information before proceeding.
   YES: Proceed.

3. Has the person advising the treatment given you clear written information about:
   the benefits to expect
   any potential risks
   how you will monitor or see them
   how long before you will see the benefits – short and/or long term
   risks of side-effects – short and/or long term
   possible complications
   what to do, who to contact if complications or side effects occur

what the costs might be in terms of money and time
NO: ask for answers before you proceed
YES: They are professional and you could proceed with
confidence, but
4   There is no harm in seeking a second opinion or checking
the information through your Down syndrome association,
the Internet, or other parents.

Questions parents should ask themselves and other members
of the family.
5   Does your child really need/want this intervention or
treatment or are the benefits really what you want?
6   Do you and your family have the resources and
commitment to carry out the intervention or treatment?
7   Does it mean that some family members may have to give
up things they want to do, and if so have they been
consulted?
8   Do all the family understand the implications of the
treatment and are they willing to proceed?

'Medical' Therapies

Cell therapy

This consists of regular injections of freeze-dried organ cells from
foetal lambs, called **sicca cells.** The theory is that the corresponding organs or parts of the brain in the child with Down syndrome
will absorb the cell material. It argues that this should compensate
for the lack of nerve cells and the difference in their outputs, which
will then improve the function of the organ, and many aspects of
physical and intellectual development.

Cell therapy has never been used alone. Additional vitamins,
minerals and enzymes are given, as well as advice on diet, educational and therapeutic treatments. It is impossible to work out
which aspect of this holistic treatment might be effective for which
of the many benefits claimed.

Proponents have reported that it accelerates growth and improves facial features, IQ, motor skills, social behaviour, language and memory. Unfortunately, the studies making these claims have problems in their method; there is little information about the background and selection of the groups given treatment, and those without treatment, used for comparison. This is important, because social and economic background, and the educational level of parents are both related to the level of development of typical children and those with Down syndrome (Chapter 10). This treatment is expensive, and it may be that more educated and well-off parents are likely to have it. Also, it is not clear which families dropped out. Parents who do not see much improvement in their child are more likely to stop.

When I looked at the data claiming benefits, I was struck by the fact that the group who had the treatment, although more able in terms of the measures of motor, social and intellectual functioning than the comparison data, still fell within the range of what is found for people with Down syndrome. Therefore they could be a group selected from the potentially 'more able' within the normal range of ability for Down syndrome.

I would be more convinced that the treatment really did affect fundamental processes, if the normal range for Down syndrome had shifted up towards the normal range for typical children. I have met parents whose children, now adults, believe the treatment really helped them, but again, these 'treated' individuals with Down syndrome were functioning in the ranges that many people with Down syndrome achieve without the treatment.

Several controlled studies failed to find significant benefits for cell therapy. Some critics feel that these studies are also flawed. In a recent retrospective study comparing people with Down syndrome who had the treatment some years before, with well-matched ones who had not, there was no evidence of a permanent or long-term gain, once the groups were matched on factors known to influence development.

New variations of cell therapy are likely, and may include the use of freeze-dried human foetal tissue. However this is currently a subject of huge debate on scientific and moral grounds.

Electrochemical (neurotransmitter) treatments

These treatments are aimed at enhancing electrochemical neuro-transmission in the nervous system. Several medications (physostigmine, tacrine, donepezil, aniracetam and piracetam) appear to have achieved some success in adults with dementia and some aspects of learning difficulties. This approach is essentially one of compensating for low levels of the chemicals. The main examples are:

5-hydroxytryptophan therapy

This treatment was explored in the 1960's and 70's. The aim was to reduce the effect of lower than ordinary levels of a neurotransmitter called **serotonin**. This is related to slower responsiveness and poorer muscle tone found in children with Down syndrome. It was argued that treatment with 5-hydroxytryptophan, a precursor in the metabolic pathway leading to serotonin, would increase levels and improve function. Some early small studies, with no comparisons with non-treated control children, suggested it might help. However, several well designed later studies, failed to find any benefits, even though the injections did improve muscle tone. This points to the need for careful scientific research before believing a cure has been discovered. Being part of the study can raise the hopes of parents and the way they interact with the child. Any perceived benefit may be due to changes in the parent, not the treatment.

Piracetam

This is a more recent stimulant of the nervous system. Some studies of typical children with specific difficulties in reading, spelling and writing found that the children given piracetam over a period of time gained higher scores than those who were not. Other studies have failed to support some of the claims. Although the higher scores were statistically significant, many people have argued that the difference was not important to the child's life. Clearly, any treatment has to be shown to be useful to that person. This drug has been studied in relation to other disorders, such as Alzheimer's disease and certain seizure disorders. The prospect of it being effective for children with Down syndrome excited many parents and professionals, but the one controlled study completed so far has not found any significant benefit in intellectual functioning.

A problem with 'neurotransmitter therapy' is that the substances taken may not be absorbed in their original form; and what might work in one person's system may not work quite the same in another. We know there are many differences in the biochemical system of people with Down syndrome (Chapter 8), not just compared to typical people, but also between people with Down syndrome. Because the level of a substance is less in some people with Down syndrome than in typical people, it does not follow that giving it to them will help. The low level might be normal to their system. Some drugs, like Deanol and Ritalin, are stimulants and have been shown to be helpful with behaviourally disturbed children and those with hyperactivity. They may help with such problems in people with Down syndrome (Chapter 9), but they are addictive and can induce seizures. They should only be considered with the specialist advice of a child neurologist.

At present there are a large number of potentially influential biochemicals, and many are being explored in different groups of people, some with Down syndrome. But so far there is no substantiated evidence of benefits for all children with Down syndrome. Efforts will certainly continue and may one day result in some effective treatment.

Can treatment prevent degeneration?

The above treatments have mainly been aimed at compensating for a deficit. A second approach is to try to protect the nerve cells from premature dysfunction or degeneration. See also the later section on nutritional supplements and folate.

Recent interest has focussed on REST, short for **repressor element-1 silencing transcription factor**. REST interacts with other chemicals to help regulate normal nerve cell growth and development. This means it is an important part of brain development, neuronal plasticity (the way the brain organises itself) and forming synapses, all of which are different in Down syndrome (Chapter 7). A recent study has suggested a link between problems with the REST factor and neurological problems in Down syndrome.

Under-activity of REST has been shown to trigger early programme cell death, which might be part of the reason for the
under-development of nerve cells, particularly the branching and
connections that are a characteristic of Down syndrome.

These advances open potentially important opportunities for
treatment. Rather than just compensating for the lack of a sufficient
amount of a particular chemical, they may prevent degeneration or
restricted growth. Thus they remedy, though don't fully cure, a
problem.

A 'MAGIC' GENE?

As I write this, another headline: 'Down Syndrome Cure' has
appeared in my local paper, followed by parents and
professionals seeking details, some of whom want to enlist in
experimental trials. A recent study using trisomic mice
(Chapter 4) identified a gene that is associated with nerve
damage and problem solving, and then found they could
reverse the damage. Potentially, this means any degeneration
might be reversible. This might enhance intellectual
functioning, but of course it will not change physical
characteristics. The article about this appeared in a
professional magazine and not in a peer reviewed academic
journal. As found in many potential cancer treatments, what
works in a mouse frequently does not work in the more
complex system of the human being. This headline emerged
before other scientists can even begin to examine the
evidence, let alone try to replicate it. But we are nudging
closer to treatments that are more fundamental than previous
attempts.

Alternative therapies

My impressions are that the use of alternative therapies such as
dietary supplements, reflexology, aromatherapy and craniosacral
therapy, is increasing. My observations suggest that many parents
who take up alternative therapies believe it will help to remedy the

child's intellectual disability, and that some have not fully come to terms with the disability or do not fully understand the nature of Down syndrome as a complex chromosomal disorder affecting many parts of the body.

Having said this, it is difficult to resist getting involved when other parents around are excited by the prospects of some new treatment. Many try it for a while, but in my experience it gradu-

---

A recent alternative treatment is being developed in India. I will describe it in some detail to illustrate how things develop in this world of Down syndrome, rather than to advise that it should be used. The product – **Learnol-Plus** (from the Dalmia Centre for Bio-Technology) is syrup containing well-known and widely used herbs (notably Brahmi) that, according to the producers, have a long history in herbal medicine in India for nervous disorders. I assume it will be attractive to many people because of the increasing interest in herbal medicine. Experimental studies in rats have shown that Brahmi prevents the loss of **acetycholine** (part of the neuro transmission system). In people, it is claimed to reduce brain overactivity and increase attention span. This is thought to slow down degenerative processes as Brahmi regulates the metabolism of biogenic amines. The manufacturers have had some studies carried out to evaluate its use for children with learning disability, including some with Down syndrome, and claim that concentration and memory was improved after 3 to 6 months of therapy in those with mild and moderate levels of disability. No differences were found for those with severe intellectual disability. It is also claimed that improvement was found in speech defects and overall mental performance, and anxiety levels were reduced in teenagers. This suggests that the effect may be to calm some children, and so improve their concentration and learning. Unfortunately, as far as I can determine at this time, there have been no independent trials about the use of Learnol-Plus with children with Down syndrome.

ally fades out – usually because the hoped for benefits have failed to emerge, or the evidence against it is more widely available. Because such treatments often ride on the back of publicity and word of mouth, what is waning in one country is often found to be starting up in another. Again, I would emphasise the importance of seeking out information from many sources before taking on any treatment.

Craniosacral therapy or cranial osteopathy

This treatment is based on the idea that the fluid-filled cavities in the brain and spinal cord represent a semi-closed hydraulic system with its own intrinsic rhythm. By gently manipulating the skull and this system, it is believed that other systems are helped such as the nervous, musculo- skeletal, endocrine and respiratory systems. I have found no studies of its use with children with Down syndrome, but some parents have tried it.

Aromatherapy and massage

These therapies are popular and are used regularly in some special schools. Again, I have found no reliable studies showing benefits or not, for children with Down syndrome. The therapies do soothe and calm, and help circulation, and are sometimes included in physiotherapy programmes, particularly for children who are not mobile.

Diet and nutritional supplements

As noted in other sections of this book, studies have shown differences in the metabolism and levels of enzymes, trace elements and some minerals of people with Down syndrome. This has led to several 'treatments' with various dietary supplements, but as we shall see, very little good scientific evidence to support them. What is worrying is that at the end of the 1990's, estimates suggested that about 20% of parents had or were using megavitamin therapy with their children with Down syndrome, and too much can be toxic.

If any child has a medical complication or is ill or less healthy, parents naturally wonder if they can do something to help, and often look at diet and supplements. Dietary supplements are becoming more popular with the general public, and so many parents of children with Down syndrome ask if such supplements are needed.

The broad answer at this time is that vitamin or mineral supplements are not needed for Down syndrome. They may be needed if the child has some additional problem. Excess supplements cause toxicity.

There are inborn errors of metabolism caused by chromosomal errors (Chapter 4) and special diets do reduce or prevent intellectual impairment in children with these conditions. However, the problem in Down syndrome is that it is not just one, but many, bio-chemicals that may differ, and we do not fully understand the complex processes that they are involved in.

> If your child is active and having a reduced calorie diet, multivitamins may help (Chapter 7). Similarly if the child has been ill a supplement may be advised, as with any child. If as a family you tend to take supplements, and understand the dangers of toxicity, then there is no reason why your child with Down syndrome should be excluded. In recent years there is a growing argument for supplements, often related to ageing and more and more research is being carried out. At the present time, there is no apparent reason why older people with Down syndrome should not take them. It is always best to double check with your medical advisor.
>
> *Using hair samples as a method of detecting problems with metabolism has been found to be unreliable. Unfortunately this method is still used by some people to determine if supplements are needed.*

What we do know about a few of them is that some are over-active and some are under-active. It may be that treating Down syndrome with high doses of vitamins will improve the function of some of the under-active bio-chemicals, but equally well, they may make some of the over-active ones even more active, which may be harmful. It is known that pyridoxine (vitamin B6) given in high doses when not needed, damages the nerve cells. Toxic states are also found from too much Vitamin A and D.

Specific vitamin and mineral therapies

The most widely used megavitamin treatment for Down syndrome, was the Turkel 'U' series starting in the 1940s. A mixture of 48 vitamins, minerals, enzymes and other drugs are prescribed, and it was claimed they diminish the 'inborn structural, functional and chemical abnormalities in Down syndrome'. A controlled study carried out in the early 1960's found no improvement in treated children compared to non-treated children. Although beneficial claims are still being made, no medical authority supports this treatment.

In studies like this, parents are often sure they have observed benefits in their child and so feel the treatment works. However, measures from the evaluation tests used fail to show benefits. It may be the measures were not tapping the things that the parents saw as beneficial. Equally, taking part in the study may have altered the parent's behaviour or way of looking at the child. Parents may have invested financial resources, time and much emotional energy in the treatment, and so be reluctant to conclude it failed.

A more recent study reported increased intellectual functioning and improved health and physical appearance after an eight-month treatment of mega doses of 11 vitamins and eight minerals. But some children dropped out of the research, and no reasons were given. They could be the ones whose parents felt that it was not working. 14 of the children were given thyroid supplements, and as noted earlier, some children have thyroid disorders (Chapter 7) and may have needed to be treated. Was it the vitamins or the thyroid supplement that was effective? Although this study was criticised for being badly designed, it received wide publicity throughout the world, mainly under the headlines of 'a cure for Down syndrome'.

Many parents started to use megavitamins. Since then, several well-controlled studies have all failed to repeat the findings and there is no scientific evidence to support the idea that this package of supplements is helpful in Down syndrome.

FUTURE POSSIBILITIES

Folate

Folate is a dietary chemical that particularly promotes growth in red blood and nerve cells. It has been found to be low in the red blood cells of people with Down syndrome and it is suggested that occasional checks in adult life and possible treatment with folate supplements may help metabolic problems (Chapter 7). As yet, I have not found any studies evaluating this idea.

Trace elements

A number of trace elements, essential in metabolism, have been found to be low in many people with Down syndrome. Many are related to problems with ageing and the defensive mechanisms of the body. There is quite a lot of research activity in this area but so far no treatment has been established as beneficial by quality research. There are ongoing studies with various supplements in infants.

Some physical programmes

Kinaesthetic Training

This is a system of motor training developed for 'clumsy' children. It is based on theories of perceptuo-motor coordination – it attempts to improve the integration of the systems and build up automatic programmes (Chapter 7). Because of similar difficulties in children with Down syndrome, it has been suggested that it may help them. There has been considerable debate about its claims of success in the scientific and clinical literature. I have not found any published studies about its use with children with Down syndrome.

My current view is that plenty of exercise involving balance and different motor practices is probably as good, and more part of an everyday life-style.

Patterning

This was initially developed by Doman and Delcato some years ago for children with severe physical and intellectual disability. It was based on taking children through the sequential order of motor development for typical children in very intensive ways. There was considerable controversy about it. The theory was questioned and the results were not replicated independently. A major problem was that it demanded so much organisation and time from parents that family life was disrupted. However, at a time when society generally held a medical model of intellectual disability (Chapter 10), the programme motivated many parents and their children profited, if not directly from the patterning then from increased stimulation and positive expectations. The programme and several derivatives are still found in many countries.

Drama Therapy

This is not an alternative therapy but a well-established approach used to help with emotions and relationships with other people. Using puppets and dolls as actors can help the child work through difficult experiences and express themselves. Many special schools and some mainstream schools, use drama to help with such emotional problems. It is also used for role-play, such as being a shop-assistant, having a job interview and so on.

Drama therapy is not just for professionals. Parents can easily learn how to use it and I am quite sure many would find it beneficial. It can seem strange at first, and everyone can feel self-conscious; but it is one of those things that can arise naturally out of early play. It is easier if it is established early on, rather than tried as something new at later ages. Most children like drama and play-acting, and young siblings are usually happy to join in.

I once observed a young man with Down syndrome and very limited language, acting out to his brother how he had had a fight in the playground. The brother then engaged in this and showed how he could defend himself. It was all quite natural. Other families have told me about how they often sit through the child acting out what has happened. My point is that this can be extended, just as we extend verbally expressed ideas in conversation.

Parents may find it useful to set up role play in which family members act out a scene and show the child with Down syndrome how they might deal with it. As noted earlier in this book, the use of drama for people with Down syndrome has a long history and was certainly recognised by Langdon Down.

Facial Cosmetic Surgery

The idea that changing the appearance of a child with Down syndrome has a substantial effect on their intellectual and social functioning is, to me, very simplistic. The characteristics of people with Down syndrome are influenced by many factors. Appearance is important, but once you get beyond it, the ability to communicate and find shared interests is what helps people engage with one another. As described in Chapter 7, studies have tried to find evidence of an association between the physical characteristics of Down syndrome, including appearance, and social skills, language, intelligence, social life and behaviour difficulties, but without success.

A survey in 1984, found that parents were far less likely than medical practitioners to regard the facial features of children with Down syndrome as unpleasant, and the practitioners were more likely to favour the use of cosmetic surgery.

The studies that have reported positive benefits of cosmetic surgery have largely relied on parents' perceptions, and have not used more objective controlled measures to prove the point. Since parents who choose cosmetic surgery are a very small and select group, and invest quite a lot of their time, emotions and money into the procedure, it is reasonable to question their perceptions of benefits.

There may be specific cases in which surgery is appropriate. The criteria for making the decision should be those that apply to any child – not just one with Down syndrome. The reduction of a very large tongue may be needed if it is causing problems with eating, breathing or speech. Such an operation can lead to more normal mouth closure, fewer respiratory infections and improved eating. Improvements in speech have not been confirmed, although this was amongst the first claims of benefit by those advocating this surgery. Speech problems are likely to have complex causes involving the mouth, tongue and lip movements.

Parents should carefully consider the advantages and disadvantages of such procedures. Children take little notice of the physical features of their fellow playmates – at least up to six to eight years of age – especially if the features are not very striking or disfiguring. Instead, they make friends and create impressions by who they are – their temperament, skills, behaviour and, when older, their interests and abilities. Although facial appearance may have a small initial effect, it is not likely to cause the major social isolation that prevents good social functioning in the early years. I have never come across research or anecdotal evidence where the appearance of children with Down syndrome has been cited as a major barrier to integration.

I believe it is more appropriate to make a concerted effort to change society's attitudes, rather than to subject these children to surgery, with the attendant risk to their physical and emotional well-being. Young children do react to the trauma of hospitalisation – especially long stays over two weeks – and separation from home. In typical children this can be associated with later disturbances in behaviour, particularly when there are difficulties in family relationships and they feel insecure. Our own research has indicated similar results with children with Down syndrome.

The case for cosmetic surgery may be different for adults. In our recent work we have found a small number of adults with Down syndrome who did not like to be associated with Down syndrome and some reacted negatively to the features of Down syndrome. I have met one young person who wanted to change some of his facial features, to make him 'more attractive to girls' and others who try to disguise their features

Cosmetic surgery is becoming quite widespread, and in developed countries, more young people are investing in cosmetic procedures. As techniques develop and become less expensive and traumatic, this is likely to increase. There is no reason why people with Down syndrome should be excluded from this, assuming they understand the risks.

Some conclusions on treatments for Down syndrome

Years of research lie ahead before the full mystery of the twenty-first chromosome will be revealed. At the end of that research, we may find that the problem is too complex ever to be put right. Meanwhile, people continue to promote treatment ideas in the hope that they will at least make the child's problems a little better. This is preferable to the alternative of ignoring the issue – and possibly the children with Down syndrome – as not worthwhile. Care is needed to assess individual treatments, remembering that they could just as easily do harm as do good to the child or to the family.

How do parents decide? As outlined in Chapter 7, where treatment has been advised for a specific problem such as a thyroid dysfunction, a specific vitamin deficiency, a hearing problem, or an extra-large tongue, there are usually very good arguments to support the treatment. The same treatments are given to other children – not just to those with Down syndrome.

When a treatment is held up as some general and all-embracing cure, little evidence is usually found to support it and there is no consensus of scientific opinion. Those who promote the treatment often do so with very generalised statements of effectiveness, and more hope than fact attached to the argument. If there is a major breakthrough on some new treatment it will quickly be circulated. But, please do not pin your hopes to a sudden discovery and breakthrough. The condition is so complex that the best we can hope for is treatments for specific aspects.

Early Interventions and Stimulation

I am talking about early intervention programmes in the first three years of life. After three years of age, pre-school education begins. There is evidence that quality pre-school education and good teaching is beneficial to all children; it is certainly important for those who find learning difficult.

In Chapter 7, I described studies showing that messages appear to take slightly longer to pass along the nerve pathways in people with Down syndrome, probably due the differences in the structure of the nervous tissue. Some of the treatments above were attempts to remedy this.

In the same way it has been argued that starting early in life and giving the infant intensive and focussed stimulation, might promote the development of nerves and nerve groupings. This would not just speed up development and learning – a sort of high practice effect – but also have a long-term effect by reducing the impairment in the nervous system. Evidence for this was generalised from studies of animals and poorly devised studies of early intervention with children with Down syndrome. As we will see, they have generally been shown to be over-optimistic.

Intensive physical training and sensory motor coordination

We tested the above ideas with several intervention studies that focussed on a weakness found in young children with Down syndrome in coordinating sensory input (vision and balance) with physical strength and coordination.

We gave one group of 12 babies with Down syndrome very intensive physical training on sitting up, and compared their progress to 12 similar babies whose parents gave them the 'regular' physical play programme. When I say we, I mean the research team devised the training exercises and the mothers did them five times a day in the intensive group.

We not only did exercises to increase the strength of the babies and overcome hypotonia (e.g., rolling over, pulling to a sit, weight-bearing on legs), we also asked parents to include 'wobblies' – for example, holding the baby firmly around the waist in a sitting position and gently wobbling from side to side and back to front to help balance. Figure 18 shows what we found. If you compare the progress of the typical babies with those with Down syndrome in the intensive group, the slower development only appears when they got to the first 'balancing alone' item. Then a slower rate of development, or a plateau, is seen until they can sit for 30 seconds or more. I think it is reasonable to assume that they consolidated the links between balance and the physical sitting programme during this period.

After this the next steps in sitting are achieved at a rate parallel to the normal pattern but at an older age. The regular group showed

The developmental sequence

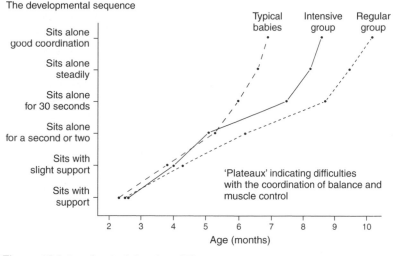

Figure 18 Intensive training for sitting

a similar pattern but the muscle strength did not seem to 'tone up' quite as quickly. Thus the intensive input compensated for the low muscle tone; it could not rectify the coordination problem, but it did speed it up compared to the regular group.

The next question was, would it have a long-term effect? If the intensive stimulation had 'corrected' the fault in coordinating strength and balance, then the children who sat up earlier should not have the same problems of coordinating balance with strength during the stages of walking. In short, they should walk earlier than the regular group. We knew the two skill areas of sitting and walking were linked because the babies in the rest of our study (not this intensive study) who sat earlier also walked earlier.

Unfortunately we did not find that the intensively trained sitting babies walked significantly earlier than the 'regulars'. It would seem that the intensive training had not had a general effect on the brain area associated with coordination. Nevertheless, they all had plenty of exercise, enjoyed wobbly games and could sit up and look at their world from a different angle sooner than they would otherwise.

It might be that our special program was not specific enough or that we needed to keep the intensive training going for longer.

We also trained the babies in the development of visually directed reaching, which again showed problems between visual and motor coordination. The same pattern was found; the intensive training got reaching started sooner, but a plateau appeared with skills requiring coordination of vision and reach. Because they could reach and play with objects earlier the 'intensive babies' did show more advanced general development than the 'regular babies'. But again, the advantage was relatively small and their success on the test could be explained by being able to do things with objects a bit sooner (see Chapter 10 on tests). We found the 'regular' infants soon caught-up and there were no long-term effects.

In another study we got mothers to encourage the primary walking reflex by gently holding the baby from behind and touching his or her feet on the floor, moving slowly forwards. In the first weeks of life, babies make reflex stepping movements. We found that if we kept these going, most of the children walked about six to eight weeks earlier than the 'regular' children without the exercise. Of course, babies are all individual, and some are not programmed to keep the walking reflex going and it disappears; we found that these babies usually crawled earlier. Yet again, we did not find any long-term benefits for the advanced walking group on running or jumping or general development at later ages.

So, mothers have to decide if the risk of backache is worth the gain of a few weeks. My view is that it is not, especially as there are other things that the baby needs as well, such as play and social interaction. We carried out similar types of studies on attention span and object permanence with similar results. In all these the intensive training had a short-term effect, but no general or long-term improvement. So we failed to show that increasing the intensity of the training had any major advantage and certainly there was no suggestion that we had substantially changed the underlying nervous system.

An overview of our research on early intervention

Our research is based on following the development of more than 160 children with Down syndrome from the first weeks of life. Some were visited every week at home, and all had at least one visit every six weeks until the age of two years, and then six monthly after that. Some of the children received very intensive stimulation as described above. Some mothers and fathers found this too much and stopped; others carried on for several months. In one group, they carried out intensive programmes for over 18 months. Other groups carried out plenty of stimulating activities but not in a very intensive way. They would try to spend time each day playing with and stimulating the baby, and planning the play to fit in with the baby's current level of development. This was all fitted into a fairly natural routine much as one would do with any baby. Another small group was only seen every six months, but used a book we had written to guide them (*Helping Your Handicapped Baby*, Souvenir Press 1978).

Our aim was to encourage quality interactions between parents and babies and for parents to have a positive attitude, and believe it was worthwhile. We developed early intervention programmes based around the behaviours described for babies found in most developmental tests.

These include programmes to help gross physical development (such as sitting, standing and walking, balance and coordination), fine motor development and visual–motor coordination (such as reaching, picking up and manipulating objects), communication skills, like listening to and following sounds, babbling and recognising first words, using gesture, saying first words and then two words together.

There were programmes to extend the babies attention span and exploring objects like putting things in or out of cups, placing pegs, playing hide and seek with objects and learning that objects can be permanent, which involves memory. It included a whole range of play and exploration ideas with objects and looking at pictures

If asked, we also helped parents with health matters, schooling, family issues and behaviour problems. We did not teach parents formal signing systems (Chapter 8), but we did encourage them to develop their own systems using gesture.

Our research results

When we compared the progress in the different groups we found:

1   Babies who had very intensive schedules were a little more
    advanced than those on more natural ones, but only during
    the intensive training period, and only on the behaviours that
    were being trained. We concluded that, in the first year or
    two of life, very intensive and highly structured training pro-
    grams like ours, do not appear to be any more beneficial than
    less intensive and more natural approaches. However, if a
    baby has a specific difficulty, like being very floppy or not
    feeding, or has a specific motor problem, then specific and
    intensive programs are needed while the problem is being
    treated.

2   Babies whose parents joined the research and began the stim-
    ulating exercises in the first month or so, were more advanced
    on the developmental assessments than babies who started
    later in the first year of life. However, all the later starters
    caught up to the early ones within a few months. The later
    ones were not that far behind on physical activities; many
    parents said they had being doing exercises with the babies
    because other parents had told them it was worthwhile. This
    suggests that changes in social attitudes were influencing the
    parents and removing 'hidden deprivation' effects (Chapter
    10). The small group who had used our book and whom we
    had visited every six months, were just as advanced in their
    development as the rest.

3   When the children were over five years of age, we compared
    them to similar children with Down syndrome whose fami-
    lies did not receive such help. We did not find any major
    differences between the two groups on mental ability or lan-
    guage tests, nor on checklists of functional development and
    attainments. We think that if these children were slower than
    our group, they soon caught up when they started to go to
    pre-school. Talking with parents led us to conclude that
    many in this comparison group had developed positive atti-
    tudes to their children, and *were* actually stimulating them in
    a natural way. We did not pick up signs of general hidden
    deprivation, although there were individual children and
    families who were deprived. Both groups were more
    advanced than would be predicted from earlier studies (see
    Table 4).

4   When we compared the children in our research group with those in the matched group, they tended to be healthier, and more had help for hearing and visual problems. We feel the interventions had alerted the parents to the likely health difficulties. It could also be that the physical exercises had kept them healthier by improving any floppiness and encouraging physical development.

5   Many parents said of the early intervention that they felt better, and more confident about the child when they were doing things, like the exercises and games for the intervention. I am quite certain the babies felt better when the parents stimulated and played with them, and had a more enjoyable day. But this does not mean parents need an early intervention programme. Feeling confident and happy with the baby is probably sufficient.

6   When applied at the right time in the child's development, training that focuses on specific activities does work from soon after birth. Children in our 'intensive' groups sat up a month earlier, and walked a month or two earlier. Children who were taught to eat or drink, to wash, or to use the toilet in a consistent and structured way, learned these skills more quickly than those not taught directly. If we target an activity that matters and is worth achieving as soon as possible, we can certainly help the child attain it, and hopefully feel more competent and self-sufficient.

Summary and current directions in early intervention

Early intervention programmes for young children with Down syndrome are well established in many countries. There are lots of variations and differences in emphasis; some visit homes, others are based at centres; some focus on training the development of the child as intensely as possible and others on a wider family perspective. The research studies available have problems and, for me, the results are not as straight forward as many people suggest. Parents will find different views from different professionals and these can be confusing.

My conclusion is that most babies and young children with Down syndrome do not need highly structured and intensive programmes, and parents who are unable to carry out such programmes should not feel they are letting the child down.

In the first year or two of life, the immediate focus should be that for any baby and family, and not on trying to remedy the disability through training some behaviours and passing test items sooner. Training to pass test items is to focus on performance, whereas improving ways of interacting with the infant and fostering self-initiation, exploration and confidence is about the processes of learning and becoming independent. Of course within this there are basic skills that need to be fostered and trained, but passing a tower building task a few weeks earlier is not that important. As noted in Chapter 8, I think parents need to learn how to interact with their infant, and how to utilise resources to maintain a balance and happy family. Many early intervention schemes take a similar view and provide access to other parents and facilities.

Overall, the evidence shows that:

- From the earliest weeks of life, babies with Down syndrome are responsive to environmental influences, and prosper best in homes that provide love, care, plenty of stimulation and a variety of experiences.
- Planning and carrying out special games and activities can be beneficial both to parents and the babies, but they need to be selected and matched to the child's level of development, be worthwhile for the child, and in everyday use at the time.
- An activity programme can help parents feel confident. It can help the parent and the child to get to know each other, make the days more satisfying and enjoyable, and prevent the possibility of slower development due to a lack of encouragement and stimulation.
- Where families have reduced resources, and there is a risk that the child will be deprived of 'good enough' care and support, the intervention should focus on getting these resources before making additional demands with child training programmes.

- The consensus from current research shows there is little benefit in carrying out intensive training regimes that may be unpleasant for the child and the parent. This can interfere with a balanced family life and the parent-child relationship.
- There is no overall intensive programme of early intervention that should be applied just because the child has Down syndrome.
- Before taking on a programme, parents should think about the costs in terms of their time, the child's time, their finances, the investment of their emotions and hope that it will work, the risks of disappointment, the feelings of their partner and other family members, and compare this to the potential benefits.

Teaching and Learning

In this section I will describe some basic principles of teaching or helping children to learn. By teaching, I mean ways of encouraging learning, not just formal instruction. I again emphasise that the parent role is far wider than the professional role (Chapter 2) and more important than just the teaching bit. There are many books available that spell out ways to help the child learn and provide specific teaching programmes (see 'Resources').

Hopefully you will feel that a lot of this section is 'common sense' and what we all naturally do. If this is so, I believe that you are more likely to feel confident about your abilities to help and engage with the child with Down syndrome. You may also feel less reliant on professionals and, by understanding the terms they use, may find it easier to engage with them.

Interacting with your child

In the first years, the emphasis is on the interactions between the child and the parent. It is best to think of these as **transactions.** In an interaction the two sides may exchange information but remain the same. In a transaction both sides change as a result of the engagement. When parents are sensitive to the child's way of interacting, and understand how to interpret the infant's actions, they are also more likely to gently direct the infant's attention to new objects and actions without dominating and taking control. Much of this was discussed in Chapter 8.

Use imitation to reflect back the child's actions, and games of turn-taking and anticipation. Try to set up games in which the child takes control and reinforce occasions when the child initiates and makes choices. Learn to 'read' the child and use eye contact. Building towers of bricks, sorting colours, posting shapes, rolling balls, singing rhymes, listening to words can all be playful games in which the processes of learning choice, self–regulation, social cooperativeness and rules of exchange can be encouraged and developed. Actually learning to post the shapes correctly and quickly is not the main aim.

We found that many mothers learnt to begin play with some good physical, boisterous activity to get the baby aroused, and then moved into a quieter style. They made fewer demands on the baby and waited for longer – often four or five seconds – before a new initiation. They imitated the responses or reacted to the babies responses rather than trying to get the baby to do things. When this happens, the babies, depending on their mood, usually do more and are more responsive.

'When I deal with Dave I keep putting myself in first gear, but then I have to change up to top when the other children come in! It can get very frustrating at the busy times of the day – like getting them off to school or around 4–6 o'clock – but it is worth it because you can see he does learn to do things and often surprises me with how much he can do'.

Helping your child learn

If a child has Down syndrome, they will need extra help when learning about every aspect of their life. Part of intellectual disability is impairment to the typical learning mechanisms. The more the

---

EXPECTATIONS ARE IMPORTANT

If the person who is talking or playing with the child with Down syndrome does not expect a reaction to a tickle or a question, and does not understand that it takes longer to get a reaction, they may not give the child enough time to respond. Then, because the child does not appear to respond, they may conclude that the child cannot respond. This then reinforces their idea and expectations.

---

impairment, the slower the learning and the more the child will rely on others to help.

In a sense they need a 24-hour curriculum; it will help them a lot if all members of the family have some idea of what they are learning and how to encourage and teach them. It also helps if what happens at school and at home support each other.

People with Down syndrome do not just find learning a skill difficult; they find consolidating the learning difficult and need a lot of repetition and practice (Chapter 7). You may teach them something, but they soon lose it unless they have opportunities to maintain it. They also find transferring their learning to new situations difficult, and need help in gaining experience of using a new skill or knowledge in different situations. For example, you may teach them about traffic lights using a book, but they are unlikely, by themselves, to adapt this to the real life road situation.

Most of the help parents and siblings give the child with Down syndrome is done in natural play situations and we are often not aware of it. Nowadays there are many 'educational' toys. Often the purpose of the toy is obvious, such as a post-box of shapes. Teaching can become rather formal and structured because the task is constrained and we fall into 'making it work'. If the person playing with the child sees the achievement of the task as the important thing, they are likely to become very focussed and instructional. In some tasks this may be the best approach, but the child needs more than just training to perform. Being able to use one toy successfully does not help with transferring the skills and using the learning adaptively. My approach would be to try to capitalise on the many opportunities that occur throughout the day, and to keep more formal type of instruction to one or two small sessions. We need to enjoy our children, and them us, and not to get too caught up with performance.

Be an opportunist

This simply means looking for and taking opportunities to teach the child as they arise in everyday situations. We need to spot that the child has an interest in something and then the possibilities of using that 'something' in teaching a new use of a skill, or a new skill. Success depends on:

- Your knowledge of child development and the 'zone' of skills and knowledge that the child is in.
- Your skill in turning a situation into a learning game.
- Your ability to observe the child and spot the opportunity.
- Your 'teaching' skill.

Here is an example of opportunist teaching described by Steve's mum.

'I am ironing and have a big basket full of clothes. I soon noticed that Steve loves looking at the clothes in the basket. He has a funny mischievous look on his face and smiles when I take some things out. I start to tell him who the clothes belong to, and pop socks, vests, scarves and other clothes on him. Now he comes to the basket and starts trying on all sorts of things, especially Dad's vest. He is always laughing and feels it's a good game to play. Every now and then I stop and just give him a little hand to get something on when he's stuck. This is good practice for dressing. Of course, I keep telling him whose things they are and what they are called, and I hope that soon he will begin to tell me!'

Some time later, this mother explained to me how she got Steve to put the clothes in groups, firstly socks, pants, shirts and then according to whose they were, starting with his own clothes. He not only had a good game and practice at dressing, but he had learnt about the classification of objects by their shape and function, and then by social features – whose clothes they were. This helped him learn about kinships, and gain a sense of self through having his things and discriminating between them and other people's things. Helping to put the clothes away in their correct places is to further adapt this knowledge.

What increases the likelihood of successful learning?

There are some general rules:

- Draw the child's attention to the relevant bit of an action, sentence, object or picture. For example, when you are modelling an action and they are imitating, exaggerate and emphasise the key part. If you are showing them a picture, point to the key bit, linger on it and repeat it.
- Give the child time to respond. Don't jump in too soon. Try to work at their pace.
- It is easy to overdo the teaching in your concern to help the child. Do a little at a time and achieve and consolidate each small step, rather than bombard the child with too much information or pushing on too quickly. Be patient.
- Give the child plenty of warning and time when switching from one activity to another.
- Stop while it is still fun. If you go on too long the child can get tired and fed up with the task. He or she may then associate the task with negative feelings and so be less willing to do it the next time you try. One method of stopping unwanted behaviour in children is to make them keep doing it until they get so fed up they never want to do it again. This works quite well with striking matches and writing on walls – but you need to plan your decorating to fit in with your behaviour programme.
- Know what it is you are trying to teach and work from the known to the unknown, building on what they can do. Have a good idea of why the child wants to do what you are trying to teach. What is the reward for them? You may know why it is important, but that may be of very little interest to the child.

Creating a learning environment

Children with intellectual disability have problems:

- breaking down and understanding tasks (analysis)
- putting skills and ideas together (synthesis)
- retaining and transferring what they know or the skills they have to new situations (adaptation).

Think about your surroundings as places to learn. Walking down the street with the infant in the pram offers a good example of how we might develop learning opportunities. The infant is usually looking around and trying to reach. They reach out to touch a hedge. This is a learning opportunity, assuming we let them. We might rightly feel it is dangerous due to the hedge being very prickly or dirty, but we need to think if we are being overly cautious and so preventing an experience that they seem interested in. We need to stop for longer to give them a chance to explore the leaves and possibly prompt them to look or touch – bringing the leaf towards them or touching their arm to provoke a reach. We also have to stop more, and repeat the experience more often than we might for a typical child.

If we surround the child with masses of toys it may be overwhelming. It is better to select one or two and change them relatively frequently using little demonstrations (modelling the behaviour) of how they might be used. This creates variety and opportunities. I often see lots of toys piled up in a deep toy box. This makes it is less likely that the child will find one they want or see differences between them.

Routines and order provide a familiar and safe base from which to explore. Try to establish routines and organise the child's space in a fairly systematic way. Provide easy *access* to toys, and order and consistency in the child's world so that he or she learns to know what to expect and why to expect it. When the skill, behaviour or knowledge is established, introduce flexibility, in small steps, to teach adaptability. For example, have all the toys in view on an accessible shelf. If the child tends to keep them in order and has a preference for certain toys, change one or two.

New things attract us all. We are born with a sharp eye for something that is different from what we expect, and we are motivated to explore it. If it is too different, we tend to ignore or avoid it. Most parents will have experienced the embarrassment of a new present from a grandparent that the child absolutely refuses to play with; it is a bit too novel, or outside their level of understanding and experience. But if you leave it aside for a few days and let the child approach it at their own pace, it can become a favourite.

A good **learning environment** will have:

- A sense of security and confidence – organisation and order.
- Easy access to experiences, toys and learning materials and opportunities for exploration and self expression
- Variety, novelty and stimulation

Successful teaching is about assisting the child in becoming more competent in their knowledge and skills. It is also about making them feel confident, successful, self-reliant, and having a positive sense of who they are. These things come from how we engage with the child – how we treat them. We can train people to do many things and perform well, but this is not the same as helping them to feel they can do it by themselves and that they want to use their new skills. I will illustrate these ideas with a teaching pro-gramme.

Putting on pants or knickers
We need to:

1. Pick them up and check that they are the right way around, and that the label is towards us, or the front panel of the underpants is facing away from us.
2. Hold them at the sides and open them up
3. Step in with one leg, and pull up – not too far, making sure that the foot is through and clear of the pants.
4. Step in with the other leg.
5. Pull the pants up to the waist. Often we need to reach around the back and pull them up – they get stuck under the but-tocks, especially if the hands have been placed too near the front and centre.
6. Then we straighten the top.

This is the plan of the task, and it gives us a good idea of what we want to teach and how to build up the skill in small steps. Most people would try to teach this in the logical sequence, 1 to 6. But if you do, the child has to take at least four major steps to complete it and is likely to meet many setbacks and failures on the way, even with the aid of your prompting. This runs the risk of both of you getting frustrated, the teaching going on too long and not being fun, and there are lots of switches of attention between steps.

These potential problems can be reduced using an approach called **backward training.**

The aim is to develop confidence and independence. The key is to help the child feel they have done it – they can put on their own pants. By starting with the last step of pulling up the pants, you always end up with them doing the task. You are working backwards through the logical sequence. So, start by having the pants high up the legs first, and then encourage the child to pull them up and straighten them. Then we can say, 'yes, you have done it yourself'. Gradually you leave them further down the leg and then only have them on one leg and so on. The point is that at every attempt the child ends up completing the task with few problems and feeling they did it themselves. Of course, there are always alternatives to every plan. In this task, if a child finds balancing on one leg difficult, we can teach the task from a sitting position – sit down, then put the pants on over the feet, pull up to the knees, and then stand and complete the task.

Working backwards through a plan also means you work from what can be done to the new step. If you start at the beginning of a task with several steps, then you have to use lots of prompts during the teaching, and so it can get very complicated.

Another example – learning to read
Similar ideas, though not quite backward training, are found in paired or guided reading. Instead of spelling out sounds and trying to teach the child to say the correct word, with the risk of them feeling a failure and not enjoying it, you read the story with them. But you read slowly so that they have a chance of reading what they can just before you. When they hit a word they are stuck on they try to work it out, but you then read it with them. They have the fun of the story, the feeling that they are reading, and they do not

suffer from constant correction. It takes a bit of practice but it works well; the great thing is when they tell you to be quiet because they can read it themselves. You have to choose books at the right level of interest for them, and not too long.

Finally, although we all say we want to learn something, the truth is we want to be able to do something. If we had a magic wand we would probably wave it and become instantly competent – we are unlikely to say we would rather go through the process of learning. Backward training almost does this.

The most effective teaching is fun and part of everyday life. The child sees it as interesting and something they want to do, and tasks or play is planned so that the child feels successful and competent.

Summary

1   There have been many hopeful therapies and treatments based on specific differences that are characteristic of Down syndrome. Most have been simplistic in their understanding of the complexity of the syndrome and when tested with quality scientific studies have failed to be supported.

2   Parents can get swept up in such treatments in their desire to do the best for their child. They need to find out about the treatments and apply a set of guidelines before getting involved.

3   Our understanding of early intervention with families of children with Down syndrome has shifted over the last 30 years. Originally it focussed on training their developmental skills and judging success by how this speeded up attainment of early skills. In a sense, it was about improving performance on some product of development. Training focussed on targeting aspects of the child seen as a specific deficit associated with the syndrome. The research has failed to support the optimistic hopes of these programmes, but has shown that the families and children do benefit from early support and structured teaching.

4 The lack of evidence and the experience gained has brought a shift away from this product model with its focus on the child or deficit. The focus is now on the family, on social aspects of development and on the processes by which children learn and achieve competence and self-regulation. This model does not imply that attaining skills and learning to do things, like putting bricks in boxes are not important. But it is not worthwhile to achieve a skill just a few weeks earlier if it produces negative reactions to learning in the child, and loss of enjoyment for parents in playing and engaging freely with the child.

5 There are established principles for teaching and fostering learning that parents find beneficial for helping their child directly and for working with professionals.

12

Working with professionals and local services

- Who are the professionals and what do they do?
- How do I establish a good working relationship with them?
- What can I do if there is a problem with a professional?
- What is the person centred approach?
- What are the issues around research and people with Down syndrome?

'At first I thought I just had to learn about the baby. I didn't take long before I realised I had to learn how to deal with professionals and services. That's one of the things that's different when your baby has a disability'.

In Chapter 1 I emphasised the importance of getting to know about and organising resources to support you, which includes building up a file of local services. Chapter 2 noted the differences between parents and professionals and why the recognition of such differences is important to any collaboration. Chapter 10 described the different 'models' of disability and how they relate to different profession.

Professionals invest much of their life in their profession. When you ask someone about themselves, the first question is often – 'what do you do?' We gain status from our profession. If it is criticised, we will tend to defend it. We are more likely to favour our professional model of disability and emphasise it when advising parents.

Different professionals may give parents conflicting advice and emphasise different things as important. Parents often find a lack of coordination between different professionals and can be overwhelmed by what they are advised to do with their child. Many find they are having to explain to different professionals what another has advised, and then deal with comments suggesting disagreement.

For example, when early intervention started, many parents were given lots of advice on things to do with their young child but did not have the resources to carry them out. The model used by these professionals focussed on the child, or that bit of the child they thought needed help, rather than on the whole family and their resources. Many parents had feelings of guilt and frustration that they were not doing the best they could.

Because of such problems and the wide range of needs of many children with disability, many professionals now work in multi-disciplinary teams made up of professionals from different areas of expertise such as therapists, teachers, social workers and medical practitioners. This is not always successful, especially if some of the team have different models of disability and needs, or are defensive. Research and experience has shown that the teams that work are those made up of professionals who respect each other, do not feel threatened, and are willing to share expertise. They actually engage in transactions and learn from each, rather than just state their opinion. The key thing is to look for a shared understanding and goal.

Parent and professional partnership

Parents will have their own model and set of goals, and the best understanding of their resources. Professionals now recognise this, and believe that that parents should be active partners in multidisciplinary teams, or in any parent–professional relationship. This shift towards 'partnership' is part of the overall shift to more democratic decision making in many societies; increasing the involvement of people in things that directly affect their lives. It is a 'consumer' model where parents and the child are seen as the consumers of services, with their needs and satisfaction with the service taking priority.

Ideally, the basis of this partnership model is that both partners respect the expertise of the other and make shared decisions. It is not about parents being the junior partner and doing what the professional thinks best, nor is it about the professional acquiescing to the demands of the parent. After all, professionals have been given the task by society to do a certain job and act professionally, which may not always fit with the understanding, aspirations or demands of individual service users. We all need to try to understand the views of others, be respectful and have negotiation skills.

Unfortunately, most parents will experience difficulties with some professionals and with getting services at some time. Sometimes it is due to incompetent professionals. Sometimes it is due to parents' unresolved feelings about the child and disability, and unrealistic expectations of what can be done (Chapter 2). Often, it is due to the pressure on resources and too few professionals trying to meet the increasing demands. For example, life–expectancy is increasing (Chapter 5), and with it demands for services for older people with Down syndrome. Our changing views of disability and living in the community, has brought increased aspirations and demand for services.

This implies that parents will need to develop their skills and compete for resources. Parents who do not have such skills can become disillusioned, antagonistic and so fail to obtain what is best for their child.

But even with the best skills and tolerance, parents are likely to meet professionals who should come with a badge stating – ' working with me may damage your health!' Some are just not very good at their job; others are not as 'committed' as parents would hope; others are more interested in their career and tend to use, rather than support, families. Some are so committed and enthusiastic that they fail to see the parent's point of view.

Fortunately, most studies find the majority of parents of children with Down syndrome are largely satisfied with the

majority of professionals they meet, although they do experience difficulties with the complexity and bureaucracy of many services.

Who are the professionals and what do they do?

An early task for parents is to find out about services and what professionals there are, and what they can and cannot offer. Sometimes a supportive friend or relative will do this. When you first meet, ask the professional what they can offer in relation to the needs you have identified. I am constantly surprised by how many parents come away from meeting a professional with little idea of what they do. Parents usually do not ask, and professionals seldom explain their role.

There are many specialities within professions. Some specialise in a particular client group, such as babies, children, adolescence, adults or older people. Others focus on parts of the person, eyes, ears, heart, brain, mental health, speech, social problems and so on. Within these areas you have more specialists such as hearing in infants and then, hearing in infants with a disability and then possibly Down syndrome. Similarly, there are child (paediatric) physiotherapists, occupational therapists and speech therapists and within this, people who specialise in intellectual disability and Down syndrome.

There are educational psychologists, child clinical psychologists, adult clinical psychologists, and within these groups, those who specialise in learning disability. The same distinctions are found in psychiatry. Like psychologists, clinical psychiatrists specialise in mental health problems, but come from a different discipline. They are medically trained and may have different 'models' and approaches to psychologists. Social workers and nurses range from those working in hospitals to those in the community with specialities across many areas. Some social workers are experts in welfare benefits advice, and others in providing counselling and emotional support.

To complicate matters further, even within a speciality the individual professional will have their own unique view of what they can or should do, and this is within the uniqueness of the service they work in. Thus a nurse specialist in learning disability in one local area may not work in the same way as one in a different area.

Given all this diversity, it is not surprising that most 'consumers' are confused about what can be done and why things are sometimes done differently in differently places. Even professionals within a service may find it difficult to accurately say what another professional actually does, except in the most general terms.

UNDERSTANDING PROFESSIONALS' ROLES

A simple way of understanding professional roles is to separate the general or mainstream services offered to most people such as the general medical practitioner, health visiting nurse, community social worker, and teacher from the specialists; early intervention home visitor, learning disability nurse, specialist psychiatrist in learning disability. The generalists are unlikely to know very much about Down syndrome. Compared with their everyday work, Down syndrome is quite rare. Don't expect these people to have all the answers about special aspects immediately. Try not to be too critical if they don't know much about Down syndrome. Work with them to find the information, and share the information you find with them.

Establishing a working relationship

At the first meeting, there is a good opportunity to establish the partnership relationship you want. Instead of waiting for the professional to ask you questions and so control the meeting and agenda, as most of us do, try starting with your questions. This can be about explaining their job and what they can and cannot do. You can do this by trying to explain to them what you think their job is and what you think you can expect from them, which gives them an opportunity to correct any misunderstanding.

If you share information, you are starting to work out a 'contract' or an understanding with the professional. Phrases like 'is there anything I can do to help you' should not just come from the professional; they emphasise that you are not a recipient of help but a partner. Your first goal is to establish a good working relationship within a partnership model. Your second goal is to ensure that you both have the same goal(s) for the child. This has to come from a shared understanding and agreement about what is best for the child and how to achieve it. This demands good communication and a sharing of information, in an atmosphere of trust. If one or other of the partnership feel they can't say certain things because they will be criticised, or even laughed at for being stupid, then there will be problems.

HOW TO MAKE A GOOD WORKING RELATIONSHIP WITH PROFESSIONALS

- Prepare your self for any meeting in advance by making a list of your needs and questions. If you can, try to find out more about the issues.
- Present the list – your agenda – to the professional(s) and make sure each point is covered.
- Don't be afraid to ask them to explain something a second time if it is unclear. It is not just what they think you should do, but sharing with you why it seems the best thing to do.
- Ask for a brief written statement of what has been discussed or advised, including the reasons for the decision.
- Keep your own file for your child; read the important information again before any meeting.
- If you feel uncomfortable, take someone with you to the meeting. This can be your partner, a relative or someone like a family support worker or social worker. Most professionals will not object to this, especially if you let them know in advance.

Parents can be embarrassed about presenting lists. Many tell me they think the professional will see them as neurotic parents, and it is true that some professionals will not react positively. Having lists and demanding written notes, however, is becoming far more common in many countries, and research is beginning to show that is very helpful to parents and professionals.

As we all know from experience, this type of negotiation is not easy. It needs skill, and the ability to be assertive but not aggressive. You need a clear idea of what you want – your agenda – and the ability not to lose sight of it when faced with a professional. Equally, it is about actively listening to others and having time to think about and reflect on difficult issues.

Understanding the professional view

Looking at things from the other person's viewpoint is usually good for relationships. Professionals often feel threatened by parents. As mentioned above, many non-specialist professionals may have very little knowledge about Down syndrome. Often a professional may agree with your assessment of your needs, but not have the resources to meet your demands. They may want to give you more time, or to discuss things beyond their job specification, but are unable.

Others may be unsure about something, but feel they have to be the 'expert', or that they need to give you reassurance by appearing confident. Somehow you have to let them know that it is all right to say ' I don't know about this, but will try to find out'. Too often, we react in a negative way because of our own stress and frustration about not knowing what to do.

What to do if there are problems

In many situations there are no simple solutions for children with severe disability. But if the professional explains things hurriedly and in jargon that you do not really understand, ask them to explain it again. If they refuse, or explain it in the same way there is a problem with that professional. If you are not in a position to seek help or information from elsewhere, you may have to engage in some 'you-me' talk about the relationship. This could be face-to-face, saying we can't manage with this way of working together, or by writing a letter. In extreme cases you may need to make a complaint. Nowadays, in the consumer–partnership model, we can expect professionals to be able to communicate reasonably well, even if they are unable to do what we want.

Many parents are concerned that if they push too hard or become critical, the professional or service may react by treating their child less well, or not providing the necessary help. I have personally never met a case when a professional has acted badly toward a child because they have problems with the parent. But it is true that most of us prefer a happy and contented day, and so will avoid people who make our lives difficult.

The Person Centred Approach

The person centred approach is a good example of the changing ideas about disability e.g. the social model (Chapter 10) and more democracy in our society.

Although most professionals would now claim they have no such power, they still largely dominate decisions about support and help, and therefore how people with disability lead their lives. To ensure the power base shifts to the people themselves, we not only need to change attitudes, but to establish ways of making these ideas work. It will be difficult, as it means changes in the training, roles and above all the 'traditional' way our professional services are structured.

Around the turn of the millennium, the UK government produced a White Paper called **Valuing People,** which was an attempt to set in motion such changes. Part of this is about **Person Centred Planning**. The formal definition is – an approach to decision-making and planning that supports a person with disability in partnership with others, to think through their aspirations and needs, identify their goals and set up strategies to achieve them. Essentially, the person with disability leads the process. It starts with finding out what they want, rather than what can be provided. The aim is that by placing the person in the central role, they become the most important or powerful member of the team, the executive decision maker. It is their dreams, needs and goals that drive the process.

To quote one young person with mild intellectual disability and trained in self-advocacy:

> 'Person centred planning is about me being in charge of my life. I plan my life the way I want it. It is about the things that are happening in my life. I don't have to do it on my own. I get other people I want and trust to help me'.

The levels at which people with intellectual disability can understand or take such actions will vary enormously. But the principle of person centred planning can be applied to everyone, whatever their disability. Only by trying, will we learn how to develop and adapt this approach to each set of unique circumstances. There is no room in this model to exclude anybody on the grounds they are not competent to engage. Everyone is capable of indicating their preferences, what gives them pleasure and whom they like. The question is how best to find out what their wishes and needs are, and which strategies are most likely to attain them.

Many local services now have care-managers whose role is to ensure the best care for an individual with a disability. This is a complex job and is relatively recent – how it is done varies from place to place. It is needed for people who may not have an appropriate carer or who are not in a position to set up a Circle of Support (see 'Principles' below). There are training programmes to help people with intellectual disability to train others in self-advocacy and in person centred planning.

As with most things in life, all this rests on money and its use. Changes are needed in who controls the money and who has the power to buy the services or desired life style. More and more people with a disability, and/or their parents, are being given the money as direct payments and vouchers. Terms like self-determination and brokerage are becoming more common, and reflect the shift of control and power from the traditional service based model.

At present, the person centred approach is mainly with adults but the ideas driving it are influencing services for children (Chapter 12). There are many implications and opportunities for parent involvement in these developments and with them the need for parents to develop their understanding, skills and knowledge.

The principles of person centred planning

Observing, listening and learning about what people want from their lives
This uses simple techniques, like making a collage of what they like, or selecting who they like from photographs, or anything that helps individuals express their wishes.

Helping people to think about what they want now and in the future

This includes showing people a wider range of possibilities and activities, as well as achieving their current goals. It involves helping people to think through their dreams and wishes (see box).

Families, friends, professionals and services working together with the person

This is the Circle of Support. The decision about who is in it comes from the person, or those who know the person best. It should not be dependent on their verbal ability; many techniques can be used including photographs, illustrations and observing the people they particularly like. It can include other people with similar disabilities.

ACHIEVING DREAMS

Often, future dreams can appear fanciful, but they still need to be taken seriously. An example of this is a young man with intellectual disability whose dream was to be in films. He expressed this in a way one would expect for a typical boy at a similar level of ability, citing several famous Hollywood actors. As part of working through this dream, he joined a drama class and did some acting. He recently appeared in a TV drama. A similar example is a young man who wanted to be a fire-fighter. After visiting fire stations to learn what it entailed, it became clear he was very happy simply being in that environment and was welcomed by the fire-fighters. He now spends much time helping with the fire engines, in a voluntary capacity, and feels he has achieved his 'dream'.

Learning Disability Partnership Boards

In order to encourage and facilitate Person Centred approaches, the UK government White Paper stated that Learning Disability Partnership Boards should be established. These are made up of different organisations and people from the community, including people with intellectual disability and carers. They make decisions about how services for people with disability are planned and run, and importantly, how the money in the local community is spent.

Research and people with Down syndrome

Because of my professional needs, I would like to make some points about getting involved with research. Most parents or carers of someone with Down syndrome are likely to be asked to take part in some sort of research at some time. This may be by a student working towards a qualification, or as part of a larger project based in a University or hospital.

Major research about Down syndrome can be divided into two types:

- Research that aims to find ways of helping people with Down syndrome, either directly through some sort of intervention, or indirectly through improving what families, carers, services, voluntary bodies or the general public do for the well-being of individuals with Down syndrome.
- Research that aims to use people with Down syndrome as a 'natural experiment' to try to understand how we all work. Experiment may sound rather cold and clinical, but it is just a scientific term that means objectively comparing two things and carefully describing their differences, or setting up a situation in order to control what is going on. A lot of this research looks at the development, behaviour, medical and physical aspects of Down syndrome in order to compare it to other types of differences, like autism, general slow development, or different syndromes caused by chromosomal errors.

In my experience the majority of parents of children with Down syndrome are very willing to take part in research. Those in our cohort have been amazingly committed and willing. The reasons they become involved, relate to the two types of research:

- The parent hopes the research will directly benefit their child
- The parents realise the research may not be of direct benefit, but take part for the good of others. They hope it will be of

benefit to other people or families with Down syndrome, or that it will add to our better understanding of people.

Unfortunately most research does not lead to immediate and major benefits. We researchers always hope it will; it is often this hope to discover something new and beneficial that starts us off and keeps us going. We have a tendency to be over enthusiastic about what we might discover, or the intervention we want to prove to be helpful. Without such enthusiasm we would not begin – it would be like a teacher trying to teach a class but either not believing they can learn or that what they are teaching is of no benefit. Of course, enthusiasm can bring problems such as over-optimism (see early education – Chapter 11). If you are a parent and are asked to take part in research, please help, but ask yourself:

- Why you are doing it and what do you expect?
- Have the researchers given you objective and full details of what they hope will be the outcome?
- Have they got ethical permission for the research? This is when the research has been assessed as of high quality, not damaging to people, respecting the rights of the people involved, and not wasting peoples' time. If there are risks, these must be carefully explained and the necessary safeguards put in place.
- Have they fully explained what it is they are going to do, and what they expect of you or your child? Have they explained your rights in terms of withdrawing, complaints and confidentiality? You and your child need to have a contract agreed by both sides as to how your partnership with the researcher will work. Also note the list at the beginning of Chapter 11 about agreeing to different treatments.

The shifts in participation between professionals and parents described above have also affected research. Nowadays, most projects involving parents of people with a disability have some parents on the steering group or as part of the development team. Similarly, people with a disability are increasingly part of research teams and are involved in defining the issues to be researched, and when appropriate, work as research assistants; interviewing other young people, for example. This inclusion of the 'consumers' of the service as participants, rather than recipients, with the right and power to determine what happens to them is part of wider changes in our society and how we view disability, described throughout this book.

13

Inclusion, integration and choosing schools

- What are the advantages and disadvantages of mainstream schools?
- What are the advantages and disadvantages of special schools?
- How many children with Down syndrome go to mainstream schools?
- Why do some move from mainstream to special schools?
- Guidelines for parents on choosing a school

Choosing the first school or pre-school, is a major task for many parents, and even more so if the child has a disability. For some parents the thought of sending the child to a special facility is very difficult. Some may have a strong 'political model' and disagree with anything that involves segregation and exclusion from mainstream life. Others may have come to terms with having a child with Down syndrome within the safety of the family and friends; but may find it difficult to cope with this publicly. Going to the local school like the other children in the neighbourhood has less 'stigma' attached to it.

If you are a parent and have such feelings, you may wish to reflect on how well you have adapted to the fact that your child has a disability (Chapter 2). If you and your child have been involved in an early intervention project emphasising specialist techniques or therapy, then sending the child to a local mainstream school with few specialist resources could seem inappropriate. What really matters is what is best for the child. Unfortunately, there is no simple solution, and we do not have sufficient quality research to provide absolute answers. This is because children with Down syndrome, or any major disability, are all different and their needs change with age. If money was no object and there were many resources and trained people, then all schools could be equipped to cope with all the children. However, this might still not solve the problem. As I will discuss below, children with disabilities can become isolated, particularly as they get older, because there are no similar children in the school.

FORCES FOR CHANGE

The change towards integration and the current emphasis on mainstream schooling were driven by two main factors:

1 **Ideology** – the argument that children should not be segregated just because they were different and that by segregating them from other children and people, it prevented society from overcoming their prejudices and fears and learning to be tolerant and understanding of differences. This was part of a strong 'political model' of disability and how societies relate to differences. In many countries today the aim, and political policy, is towards inclusive societies.

2 **Benefits for the child** – this argues that most children with Down syndrome gain from being with typical children more than being with others with disability – especially in terms of their social skills (Chapter 8).

Most parents would probably agree that the second point is more important, but ideology often drives the major changes in society, to the detriment of some individuals.

A Brief History

Chapter 10 outlines shift in ideas and practice from segregating individuals with Down syndrome to them remaining in their families and local communities. The changes in schooling were part of this.

In the UK in the 1950's all children went through a selection process at 11 years using IQ and normative tests of ability (Chapter 10). They then went to different types of school, which provided an education thought to be best suited their abilities – as measured by these tests. There were many problems with such tests and the idea of segregating at this age. Selection was largely dropped and schools became more comprehensive, taking all typical children in their area. Children designated as intellectual disabled were not included and in the late 1960's to the early 1970's there was an expansion of special schools and in the training of special education teachers. At this time, it was also generally felt that children with Down syndrome needed specialist help and would not benefit from mixing with typical children. Often both parents and teachers in mainstream schools objected on the grounds of the lack of resources, including specialist training, and potential 'dangers' to, and slowing the progress of other children.

Children with Down syndrome gradually began to attend preschool facilities with typical children. Some of the first were called 'opportunity groups' and were mainly attended by the siblings and children of family friends, as well as by the children with disability. Others were typical nurseries or schools with enlightened staff who responded to parent's requests, and depending on their progress transferred into the primary school with their friends. Others started at schools for moderate learning disability, rather than automatically being placed in schools for severe learning disability (see Chapter 10 – terminology).

The first children with Down syndrome going into these schools were the more able with no behaviour problems. We used the IQ test scores of several in our research group to argue that they did not fall into the severe category, and so should not be placed in a special school – just because they had Down syndrome. Such experiences supported the changing ideas about intellectual disability and fitted in with a more inclusive and self-determining society. The image of 'Down syndrome' was becoming more positive through the activities of voluntary organisations, and stories and articles in newspapers and popular magazines.

Increasing numbers of children with Down syndrome began their school career in a mainstream pre-school school and continued in the mainstream schools for longer. Some areas began to phase out special schools for younger children, and have special units within the mainstream school. Many special schools started to develop programmes and policies to try to integrate the children into mainstream schools. This involved visits between schools, integration into some classes, and finally, transfer to the mainstream.

During the 1980's this movement was brought together in legislation in the UK. Local Education Authorities had a legal duty to issue a **Statement of Special Needs** (other countries use different terms). This demanded a thorough assessment by all concerned; the parent(s), a medical officer, educational psychologist, any therapists involved, nursery teachers and any other professional involved. From these assessments a list of the child's special needs was drawn up. These were needs that were additional to the majority of children in mainstream school. The resources to meet these needs where then stated. The basic principle was that children with a disability should be provided with the resources to attend the 'least restrictive environment'. In other words as inclusive within normal life as possible. Of course authorities had the right to decide if these extra resources were beyond what they could afford.

The Local Authority has to be mindful of its resources, and how they are best used to meet the needs of all children. This shift in thinking required massive changes in services and resources. Authorities that had invested in special schools found it difficult to maintain them as well as finding resources to support children with special needs in the mainstream. Providing choice is always costly. In Italy, all special schools were closed and all resources transferred into mainstream schools.

Parents in some places found it difficult to get the child into mainstream schools; in other areas special nurseries and junior schools began to be phased out. More children attended mainstream schools in education authorities that had a policy of integration. This has resulted in the closure or amalgamation of special schools because of the fall in the numbers of children. The same has happened in mainstream schools with changes in birth rates and in rural areas, as younger people migrate to cities.

While in the recent past, parents felt they had little choice but to send their child with Down syndrome to a special school, there is now some concern that they have little choice if they feel a mainstream school is not the best place for the child. Others find they have to fight hard to ensure that additional resources are provided at the mainstream school.

What are the advantages and disadvantages of different schools?

The best school for a child is a good school. Going to a bad mainstream school will serve the child less well than going to a reasonable special school, and vice-versa. There is some evidence that having a child with a disability in a mainstream class helps the other children to become more tolerant and understanding. This depends on the characteristics of the child with the disability. If they have behaviour problems or fail to engage with the other children it can have the opposite effect.

Travel and local contacts

A major disadvantage of special schools has been that the children have to travel longer distances and spend a lot of time getting to school. As the number of special schools has reduced, the distances involved have increased; this brings problems for parents in maintaining out-of-school contact with friends. Children of families with resources, or those who live near the school, tend to have more contacts. Those children attending the local mainstream school, especially the younger ones, usually have more social contacts with other neighbourhood children. Another advantage is that the parent has more chance to meet other young parents at the school and form their own networks and potential support. But if they want to meet other parents of children with Down syndrome they need to find them through other services or the Down syndrome Association.

Learning from the other children

Studies of the developmental progress of typical children have shown that through the 2 to 4 year age range, they benefit from being in a group of mixed ages (such as under 2 to over 5 years) rather than the same age. By 4 to 5 years however, the children progress more when with children of the same age or slightly older. The 'advantages' do not appear that large, and by the time they are in mid-childhood there is no strong evidence that any advantages are still detectable.

These advantages seen in the younger children are more initiation of activities, more social pretend play and higher socialisation skills. Much of this is because young children perceive older children to be more competent. Just as they have inbuilt motivations to master their environment (Chapter 10), they aspire to competence and are more likely to imitate the actions of older children, or any behaviour they see as desirable. But it is behaviours or skills within their zone of ability. They cannot imitate that which they fail to comprehend or don't have the skills to master relatively quickly.

Older children tend to help younger children, who they see as less competent, and so act as teachers and tutors. The learning and play environment created by older children tends to be more stimulating. They are more likely to have a bigger repertoire of behaviours and ideas to use in play and when exploring objects. This provides a wider range of models for the younger children. This may also explain why 4 to 5 year olds tend to show less progress when largely mixing with young children – they do not have the benefits of the older and more competent models.

Children with Down syndrome should benefit in the same; they are smaller, look and act younger. Many have good imitation skills and are sociable. However others may have behaviour problems or additional disorders (Chapter 9) that prevent useful engagements with others. Some may be so slow in their reactions, or have such major impairments in their communication skills, that other children do not engage with them. This is part of the constant debate about inclusion; merely placing a child with intellectual disability in a mainstream facility will not be beneficial if they need specialist help to overcome their learning difficulties and acquire skills. It is called locational integration – they are in the physical space but fail to engage.

Social contacts and socialisation

What about the social contacts? Do typical children play and engage with children with Down syndrome. Children of 3 to 4 years of age become aware of gender, physical and behavioural differences in others. At this time they also begin to show preferences for other children 'like me'; they choose playmates and friends with similar interests and abilities. They avoid those who seem threatening or strange, and ignore a younger child if a same-age or slightly older playmate is around. The same thing seems to work throughout life. We all tend to choose people to be with who have similar abilities and interests to ourselves. It is very rare to find lasting relationship where the two people vary greatly in their competence or have major differences of opinion on key issues. In a sense there is a zone of physical, cognitive and social competence for each of us in which we are more likely to operate with others and it is seen from early childhood. Those outside the zone will receive less attention and in extreme cases, hostility (Chapter 8 – society and differences).

Studies of integration of children with disability, including Down syndrome, have mainly found the same. In pre-school settings children with intellectual disability are gradually chosen less as playmates and 'best' friends as their slower development becomes more marked. They appear more isolated in the classroom. The greater the 'difference' in their levels of competence and behaviour, the more likely typical children are to ignore or actively exclude them from their activities. This continues throughout their school career.

Parents describe how the neighbourhood children gradual 'outgrow' the child with Down syndrome and come to call less often. The child then begins to make friends with younger children, but the same thing happens, and gradually they become more isolated. Some parents have moved the child from mainstream school to special school because they had no friends and few social contacts. The exceptions, and for those who tend to remain in mainstream school for longer, are usually those who have easy personalities and reasonable social skills. Academic competence or physical ability appears to be less influential but does restrict the types of things they do. Children who live in areas with lots of other children tend to have more social contacts and maintain friends for longer, especially if they have a shared interest like music or dancing. Parents will recognise that much of this is what we observe in all our children.

Social engagement is also higher when the parents of the typical children at the school or in the neighbourhood have positive attitudes, and when the school ethos is good and the teachers facilitate contacts and interactions. However by the teenage years most children with Down syndrome have fewer and fewer friends or contacts with typical children and can become isolated.

There are exceptions. These are usually the more able child and those with an attractive, lively personality. They also tend to live within easy reach of their school friends.

Skills and attainments

Do children with Down syndrome make better progress in mainstream or in special school? I have discussed some of the factors influencing development, including mainstream school in Chapters 8 and 10. There are three aspects: progress in their social skills and sense of self, progress in self-sufficiency skills, and progress in their academic skills and knowledge.

Social skills and sense of self

Unfortunately there are no quality studies on social skills including things like self-esteem and happiness. There are anecdotal reports that those attending mainstream schools feel 'normal' and are less aware of being different, but it applies to small numbers and specific cases. It is suggested when they leave mainstream school, some find it difficult to come to terms with their limitations and the realisation that they are seen as different (Chapter 8). In contrast, it is argued that those in special school are 'cocooned' and protected and then find it difficult when they enter the 'real' world and have to face the fact that they are different. My view is based on our recent work showing that the understanding of self is closely associated with cognitive development and not just social experiences (Chapter 8). It suggests that attending a mainstream or special school is not that influential for the majority of children with Down syndrome as is often proposed. I *believe* that in the early years attending mainstream facilities does help social skills and increases the chances of more local contacts and friends, and so a better quality of life.

Self-help skills

Studies indicate that when you match children on ability, their competence in self-help skills is about the same whether they attend a mainstream or special school. The curriculum in special schools often places more emphasis on such skills, and is one reason used in deciding if the child would be better served in a special school. Of course, it may be that the main influence is not the school but parents and carers who teach these skills at home. It may be that parents can construct a life–style for their child with Down syndrome that provides sufficient variety and quality of interaction, so that the type of school they attend is of less importance.

Academic skills

There is limited but consistent findings that children with Down syndrome who attend a mainstream school are more advanced in reading, writing and arithmetic than children of similar ability, personality and family background who attend special school. The difference is small, and some children in mainstream appear to do less well than some children in special school. It is thought the benefit is because mainstream schools give more emphasis to this part of the curriculum. But it might also be that parents who choose mainstream schools also put more emphasis and effort into these skills.

When the children with Down syndrome in our study were between 5 to 8 years of age, we looked to see if those that had received early intervention (Chapter 11) and then attended mainstream pre-schools and primary schools were more advanced than those who had gone into special school at the nursery level. We found no differences in their development and intelligence scores. There was an emerging difference in their basic skills and this was significant for those who continued in mainstream schools (Chapter 10). The children in our study did not get special training in language and social skills in the pre-school and nursery. One study has found that those given such specialist training in the early years appear to be more advanced in their expressive language than similar children with Down syndrome not given the programme. Again the size of the difference is relatively small and there is no information on whether the apparent benefits lasted over the years.

Starting and continuing an educational career in mainstream

In the late 1990's we reviewed all the available studies, including our own, about the numbers of children with Down syndrome who went to mainstream pre-schools and schools, and the characteristics of those who started and remained in the school for varying periods and why they moved into a special facility. Not surprisingly we found that more children started in and attended mainstream schools for longer if the Local Education Authority had a positive policy of inclusion.

As such policies develop and resources are put into mainstream situations, I expect the upper levels of the figures below are a better indication.

Pre-school (2 to 5 years)

From our earlier work and using the child's ability and behaviour, we estimated that at least 80% of young children with Down syndrome could be happily integrated into mainstream pre-schools; recent studies report that between 60 to 80% did so by the 1990's. Problems occurred for those children with major health problems, very slow development and difficult behaviour. Initially some facilities would not accept the child until they were toilet trained, but with the introduction of disposable nappies and changes in early childcare needs for many mothers who have to work, this barrier has reduced.

Infant classes (5 to 7 years)

In some authorities up to 80% of children with Down syndrome started in the reception class of their local primary school. About 50 to 60% appear to cope up to the 7 years level. The figures are higher in authorities that have reduced special schools and put resources into mainstream schools. These 'resourced' schools may not be the local school, and problems can occur when parents prefer all their children to attend the same school. In some places nearly every child with Down syndrome will attend a mainstream school, but it may be in a special unit. The issue then is the extent to which they mix with typical children. Just because they are in the same location, does not guarantee that the benefits of mixing with other children will be found. They do have a higher chance of making friends, because there are more children of similar competences and interests. This is something to look for when visiting schools.

Junior (7 to 11 years)

About 40% completed their education in a mainstream junior school. This was more likely in schools with good resources and when authorities provided support for the child.

Secondary (11 to 16/18 years)

In our cohort during the 1980's, about 15% started in mainstream secondary school and 10% completed their educational career in the school. These were children who would be classified in the moderate and mild levels of intellectual ability (Chapter 10), had a good attention span and concentration and did not have excitable temperaments. They were not disruptive and were relatively easy to manage. Using these characteristics we estimated that at least 20% of our group could have attended and completed their education in these mainstream schools. Higher figures would be expected from well resourced secondary schools. The advantage is that the children get specialist help and the opportunity to engage in typical activities with others. This does need to be structured within the school otherwise the children can just be isolated. Many of these young people were aware of their difference but equally felt part of the mainstream community of the school. Some became stressed and isolated at mainstream school and transferred to a special school.

The overall pattern therefore, is that children who transfer out of mainstream school, or move into special classes within a school, tend to do so at the ages 5, 7–9, 11–12 and 14 years. This corresponds to the curriculum and the main transitions in school life. It also approximates the developmental stages described in Chapter 10 and getting stuck at the stage is a possible reason for transfer.

Why do children with Down syndrome move from mainstream schools?

Isolation and stress

Usually parents, but sometimes the school, feel the child is simply becoming very isolated and needs to be with more children operating within their 'zone'. Other parents have seen signs of stress in their child and felt this was because of the pressure in keeping up and learning, or because the life of the school is just too busy and complex.

Slow progress and unmet needs
A common reason put forward by some schools is the slow progress of the child; the teachers feel they are not meeting the child's needs. This can reflect the focus and priorities of the school, for example, some value competition and achievement from an early age and the style of teaching is more formal and structured.

The demands of the curriculum
In the UK academic curriculum demands are now being applied to 5 to 7 years olds, and at around 4 years of age, some pre-schools are beginning to prepare the children for this approach. One consequence of this is more structure and formality in the curriculum. In contrast, some other countries perceive 5 to 7 year olds differently, and believe that they benefit from a less formal system. Systems that are less formal tend be more adaptable to individual differences and offer more possibilities for play, social engagement and exploration. My impression is that children with Down syndrome appear to cope and engage socially for longer in these less formal systems – as they do in play-groups. A common curriculum with a focus on academic achievement does inevitably mean the school becomes for formal, but it does have resource implications. Well-resourced schools offer variety and provide special teaching in small groups for academic skills, as well as integrating the children in other activities for social skills.

Holding back in younger age groups
To overcome the problem of an increasing difference in competence, some children with Down syndrome are kept in the pre-school a year longer, or kept a year back in the primary school. In the UK, five years is the age when most children move from pre-school to primary. At this age a large number of children with Down syndrome are around the two and a half to three year level of competence. This is when we believe the typical child is most likely to benefit from a less formal and more social curriculum. Children

with Down syndrome often transfer to special classes at this time. The gap between the children is becoming obvious and the amount of engagement with the child with Down syndrome is reducing. However the move often coincides with the child at the transition to the stage when children begin to engage with each other. If we think being with typical children at this stage of development is beneficial, then holding the child back is well worth considering.

Behaviour problems

A frequent reason for not integrating, or transferring the child to a specialist school is that the mainstream school find they cannot manage the child's behaviour. This often happens when the child with Down syndrome has attentional and concentration problems and is overactive, and has behaviour such as running away (Chapter 9). The school may not have the resources for the levels of supervision required. There are instances of older children becoming aggressive and hostile; sometimes as a result of being teased by other children. This is relatively rare in primary school.

School resources

Schools that have higher adult to child ratios, specialist staff or specialist support, cope better. Children remain there for longer, or for their whole career. Many children with Down syndrome have an adult assistant for varying amounts of time, and this is recorded in their Statement of Educational Needs. With the more able and calmer child, these assistants can help with one-to-one teaching, or by looking after other children in the class to release teacher time to work more intensively with the child with Down syndrome. As the child's needs become more extreme, and especially if they have major behaviour problems, these assistants can spend much of their time containing the child, and the two can become an isolated unit within the mainstream school. In this situation the child is not receiving specialist input from a qualified specialist teacher, nor benefiting from being in a mainstream environment. Transfer to a special school is the better option.

Conclusion

The message I take from this is that for most children with Down syndrome the best approach is to:

- Avoid strong beliefs or statements like 'my child will always be in mainstream school'. These are more 'political' statements than reflecting what is best for the child. With a number of factors to consider, like the nature of the child, the nature of the available schools, where you live and the neighbourhood, any dogmatic statement is likely to need qualifying when the actual decisions have to be made.
- It would seem sensible to start the child's educational career in a mainstream setting such as a local play-group or pre-school. Even earlier, take them to swimming, to mother-baby and toddler groups.
- Have a clear idea of what you want for the child. Is your priority academic attainments or socialisation? Is it attendance at the local school with the child's current friends and siblings? Is your priority the child's health or problems with their behaviour and personality? From this you can begin to form a set of ideas or criteria to judge whether a particular school is more or less likely to meet your needs. You will need to present this analysis during the Statementing Process in the UK, or when putting your case to the school or educational authorities.

Guidelines for parents choosing a school

1 About six to nine months before you intend to send the child to a pre-school or school:
   - Find out what is available locally or within a comfortable travel distance. The best source of information is other parents, the Local Education Authority (Parent Advisor), Social Services, or the Pre-School Learning Alliance.
   - Find out the name of the Education Officer responsible for Special Education. Make contact and ask about facilities for children with Down syndrome, other children with Down syndrome in the area, and which schools they

attend. Ask for a copy of their policy on Special
Education and information on the Statementing Process.
Ask if there is a Parent Advisor or a named person under
the Code of Practice (UK). In the UK you can get help
about a statement and integration from a voluntary association called IPSEA via the Down syndrome Association.
The paediatrician has a duty to inform the education
authorities about children that may need statementing,
and usually does this in the first year of life for those with
recognised conditions like Down syndrome.

2 Prepare yourself before visiting the school.
   There are three groups of questions:
   • Questions of **policy.** Ask about their attitudes and think-
     ing about children with special needs. When the head
     teacher and teaching staff have a positive attitude toward
     having children with differences in their school, integrat-
     ing a child with additional needs is more likely to be
     successful. Find out if they have a written policy. It should
     be in the school handbook. What experience do they
     have of children with additional needs and are there chil-
     dren already at the school? Most important is what the
     school's priorities and aims are for the child with addi-
     tional needs. If you and the school can agree on the
     priorities and how you will monitor them, a lot of poten-
     tial conflict will be avoided.
   • Questions of **process.** What plans do they have to ensure
     the successful integration of the child? For example, how
     would they explain to the other children about the child's
     differences? With older children it can help if the class is
     prepared and has an understanding. Sometimes parents do
     this themselves. Do they use home–school diaries so that
     school and home can keep in touch and reinforce the
     child's learning?
   • Questions about **resources.** What resources does the
     school have for a child like yours? Are there extra
     resources they may need? How will the school try to get
     these? What can you do to help? How can you be
     involved? What would the school like you to do to help?
     How will they keep you informed about progress?

In a sense you will be setting up a **contract** with the school – agreed aims and objectives, systems for communication, what is expected from each of the parties and how you will monitor progress on the agreed priorities both at home and at school.

3   When you have thought through these questions and made a list to remind you of what to ask and look for, go and look at the available pre-schools and schools and make a judgement about the ethos or character of each. Are the children happy? Are teachers and other members of staff cheerful? Is there a busy feeling and a sense of purpose? Look at the wall displays; are they new and fresh? Is there a positive feel about them? Look at the equipment. If you like the feel of the school, try to arrange to meet with the teacher (s) of the class or group your child would be with.

4   When you get home ask yourself:
   • Was it a **caring** school? Did you feel welcomed? Did the staff have positive attitudes to children with Down syndrome?
   • Was it well **managed?** Did the arrangements for the visit go smoothly? Was information to hand and given to you? Did you feel your questions were answered and well explained? Did you come away from the school with a clear plan of what would happen next and what you might need to do?
   • Was it well resourced to meet the needs of your child with Down syndrome?
   • Did you feel you gave the pre-school or school enough information about your child's ability and personality and your own hopes and priorities? Are you sure that what you want and what the school wants for the child are the same?

From my experience and reading, I would estimate that 60 to 70% of parents find the process of choosing a pre-school and school and the child's progress through the education system is without major problems.

Summary

Underlying these practical hints are themes that have run throughout the book. The two key ones are that children with Down syndrome benefit most if:

- their parents take an active problem solving approach to issues and
- have the belief and attitude that the child's life can be fulfilled and meaningful. They value the child.

These benefits are not dependent on the severity of disability of the child. Even the most severely impaired child has a better life with parents or carers who are positive and active.

We are not patients or clients– passive recipients of other's expertise. We are consumers, customers and partners. When it comes to our lives and our children we have expertise and rights.

A parent is the child's best advocate and advocacy is not a passive activity. Adults and older children can be advocates for themselves, but need the support and environment to promote choice and decision making.

Just as the baby is not a passive recipient of care and stimulation but an active participant in their learning and development, programmed for this before leaving womb, so we parents need to be participants not recipients; to be proactive not reactive.

Of course this comes easier to some than others, and depends on circumstances and resources. We need a sense of balance and should not neglect ourselves and other family members in trying to help the child with Down syndrome. Healthy and happy parents make for healthy and happy children. So there are times when we should relax; we need to marshal our resources and support so that the energy and expertise of others is brought into our agenda. In forming the agenda we need to be open and to listen.

My belief is that this approach is more likely to happen if we really value the child, come to terms with disability and complex questions about our values and the meaning of our lives, and take a proactive and participatory approach. This belief comes from growing up with the families with Down syndrome in our research and listening and observing and asking the question, 'what is helping them, and what is benefiting their child with Down syndrome?'

Concluding comments

I find it difficult to end this book, because it is really only a beginning. As I said in the introduction, it is an attempt to provide answers to the immediate questions asked by many parents. It covers the first period of adjustment to the diagnosis of Down syndrome, and hopefully prepares for the day-to-day business of living with, and learning about their child. But as I said at the beginning, it is about the probabilities of what might be needed and what might happen because of the Down syndrome. The reality of the unique child and the family they live in will only emerge with time. My hope is that the information provided in the book will help parents on that path of discovery; that it will allow them to put aside many questions and worries about what might happen and see through the label to the child. I think the joy of parenting, is seeing how the new person grows and develops, and having that unique relationship with them, which makes you an integral part of the process of them becoming a person. It is being able to share their delight in new discoveries and take pride in their achievements, not because it might reflect on you – although we all want to feel we did a good job – but for their own sake. If we can't respect them and treat them respectfully, they have less chance of growing up feeling self-respect. The chances are that more families will enjoy and feel strengthened because the child has Down syndrome, than will find it a difficult burden.

I have tried to show how things have changed and will change in our society (social, educational, economic, political, health and medical) and how they have resulted in a better quality of life for individuals with Down syndrome and intellectual disability. My belief is that to-days parents, once over the initial shock, will see a positive and worthwhile future for their child with Down syndrome. But like past parents, they will have to be vigilant in defending the advances made and bringing about further changes.

There are many aspects that I have not covered in the book such as details about the law, benefits, and future issues of care. For example I am aware that I have not discussed the question that is a constant worry for most parents of 'What will happen when I die?' It includes how to help the person understand death as well as securing a safe future for them. I think it is best to focus on the immediate needs and avoid worrying about things that might never arise, or that can be dealt with when they arise.

I shall end this book by returning to the main theme. The birth of a child with Down syndrome is a great shock for most parents. No matter what happens after the birth, it is an event in your life that will always be with you and must produce changes. It is a challenge.

Bringing up any child is a challenge. Whether bringing up a child with a disability is a greater challenge, or just a different challenge from bringing up a typical child, is a matter of opinion. But bringing up a child with Down syndrome is not only a challenge to cope, and to provide the child with the best available opportunities to grow and develop, it is a challenge to the set of values by which we judge others, and decide what we want from life.

I look forward to the day when a father and mother can be given assurances that they will not have a baby with a disability. But I am not sure whether such a day will be to the benefit of our society as a whole. Those members of our society who are disabled are a constant challenge to society; they cause us to question our values, they test our compassion, and they remind us that ability is not all.

Resources

Most countries now have a Down syndrome Association and most parents will be given the address of their Association when informed the baby has Down syndrome. These associations keep abreast of changes and can provide magazines for parents and list of books, information of local resources, the addresses of allied associations for intellectual disability, and Down syndrome Associations in other countries. They can also give lists of websites. Any interested person can contact these Associations.

My selection of information sources will hopefully be sufficient for anyone wishing to explore further. I have also included those that I have mostly used in preparing this new edition.

These associations also provide many of their own publications and support packs for professionals and parents. As one might expect being produced by parents or people with Down syndrome, they are generally very practical and useful. However the Association's literature and policies reflect the view of Down syndrome of the parents who run them, and many parents have different views on some issues e.g. prenatal screening, mainstream schools, the intensity of early intervention, various medical treatments. In some countries, there are separate associations for children with Down syndrome who have additional problems, such as severe heart conditions.

Addresses

Down Syndrome Association
Langdon Down Centre
2A Langdon Park
Teddington, Middlesex
TW11 9PS

Down Syndrome Scotland
158–160 Balgreen Road
Edinburgh EH 11 3AU

Down syndrome Northern Ireland
Graham House
Knockbracken Healthcare Park
Saintfield Road
Belfast BT8 8BH

Down Syndrome Ireland
41 Lower Dominick Street
Dublin 1

British Institute of Learning Disabilities
Campion House
Green Street, Kidderminster
Worchestershire DY10 1JL
www.bild.org.uk
Provides an excellent range of publications on most aspects of intellectual (learning) disability, including a new one this year on Down syndrome and Dementia.

Down's Heart Group
17 Cantilupe Close
Eaton Bray
Dunstable, Beds.
LU6 2EA

Down Syndrome Educational Trust
Sarah Duffen Centre
Belmont Street
Southsea, Hants PO5 1NA
www.downsed.org

Promotes education and development of children with Down syndrome through research and information. A wide range of written material, research journal, newsletter and provides consultations and training workshops for parents and professionals.

Mencap
123 Golden Lane
London EC1Y ORT

The Department of Health
PO Box 777
London SE1 6XH
e-mail doh@prolog.uk.com
Has a range of documents on current policy and services – mostly are free and user friendly – including some for people with intellectual disability.

Websites

Down syndrome World Wide Web Page, Organisations and Associations
www.nas.com/downsyn/index.htmi
www.nas.com/downsyn/org.htmi

A comprehensive set of addresses and links for Down syndrome in the UK.
www.43green.freeserve.co.uk/uk–downs–syndrome/ukdsinfo.html

Independent Panel for Special Education Advice (IPSEA)
IPSEA offers free and independent advice on Local Education Authorities' legal duties to assess and provide for children with special educational needs.
www.ipsea.org.uk

UK People First Organisation
People First is run and controlled by people with learning difficulties.
www.peoplefirst.org.uk

Information for medical professionals and students
A website developed and managed by the Down Syndrome Association in conjunction with St. George's Hospital Medical School.
www.intellectualdisabolity.info/home.htm

Len Leshin
Medical advice on a wide range of subjects and links to international related sites.
www.ds–health.com

Mosaic Down Syndrome
Site for specific information on Mosaic Down syndrome
www.mosaicdownsyndrome.com

The Down's Syndrome Medical Interest Group (DSMIG)
A network of doctors from the UK and the Republic of Ireland with special interest in Down syndrome. Very useful site for medical information.
www.dsmig.org.uk

Books by parents and people with Down syndrome

There are many books written by parents about their experiences. The first I read was by Pearl Buck, the well-known American writer in 1951. They are the individual stories of the family and the person with Down syndrome, and can give the impression that this is Down syndrome for everyone. Hence some seem overly optimistic and others a bit gloomy. What I have taken from them is the many similar points and shared feelings despite being written at different times and in different countries about individual families *who have one thing in common –* a child with Down syndrome.

Books by people with Down syndrome.

The World of Nigel Hunt: The diary of a Mongoloid Youth. Hunt, N. Beaconsfield: Darwen Finlayson 1967
The first book by a young man with Down syndrome and still worth reading.

Count Us In: Growing Up with Down syndrome. Kingsley, J and Levitz M. Harcourt Brace and Co.1994
A really good antidote to reading books by professionals and some parents. It puts the issues into a different perspective, and for me, a reminder that we are all people with differences.

Why me? 'Autobiography' of Sheenagh Hardie, a Down's Syndrome Girl. Hardie, S. (assisted by her parents Helen and Alistair Hardie). London: Excalibur Press 1990

Books by parents or friends.

My Friend David. Edwards, J & Dawson, D Ednick. Communications Inc. Oregeon 1984

Life as We Know It: A Father and an Exceptional Child. Berube M . New York: Vintage Books 1998
Of the recent books I found this the most positive.

Karina Has Down syndrome. Rogers C and Dolva G Lismore: Southern Cross University Press,1998

Down syndrome: How One Family Coped with the Challenge. Kaly S. Sydney: Wild and Woolley, 1998

Books written for parents and carers

In the United States of America, The Woodbine House publishing company have a recent series of *Topics in Down Syndrome.* Most are guides for parents and professionals. The topics include Reading, Language, Fine Motor skills, Gross Motor skills, Medical Care and Nutrition, and an Introduction to the Baby with Down syndrome. They are easy to read and comprehensive. However, they add up to thousands of pages and quite a lot of replication. I felt overwhelmed and am sure many parents would feel the same, but never the less an excellent resource to consult. The full list and details can be found on their website:
e- mail: info@woodbinehouse.com
www.woodbinebouse.com

Here are some titles
The Down syndrome Nutrition Handbook: A Guide to Promoting Healthy Lifestyles. Guthrie Medlan, J.E. Woodbine House 2002.
Written by a mother of a child with Down syndrome and a nutrition-ist. Provides a thorough overview of nutrition for all children and potential issues for those with Down syndrome.

Babies with Down syndrome: A New Parents Guide (Second Edition). Stray-Gunderson, K. Woodbine House 1995

Early Communication Skills for Children with Down's Syndrome: A Guide for Parents and Professionals. Libby Kumin . Woodbine House 1997

Two easy to read and useful books by a father and eminent medical doctor who has done extensive research into Down syndrome:
A Parent's Guide to Down Syndrome: Towards a Brighter Future. (Revised Edition). Pueschel S.M. Paul Brookes 2001

Adolescents with Down Syndome. S.M. Pueschel & M. Sustrova. Paul Brookes 1997

Down's Syndrome and Health Care. Vee Prasher and Beryl Smith. BILD Publications 2002
Comprehensive and straightforward and covers most aspects of physical and mental health.

Down's Syndrome; The Facts. Mark Selikowitz. Oxford University Press 1997
An excellent and easy to read introduction by a medical paediatric specialist.

The Down's Syndrome Handbook. A practical guide for parents and carers. Richard Newton. Vermilion 2004
Produced in association with the DSA (England and Wales) by a paediatric neurologist who is also a father of young man with Down syndrome and researcher in medical aspects of Down syndrome.

Down's Syndrome. Past, Present and Future. Stratford, B. Penguin Books 1989.
The early chapters provide a fascinating historical perspective.

An Activity-Based Approach to Early Intervention (Third Edition). Pretti-Frontczak K and Bricker D. Paul Brookes 2004.
Good practical ideas for young children with intellectual disability, by very experienced people. Although aimed at professionals, it easy to use for parents. It has certainly stood the test of time and for me, is sensible and practical.

Steps to Independence: Teaching Everyday Skills to Children with Special

Needs (Fourth Edition). Baker BL and Brightman A J and several others. Paul Brookes 2004
Another practical book that has stood the test of time. User friendly and covers basic approaches to teaching and many step-by-step programmes on a wide range of self-help skills starting in the early years, plus advice on working with professionals, information seeking and managing behaviour.

Technical books

I have selected more recent ones and those I have referred to in this book.
Down Syndrome: A Promising Future Together. Edited by Hassold, T.J and Patterson D (EDS) New York: Wiley–Liss 1999
Chapters by different authors of mixed readability and technical level. There is a very good section written by people with Down syndrome.

New Approaches to Down Syndrome. Edited by Stratford B & Gunn P. Cassell 1996
A set of comprehensive and well written chapters by specialists in their own field.

Simple Beginnings in the Training of Mentally Defective Children. MacDowall M. Law and Local Government Publications 1930
Not easily available, but a must for any one interested in the history of education for children with intellectual disabilities.

Down's Syndrome. Children Growing Up. Carr. J. Cambridge University Press.1995
A report on her cohort born in 1963–4, and followed up regularly to adulthood, and providing a natural history of the children and young people and their families.

Growing up with Down's syndrome. Shepperdson B. Cassell 1988
Like Janet Carr this is another detailed longitudinal study, describing two small cohorts from South Wales in the 1970's and 80's and by contrasting the two, describes the effects of changes in ideology and services on the children and their families.

Down's Syndrome: The Psychology of Mongolism. Gibson, D. Cambridge University. Cambridge Press 1978

A thorough review of early work. Very technical.

Children with Down Syndrome. Edited by Cicchetti, D & Beeghly, M. Cambridge University Press 1990
A series of theoretical and review papers about development in children with Down syndrome. Very comprehensive and thought provoking, but very technical.

Development and Disability. Lewis V. Blackwell 2003
Excellent review on different disabilities, including a chapter on Down syndrome. Technical.

The next three editions are reports from recent international conferences on Down syndrome.
Down's Syndrome. Psychological, Psychobiological and Socio – Educational Perspectives. Edited by Rondal, J, Perera, J, Nadel, L & Comblain. A. Whurr Publishers Ltd. 1996

Down Syndrome. A Review of Current Knowledge. Edited by Rondal J, Perera J & Nadel L. Whurr Publishers Ltd. 1999

Down Syndrome. Across the Lifespan. Edited by Cuskelly, M, Jobling, A & Buckley. S Whurr Publishers Ltd. 2002.

Living in the Real World. Goode C. Twenty-one Press, London. 1991
An excellent collection of the views of parents of young children with Down syndrome. Fascinating and easy to read.

Books for people with intellectual disability

Books Beyond Words. Published jointly by the Royal College of Psychiatrists and St. Georges Hospital Medical School
www.rcpsych.ac.uk/publications /bbw
A series of booklets about difficult subjects.

Index